THE LEGAL
ASPECTS OF
CHILD HEALTH
CARE

THE LEGAL ASPECTS OF CHILD HEALTH CARE

Bridgit Dimond
MA, LLB, DSA, AHSM
Barrister-at-Law and
Emeritus Professor
University of Glamorgan
Pontypridd, Mid Glamorgan

Foreword by

Elizabeth Fradd
SRN, RSCN, SCM, HVCERT
Regional Nurse Director
NHS Executive West Midlands
Birmingham

London Baltimore Barcelona Bogotá Boston Buenos Aires Caracas Carlsbad, CA Chicago Madrid Mexico City
Milan Naples, FL New York Philadelphia St. Louis Seoul Singapore Sydney Taipei Tokyo Toronto Wiesbaden

To cystic fibrosis sufferers and their carers

Project Manager:	Nigel Wetters
Editorial Assistant:	Hannah Tudge
Cover Design:	Lara Last
Production:	Mike Heath
Index:	Jill Halliday
Publisher:	Nicola Horton

Copyright © 1996 Bridgit C Dimond.

Published in 1996 by Mosby, an imprint of Times Mirror International Publishers Limited.

Printed by Arrowsmith, UK.

ISBN 0 7234 22125

For full details of all Times Mirror International Publishers Limited titles, please write to Times Mirror International Publishers Limited, Lynton House, 7–12 Tavistock Square, London WC1H 9LB, England.

A CIP catalogue record for this book is available from the British Library.

Contents

Preface

I wrote this book primarily for those health professionals who care for children, but it will also be useful as a companion to the child branch of the Project 2000 course. Although there is a chapter covering the principles of the Children Act 1989, I have emphasized in the book those aspects which concern the sick child being cared for in hospital or in the community, rather than concentrating on the law relating to child care and the powers and duties of local authorities.

Stressing practical aspects of the law wherever possible, I have shown the application of the law in case studies and examples. In this way, the reader can move from the specific to the general and later apply these basic principles to his or her own circumstances.

In many ways, this is only an introduction to some complex and developing areas of law. It describes the laws of England and Wales which, for the most part, are applicable to the whole of the UK; readers in Scotland and Northern Ireland, however, should be aware that there may be some significant differences.

LAW AND ETHICS

Every situation that confronts the health professional caring for a child has both legal and ethical dimensions; although these often overlap, the professional should note that law and ethics are distinct fields, which may conflict. This book focuses on how the law relates to specific situations, drawing on case studies and examples cited in *Ethical Issues in Child Health Care* by Jim Richardson and Irene Webber (Mosby, 1995). I have used these case studies here so that the reader may compare legal and ethical issues within a wider legal framework. In this way, the health professional should gain an understanding of two different perspectives that we use when making decisions.

ACKNOWLEDGEMENTS

I wish to acknowledge the help of many people in the preparation of this book. It is invidious to pick out certain names from the mass of people who assisted, but I must acknowledge the help in particular of Jean Jones, Lorraine Moran, Isobel Puscas, Sue Barr and her colleagues.

My gratitude to Tessa Shellen's solicitor, Bevan Ashford, is immense. Not only did she read the text offering helpful comments, but also she supplied the practical advice for health professionals dealing with child abuse (Chapter 9).

Copyright is acknowledged to HMSO (for statutes), Butterworths (for All England Reports), and the RCN (for various educational pamphlets).

Finally as always I thank my family and friends for their support and encouragement.

I have dedicated this book to the many cystic fibrosis sufferers whom I have met, whose courage and absence of self-pity is a lesson to us all.

About the author

Professor Bridgit Dimond, formerly Assistant Director and Dean of the Faculty of Professional Studies at the University of Glamorgan, is an experienced health service manager and lecturer in health service law and management. She is currently the Chairman of the Mid Glamorgan Family Health Services Authority and a former member of the Mental Health Act Commission. Her previous publications include *The Legal Aspects of Nursing 2nd Ed.* (Prentice Hall, 1995), *Accountability and the Nurse* (South Bank Distance Learning Centre), *Health Service Law* (Churchill Livingstone, 1995), *Patients' Rights, Responsibilities and the Nurse* (Quay, 1993), *The Legal Aspects of Midwifery* (Books for Midwives, 1994), *Mental Health Law and the Nurse* (Blackwell, 1996), and many articles on all aspects of professional accountability and patients' rights.

Foreword

The care of children with health needs has changed markedly over the last decade – new health technologies, increased consumer demand, reconfiguration of services, and improved professional skill and knowledge have all played their part. At the same time, the laws concerning children have changed. A greater weight has been placed on the need for children's rights to be considered as paramount, and for all professionals to act in their best interests. The Children Act 1989 firmly established that the ascertainable wishes and feelings of the child must be considered in the light of his or her age and understanding.

The consequence is a complex, demanding workplace in which professionals face moral and ethical dilemmas alongside the rights and responsibilities of their daily practice. Bridgit Dimond's book, therefore, is a particularly important addition to nursing literature. It is a practical, well-referenced guide to both common and unusual issues that result from current health-care programmes; examples include her advice on the actions that should be taken to secure the welfare of a child 'out of hours', the excellent guidelines to assist health professionals through the complex area of consent, the simple explanations of complex law concerning the protection of children in the hospital environment, and the helpful explanation of the important role of professional decision making at case conferences.

There are a number of references in the book to the professional responsibilities associated with health and safety. Practical, believable examples, such as the nurse who failed to supervise a child in a kitchen, which resulted in the scalding of a ward orderly, bring the reader repeatedly back to everyday practices. I found particularly helpful the suggested 'acceptable and unacceptable defences' which may be used in the case of an employer being charged with causing harm to a child in his or her professional care.

Some of the practical suggestions have a particular impact for managers and senior staff; examples include how to provide documentary evidence in a case involving a drug overdose, and the need for employers to draw up a procedure to protect both the child and the health professional in relation to the use of complementary therapies.

The discussion and related case law in the book ranges from the care of children in high-tech acute units to the management of children with mental health problems, and should assist practitioners in a wide range of settings. The author seeks to reinforce the good practice standards set by the Department of Health, the Royal College of Nursing, the British Paediatric Association, Action for Sick Children, and others. Throughout, excellent use is made of check lists, which act as easy reference points for action.

The law is complex for many health care professionals. Bridgit Dimond has made full use of her logical style and ensured the continued attention of the reader. Different perspectives for decision making are explored, accommodating health professionals at all levels of practice.

The text provides excellent opportunities for current issues to be considered. For example, the section about the duties placed upon the Secretary of State for Health to provide services includes mention of the new arrangements for Health Authorities in April 1996. The efficient and effective use of resources is discussed – especially important as medical technology develops. The stark choices that practitioners sometimes have to make are reflected in the section discussing the gap between resource and demand. Never has this been more pertinent than when discussing new fields (such as multiple organ donation, human fertilization and embryology), new nursing roles and the implications of vicarious liability, all of which are explored by the author.

Throughout the book the reader is reminded of that which is considered good practice and the consequences of not fulfilling expectation. The author attempts to make the distinction between that which is lawful and that which is ethically correct. On each occasion, she provides examples of recent case law. Practitioners working with children are required to understand the needs of both the child and their family in a wide range of settings. This book offers additional knowledge (in the field of law), in a format that is applicable to everyday practice, and that will assist practitioners to more fully meet the health needs of children.

Elizabeth Fradd

Table of cases

Table of statutes

PART I

THE CONTEXT OF CARE AND DEFINITIONS

The child, the parent, the legal framework, and the professional

In this first part of the book we consider some of the basic principles of law relating to the child. The first chapter considers what is meant by a child and how the law treats such a person, the second chapter looks at the parent and other persons involved with the child in a legal context, the third considers the legal framework provided by the Children Act 1989, and finally, in the fourth chapter the professional responsibilities of the many groups involved in child health care are described.

CHAPTER
1

The child and the law

There are many ways in which the law takes account of minors – as the child or young person is known – and it is the aim of this introductory chapter to spell out how a child could maintain a legal action and the significance of being a child in civil and criminal law, and at the same time to explain the main principles of the English legal system.

DEFINITION OF A CHILD

In general, adulthood begins at the age of 18 years (under section 1(1) of the Family Law Reform Act 1969 a person ceases to be a minor at 18 years), but specific rights or duties may have different commencement dates. Thus, although a statutory right is given to the child aged 16 years and over to give consent to treatment, and to access his or her health records held in manual form (see Chapter 8), a child is considered able to form the requisite mental intent to commit a crime at the age of 14 years and this presumption is rebuttable between the ages of 10 and 14 years (see below).

Terminology

For the sake of clarity and consistency, the term 'child' will be used in this book to cover a person under 18 years of age, though the cases and situations cited might refer to such a person as a young person, adolescent or minor.

THE LEGAL SYSTEM

The law derives from two main sources: statute law and the common law. These are illustrated in **Figure 1.1**.

Statute law is based on legislation passed through the agreed constitutional process. Legislation of the European Community now takes precedence over Acts of Parliament of the UK Government. Statutory Instruments are drawn up on the basis of powers delegated to Ministers and others supplement Acts of Parliament.

Decisions by judges in courts create what is known as the common law. A recognized hierarchy of the courts determines which previous decisions are binding on courts hearing similar cases.

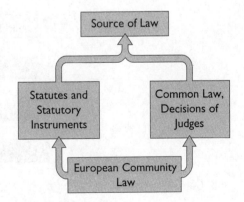

Fig. 1.1 Sources of law.

3

Figures 1.2 and **1.3** illustrate the civil court and the criminal court systems, respectively.

A recognized system for the reporting of judges' decisions means that one can be certain about what was stated and the facts of the cases. It may be possible for judges to 'distinguish' previous cases and not follow them on the grounds that the facts are significantly different, or that the decisions are from a court that is not binding on them.

Judges are, however, bound by statutes and if these result in an unsatisfactory situation, this may be remedied by new amending legislation. Thus in a recent case[1] discussed below the House of Lords recognized that the law relating to the legal age of capacity for a child to be guilty of a crime was unsatisfactory and called upon Parliament to consider reforming the law.

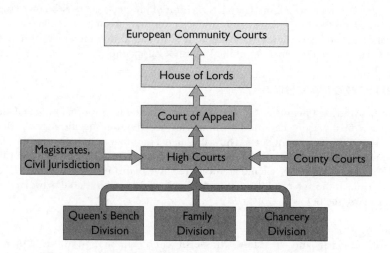

Fig. 1.2 Civil courts.

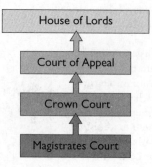

Fig. 1.3 Criminal courts.

THE PRINCIPLES OF THE CHILDREN ACT 1989

The principles of the Children Act 1989 are in force and must be followed by the courts in exercising their jurisdiction over children. They are set out below. The Act sets out as the basic principle applying to any question about the upbringing of a child or the administration of a child's property or the use of income from it that: 'The child's welfare shall be the court's paramount consideration.' This term is not further defined in the Act.

In any proceedings relating to the upbringing of a child, the court should respect the general principle that any delay in determining the question is likely to prejudice the welfare of the child.

If the court is considering making an order for residence, contact, a prohibited steps order or a specific issue order (i.e. an order under section 8), the court must take into account the following circumstances set out in Section 1(3):

- the ascertainable wishes and feelings of the child concerned (considered in the light of his age and understanding);
- his physical, emotional, and educational needs;
- the likely effect on the child of any change in their circumstances;
- the age, sex, background, and any characteristics of the child that the court considers relevant;
- any harm which he has suffered or is at risk of suffering;
- how capable each of the child's parents, and any other person in relation to whom the court considers the question to be relevant, is of meeting the needs of the child; and
- the range of powers available to the court under this Act in the proceedings in question.

Finally, in deciding whether or not to make an order, the court 'shall not make the order or any of the orders unless it considers that doing so would be better for the child than making no order at all.'

Chapter 3 considers the framework provided by the Children Act.

CHARTERS AND THEIR LEGAL STATUS

There are in existence several charters relating to the rights of the child; these are discussed below and have variable legal force. In addition, children are entitled to benefit from general declarations of human rights. For example the European Convention on Human Rights provides protection for the fundamental rights and freedoms of all people, including children and young people.[2] It is enforced through the European Commission and the European Court on Human Rights in Strasbourg. The decisions of the Court are binding on all those countries that are signatories of the Convention, of which the UK is one. It is not confined to European countries who are members of the European Community; Norway, for example, is a signatory to the European Commission on Human Rights but not a member of the European Community. Unlike some other countries, the UK, although a signatory, has not incorporated the Convention into UK law. Applicants who allege a breach of the articles must therefore apply initially to the European Commission, which examines the admissibility of the allegation and, if admissible, attempts to establish the facts and then reach a friendly settlement. A report is subsequently made to the Committee of Ministers and, if the allegation comes within the jurisdiction of the European Court of Human Rights, a hearing will take place. After the judgment, the Committee of Ministers supervises the applications of the decisions. The situation in the UK is unsatisfactory and there has been a recent call for the adoption in the UK of a Bill of Rights which would include the European Convention on Human Rights. The latter would therefore be part of UK law and would automatically be applied by the judges when hearing cases.

CHARTERS FOR THE CHILD AND YOUNG PERSON

The Royal College of Nursing has given its support to the following documents in addition to its support for the principles of the Children Act 1989.[3]

The UN Convention on the Rights of the Child

The UN Convention on the Rights of the Child was adopted on 20 November 1989.[4] When the Convention has been ratified by 20 countries, it will become international law and binding on those countries which have signed. However, unlike the European Convention on Human Rights with its court in Strasbourg, there is no judicial machinery to enforce the law and no right of individual complaint. The Convention is not directly implemented in the English courts. As a signatory, the UK would be expected to publicize the articles in the Convention and monitor progress in fulfilling the obligations, reporting to the specially constituted committee of the UN. The first report of the UK to the UN Committee on the Rights of the Child was published in February 1994.[5] It analyses article by article the progress that the UK has made in implementing the Convention. In its guidance on child health in the community the Department of Health[6] stated that purchasers should take account of the provision of the UN Convention on the Rights of the Child in considering the principles upon which they might base their contracts for child health services. Thus, even though at present they have no statutory force, the articles should be the basis of the purchase and provision of child health services.

The Resolution of the European Parliament on a Charter for Children in Hospital (1986)

In 1979 the Parliamentary Assembly of the Council of Europe debated a report from the Committee on Social and Health Questions. It supported a charter covering general principles, setting out the legal position of the child, including abuse, prostitution and pornography, child labour, social and medical protection, and sports. It recommended that the Committee of Ministers consult the Parliamentary Assembly on the content of the proposed charter on the Rights of the Child.[7] The statement on social and medical protection, that is, the Charter of the Council of Europe is given below.

- The rights of every child to life from the moment of conception, to shelter, adequate food, and a congenial environment should be recognized, and national governments should accept as an obligation the task of providing for full realization of such rights.
- The right to adequate care, including effective measures against disease and accidents, and adequate medical attention should be ensured.
- All member governments should establish systems of obligatory free medical examination of children.
- Due attention should be paid to protection against abuse of drugs, smoking, and alcohol, and advertising for these products in broadcasting.
- The right of handicapped children to be properly looked after and to be given adequate training and education should be guaranteed; urgent attention should be given to the problem of the child kept in hospital on a long-term basis; the organization of voluntary visiting schemes should be considered, using media publicity and other methods.

These principles have not yet been adopted as part of the law of the European Community nor accepted within the UK as law.

European Charter for Children in Hospital

In May 1988 individuals from 12 European countries met for the first European Conference on Children in Hospital to formalize their commitment to quality for children in hospitals and their families. A charter was agreed by participants from Belgium, Denmark, England, Finland, France, Iceland, the Netherlands, Norway, the Federal Republic of Germany, Sweden, and Switzerland. It contained the following clauses.

- The right to the best possible medical treatment is a fundamental right especially for children.
- Children should be admitted to hospital only if the care they require cannot be equally well provided at home or on an outpatient basis.
- Children in hospital should have the right to have their parents or parent substitute with them at all times.
- Accommodation should be offered to all parents, and they should be helped and encouraged to stay; parents should not need to incur additional costs or suffer loss of income; in order to share in the care of their child, parents should be kept informed about ward routine and their active participation encouraged.
- Children and parents should have the right to be informed in a manner appropriate to age and understanding; steps should be taken to mitigate physical and emotional stress.
- Children and parents have the right to informed participation in all decisions involving the child's health care; every child should be protected from unnecessary medical treatment and investigation.
- Children should be cared for with other children who have the same developmental needs and should not be admitted to adult wards; there should be no age restriction for visitors to children in hospitals.
- Children should have full access to play, recreation, and education suited to their age and condition and should be in an environment designed, furnished, staffed, and equipped to meet their needs.
- Children should be cared for by staff whose training and skills enable them to respond to the physical, emotional, and developmental needs of children and their families.
- Continuity of care should be ensured by the team caring for the child.
- Children should be treated with tact and understanding and their privacy should be respected at all times.

Charter of the National Association for the Welfare of Children in Hospital

The Charter of the National Association for the Welfare of Children in Hospital (NAWCH, now Action for Sick Children) has no direct legal force except for those provisions which are already part of the law, such as case law or statute law. Its 10 principles are set out below.

- All children should have equal access to the best clinical care.
- Parents are responsible for their children and should receive positive and appropriate support to care for their sick child at home and in hospital.
- Children and their parents should be given full information about their treatment and participate in all decisions.
- Whenever possible sick children should be cared for at home, unless the care they require can only be provided in hospital.
- Staff caring for children, whether in hospital or in the community, should be specifically trained and fully aware of children's emotional and developmental needs.
- Children should be cared for in an environment furnished and equipped to meet their requirements, whether in a hospital department or in the community.
- No child should be cared for in an adult ward.
- Every hospital admitting children should provide overnight accommodation free of charge.
- Parents should be positively encouraged to be with their child in hospital at all times and participate free of charge.
- Every child in hospital should have full opportunity for play, recreation, and education.

The Department of Health's guidance document 'Welfare of Children and Young People in Hospital' (1991)

The Department of Health's guidance document 'Welfare of Children and Young People in Hospital' (1991) sets out the standards that should be followed in providing hospital care for children and young people. It reflects many of the principles set out in the charters discussed above. Although the guidance has no direct legal force, it would be good practice to follow its principles. Failure to implement the guidance would not, however, lead to legal action unless the failures related to activities or omissions for which there already exists a remedy in law. For example it is good practice for a child to be cared for on a children's ward rather than an adult ward, but were a child to be placed on an adult ward in an emergency situation, the parents would have no redress on behalf of the child, other than the right to complain. This Department of Health guidance document is referred to throughout this book.

SIGNIFICANCE OF THE CHARTERS

These charters are not in themselves legally enforceable. Some of the rights which they state duplicate already existing rights (such as the right of the child to be involved in the decision-making concerning his or her care). The principles stated in them should, however, be followed by the health professional and they will increasingly figure as requirements in NHS agreements between purchasers and providers (see Chapter 5). Many trusts have now produced their own charter, such as 'The Child and Family Charter' prepared by the Royal Berkshire and Battle Hospitals. The implementation of these can be monitored as part of quality assurance but they do not give the child or family enforceable legal rights. (This is further discussed in Chapter 5.)

A BILL OF RIGHTS

This country has resisted the adoption of a Bill of Rights which would be supreme over Parliament and could only be changed by a specified procedure. Instead the UK has what is called an 'unwritten constitution' and principles of law are derived from the statute laws or the common law (see above and glossary). However, our membership of the European Community has meant that we are increasingly required to implement European Directives which recognize the basic principles set out in the Convention and charters described above. It is possible that over the next few years most of the contents of these charters will be directly enforceable in the English courts.

THE CHILD AND LEGAL PROCEEDINGS

The child may be represented in both civil and criminal proceedings. First these terms will be explained.

Civil and criminal law

The civil law covers the law which governs disputes between private citizens (including corporate bodies) or between citizens and the state. Thus contract law and the law of torts (civil wrongs excluding breach of contract), rights over property, marital disputes, and wrongful exercise of power by a statutory authority, come under the civil law.

Criminal law relates to actions which can be followed by criminal proceedings, in which an accused is prosecuted. The sources of criminal law are both statutory and common law; for example the definition of murder derives from a decision of the courts in the seventeenth century, whereas theft is defined by an Act of Parliament of 1967 as amended by subsequent legislation.

An illustration of some of the principal differences between a civil case and a criminal case is shown in **Figure 1.4**.

There is an overlap between civil and criminal wrongs; touching a person without their consent may be a civil wrong (trespass to the person) and also a crime (an assault or battery). Similarly, driving a car carelessly may lead to criminal proceedings for driving without due care and attention. It may also be a civil wrong of negligence if it can be established that the driver was in breach of a duty of care owed to the person who was injured as a result. In a case in which an anaesthetist failed to realize that a tube had become disconnected, the anaesthetist was prosecuted in the criminal courts and convicted of manslaughter; there would also be liability on his employers in the civil courts for his negligence in causing the death of the patient.

Both criminal proceedings and civil proceedings could thus take place.

Public and private law
Another distinction in the classification of laws is that of public and private law. **Figure 1.5** illustrates the difference between the two.

Fig. 1.4 CRIMINAL AND CIVIL PROCEDURES

Criminal	Civil
A prosecution is brought in relation to a charge of criminal conduct and heard in the criminal courts where the standard of proof of guilt is beyond reasonable doubt.	An action is brought in relation to a civil wrong by a plaintiff against an individual organization in the civil courts where the standard of proof is on a balance of possibilities.

Fig. 1.5 DIFFERENCES BETWEEN PUBLIC AND PRIVATE LAW

Public law	Private law
Relates to intervention on a matter relating to the public concern; for example, the protection of children or vulnerable adults, the carrying out of statutory duties.	The law pertaining to the rights of individuals and organizations, and the relationships between them; for example, purchasing a house, suing for negligence or breaches of contract.

Public law deals with those areas of law in which society intervenes in the actions of individuals. In contrast, private law is concerned with the behaviour of individuals to each other. The Children Act 1989 covers both private law and public law relating to children. Care proceedings, protection orders, and child assessment orders are part of the public law; orders in relation to children made after divorce or nullity, such as with whom the child is to live, are part of private law. (see Part II of the Act discussed in Chapter 3). Thus the Cleveland Report was concerned with the public law: the duty of the Social Services Department to take action to protect children. In contrast, a dispute over whether consent has been given for a child to have treatment would be part of private law.

Family proceedings are defined in section 8(3) and discussed in Chapter 3.

The child and civil wrongs (excluding breach of contract)

AS PLAINTIFF (BRINGING THE ACTION)

If the child has been harmed and wishes to seek compensation, the action must be brought in his or her name until they are 18 years of age. They therefore sue through an adult who is known as the 'next friend'. The next friend is liable for any costs awarded against the minor in the action, though the child must indemnify him or her, and would usually be the parent. Unlike an adult, however, the child cannot settle their action except by leave of court.

If negligence is alleged, the child can sue either parent, though this is unlikely if the parent does not have insurance cover. If, however, a child is injured in a car crash as a result of careless driving by the parent, the child can sue that parent for compensation and the award would be paid by the insurance company.

If a child has suffered personal injuries, the time within which the court action must be commenced will be 3 years from his eighteenth birthday unless he is mentally retarded, in which case there is no time limit so long as the incapacity exists. The rules for the defence of contributory negligence also vary (see Chapter 13).

The Congenital Disabilities (Civil Liability) Act 1976 enables a child once born to sue in respect of harm which occurred prenatally as a result of a civil wrong against the father or mother. This right is also recognized at common law. The child cannot sue his or her mother under this Act unless he or she has suffered harm as a result of her driving a car while pregnant with her or him.

AS DEFENDANT

If the child is responsible for causing harm to another, he or she can be liable in the law of tort, but this liability will depend upon the plaintiff being able to show that the child had the necessary mental element to commit the civil wrong. Consequently, a child who ran out onto a road from a nursery school, thus causing a road accident and the death of an oncoming driver who tried to avoid a collision, would not necessarily be at fault himself, but the teachers or carers who failed to take sufficient care may be. The standard of care in the tort (i.e. civil wrong excluding breach of contract) of negligence which is expected of a child may be very different from that expected of an adult in the same circumstances.

In a recent case a driver sued a 9-year-old boy for the damage which resulted to her car when the boy negligently walked into the path of the oncoming car. An anonymous donor paid the £200 repair bill and the action was adjourned indefinitely. The parents then sued the driver for the injuries that the boy suffered and £3500 was awarded in the County court.[8]

A parent is not vicariously liable for the torts of his or her children unless, he or she authorized them, or stands in an employer–employee relationship or principal–agent relationship with the children. However, there may be direct liability of the parent or other adult for lack of appropriate supervision, delegation, training, and so forth (see Chapter 14).

The child would defend the action through a guardian *ad litem* who is not liable for costs. This person would usually be the mother or father of the child.

(This is further discussed in Chapter 13.)

Children and the law of contract

The Minor's Contracts Act 1987 which came into force on 9 June 1987 amended the Infants Relief Act 1874 and the common law in relation to the liability and ability of a child under contract. The position now is as follows.

- A child can make a valid contract for the purchase of necessaries; the child can also make a valid contract for services for their benefit, such as apprenticeship and education.
- Contracts for loans and goods that are not necessary are not binding upon the child unless they are ratified after the child reaches the age of 18 years.
- Other contracts are binding unless repudiated; these are known as voidable contracts.

THE APPLICATION FOR HEALTH CARE

It would be possible for a child to agree to enter into a contract for the supply of private health services. Such a contract would probably be regarded as one that is for the child's benefit. It would therefore be valid. If the child failed to pay for the services, then it would be enforceable against him and he would have to pay a reasonable price, which may not necessarily be the agreed price.

The child and the criminal law

CHILDREN AGED 10 YEARS OR LESS

Children under the age of 10 years are presumed to be incapable of any crime (section 16, Children and Young Persons Act 1963). This presumption is irrebuttable. This means that they are immune from prosecution. They are known as 'doli incapax'.

CHILDREN AGED BETWEEN 10 AND 14 YEARS

Children aged between 10 and 14 years are presumed to be incapable of forming the mental intent to commit a crime, but this presumption is rebuttable. If, therefore, it can be shown that the child has a 'mischievous discretion' or an appreciation of the wrong-doing, then, if all the other ingredients of the crime can be proved, a conviction can be made. In one case[9] a 10-year-old boy took some items from an ambulance which was parked in hospital grounds. He threw a first-aid box over a wall and climbed over after it. He was caught in possession of the box and said to the police: 'It ain't nothing to do with me, I didn't steal it.' He was convicted of theft and it was held on appeal that there was sufficient evidence that he knew what he was doing, with the result that his conviction was affirmed. The boy had indicated by his words that he knew about theft and that it was wrong.

The principle has been confirmed by the House of Lords in a recent case.[1] A boy had been convicted by the Magistrates of interfering with a motor cycle with intent to drive away. He was just under the age of 13 years at the time of the offence. His conviction was upheld by the Queen's Bench Division on the grounds that the presumption that a child aged between 10 and 14 years was not able to be convicted of a criminal offence unless it was clearly established that he knew his act was seriously wrong, was no longer the law. The High Court certified that a point of law of general public importance was involved for consideration by the House of Lords. The House of Lords, in confirming that the principle was still law, set out two propositions:

- that the prosecution had to prove that the child defendant did the act charged and that when doing that act he knew that it was a wrong act as distinct from an act of mere naughtiness or childish mischief. The criminal standard of proof applied; and

- that evidence to prove the defendant's guilty knowledge had not to be the mere proof of the doing of the act charged, however horrifying or obviously wrong that act might be.

The House of Lords therefore allowed the appeal and the case was remitted to the High Court so that the Magistrates could be directed to dismiss the charge.

The House of Lords, however, called upon Parliament to reform the serious shortcomings of this doctrine. They stated that it appeared to have been inconsistently applied and was certainly capable of producing inconsistent results according to the way in which the courts treated the presumption and depending upon the evidence which was available to rebut it.

CHILDREN AGED OVER 14 YEARS

Children older than 14 years are fully liable for their crimes but the punishments which are available to the court and the procedure which must be followed differ from those for an adult.

Other rights and powers of a child

Below is a list of the rights in law that a child has at certain ages.

AT BIRTH
- to hold a passport
- to sue (through next friend)
- to have a deposit or bank account
- to make contracts for necessities
- to be taxed

AT 5 YEARS OF AGE
- to be obliged to attend school

AT 10 YEARS OF AGE
- to be convicted of a criminal offence (if knows difference of right from wrong)

AT 14 YEARS OF AGE
- to be convicted of a criminal offence without it being established that he knew right from wrong

AT 16 YEARS OF AGE
- to leave school
- to marry with parental consent
- to consent to medical, surgical or dental treatment (see Chapter 6)
- to consent to heterosexual intercourse

AT 17 YEARS OF AGE
- to hold a driving license for a car

AT 18 YEARS OF AGE
- to marry without parental consent
- to vote in local and general election
- to make a will
- to buy a drink in a bar
- to hold a driving licence
- to sue and be sued in his or her own name
- to be a blood donor

- to be tattooed. (The Tattooing of Minors Act 1969 makes it an offence, punishable by fine, for a person other than a duly qualified medical practitioner to tattoo a person under the age of 18 years. The person charged with the offence will have a defence if he can show that at the time he had reasonable cause to believe that the person tattooed was 18 years of age or over.)

AT 21 YEARS OF AGE
- to stand for election to central and local government
- to apply to adopt a child

Evidence in court

CIVIL PROCEEDINGS

Until recently a child who did not understand the nature of an oath was incompetent to testify and could not be called as a witness. However, section 96 of the Children Act 1989 has made significant changes and is set out below.

- Subsection (2) applies if a child who is called as a witness in any civil proceedings does not, in the opinion of the court, understand the nature of an oath.
- The child's evidence may be heard by the court if, in its opinion (a) he understands that it is his duty to speak the truth, and (b) he has sufficient understanding to justify his evidence being heard.
- Under subsection (3) the Lord Chancellor may by order make provision for the admissibility of evidence which would otherwise be inadmissible under any rule of law relating to hearsay.
- An order under subsection (3) may only be made with respect to (a) civil proceedings in general or such civil proceedings, or class of civil proceedings, as may be prescribed, and (b) evidence in connection with the upbringing, maintenance or welfare of a child.

The judge can determine the competence of the child to give evidence and would ask the child questions to form an opinion.

Criminal proceedings

A child aged 14 years or more is considered competent to give sworn evidence, unless they are unable to understand the nature of the oath by reason of unsound mind or unable to communicate in a rational, intelligible and coherent manner.

Children under the age of 14 years shall give evidence in criminal proceedings unsworn (section 52(1) Criminal Justice Act 1991). The judge's power to determine whether a particular person is not competent to give evidence applies to children of tender years as it applies to other persons. Unsworn evidence admitted under section 52 may corroborate evidence, whether sworn or unsworn, given by any other person. Reference should be made to the publications of the Children's Legal Centre for more detail.[10]

REFERENCES

1 C (a minor) *v* Director of Public Prosecutions. *Times,* Law Report; 17 March 1995.
2 See briefing note prepared by the Children's Legal Centre.
3 Royal College of Nursing: *Issues in Nursing and Health, No. 10.* London: RCN; February 1992.
4 See briefing note prepared by the Children's Legal Centre.
5 *First Report of the UK to the UN Committee on the Rights of the Child.* London: HMSO; February 1994.
6 Department of Health: *Child Health in the Community: A Guide to Good Practice* (Consultation draft March 1995). London: HMSO; 1995.
7 Thirty-first ordinary session Recommendation 874(1979) on a European Charter on the Rights of the Child.

8   Biggs *v* Dowson. *Times,* News Report; 17 March 1995.
9   I *v* Director of Public Prosecutions [1989] Criminal Law Report 498.
10 Harbour A, Ayotte W (Editors): *Children's Legal Centre Mental Health Handbook: A Guide to the Law Affecting Children and Young People. Edn 2.* London: Legal Centre; 1994.

Representatives of the child

In this chapter we consider the definitions of the various persons who may be involved in caring for the child, accompanying him or her to hospital or representing the child in different court hearings, and we look at their legal status and functions.[1]

PARENTAL RESPONSIBILITIES

The emphasis in the Children Act 1989 is on the responsibilities rather than the rights of parents. The Children Act 1989 lays down basic principles defining those who have parental responsibilities and the phrase itself.

Section 2 of the 1989 Act, that addresses parental responsibility for children, is listed below in its subsections.

1   If a child's father and mother were married to each other at the time of the birth, they shall each have parental responsibility for the child.
2   If a child's father and mother were not married to each other at the time of the birth, (a) the mother shall have parental responsibility for the child, and (b) the father shall not have parental responsibility for the child, unless he acquires it in accordance with the provisions of this Act.
3   References in this Act to a child whose father and mother were, or were not, married to each other at the time of his or her birth must be read with section 1 of the Family Law Reform Act 1987 (which extends their meaning).
4   The rule of law is abolished that the father is the natural guardian of his legitimate children.
5   More than one parent can have responsibility at the same time.
6   A person who has parental responsibility for a child at any time shall not cease to have that responsibility solely because some other person subsequently acquires parental responsibility for the child.
7   Where more than one person has parental responsibility for a child, each of them may act alone and without the other (or others) in meeting that responsibility; but nothing in this Part shall be taken to affect the operation of any enactment which requires the consent of more than one person in a matter affecting the child.
8   The fact that a person has parental responsibility for a child shall not entitle him to act in any way which would be incompatible with any order made with respect to the child under this Act.
9   A person who has parental responsibility for a child may not surrender or transfer any part of that responsibility to another but may arrange for some or all of it to be met by one or more persons acting on his or her behalf.

10 The person with whom such arrangement is made may himself be a person who already has parental responsibility for the child concerned.

11 The making of any such arrangement shall not affect any liability of the person making it which may arise from any failure to meet any part of his or her parental responsibility for the child concerned.

The effect of section 2 is to give parental responsibilities to both parents of legitimate children and to the mother of an illegitimate child, and to ensure that they retain these responsibilities whatever happens unless the child is adopted. Anyone with parental responsibility can act alone unless the consent of more than one person is required. This is discussed below. Although arrangements can be made for others to act on behalf of a person with responsibility, this arrangement will not transfer parental responsibilities nor will it affect the liability of the parent.

The way in which a father who was not married to the mother at the time of the birth acquires parental responsibility is set out in section 4. This can be done by order of the court or by a parental responsibility arrangement made between mother and father in the form prescribed by the Lord Chancellor.

Thus once parental responsibilities are acquired they remain, unless the child is adopted, until the child becomes an adult. This applies even if the local authority makes a care order in respect of the child. What then does parental responsibility mean?

Definition of parental responsibility

Parental responsibility is defined in section 3(1) as 'all the rights, duties, powers, responsibilities and authority which by law a parent of a child has in relation to the child and his property.' This also includes 'the rights, powers and duties which a guardian of the child's estate (appointed, before the commencement of section 5, to act generally) would have had in relation to the child and his property.'

The existence or otherwise of parental responsibilities does not affect any obligation which a person may have in relation to the child (such as a statutory duty to maintain the child) or any rights after the child's death in their property.

The Act makes no attempt to list all the kinds of rights, duties, powers, and responsibilities which are covered by the concept of 'parental responsibilities'. As will be seen in Chapter 6 relating to consent and the Gillick-competent child, the powers of the parent will vary according to the age and level of maturity of the child (see **Fig. 6.1**, Chapter 6).

PARENT BY ADOPTION

Adoption is now the only legal mechanism for terminating the parental responsibility of a parent and transferring it to another. The law is governed by the Adoption Act 1976 as amended by the Children Act 1989. Under the Adoption Act 1976 it is a criminal offence for anyone other than an adoption agency to make arrangements for the adoption of a child or to make a placement unless the individual concerned is a relative of the child or is acting with the authority of a High Court order. The Act also makes it a criminal offence to offer a reward to secure an adoption. The court does, however, have power to authorize retrospective payments where appropriate.

An application for adoption can be made by a person over the age of 21 years. It can be made by a single person or jointly by a couple provided they are married. An adoption order can also be made on the application of a married couple where one spouse is the father or mother of the child and aged at least 18 years and the other spouse is aged at least 21 years. Before an order for adoption is made by the court, either the parents must consent or this consent can be dispensed with by the court if specific statutory grounds are present and on proof that adoption is in the best interests of the child.

The legal effect of the adoption is that the child is treated in law for almost all purposes as if he or she were a child of the adopters' marriage. The legal responsibilities of the birth parents are irrevocably ended.

It is clear in the context of health care that the fact that parents are parents by adoption may not come to the notice of health professionals. Should they become aware of this information, they should not reveal it to the child without the consent of the adoptive parents. If parents are known to be by adoption, this will not in any way affect the legal responsibilities that they have to the child. The health professional may, however, become involved if the child is anxious to seek his or her natural parents.

Under the Children Act 1989 an Adoption Contact Register has been established to enable adopted children to discover whether attempts to contact relatives would be welcome and, if this is the case, to provide them with factual information which may enable them to do so. Access to this Register is discussed in Chapter 8.

DE FACTO CARERS

The term 'de facto carers' covers a wide range of persons who are currently in charge of the child but have no parental responsibility for that child. De facto means 'in practice' or 'in fact' as opposed to 'in law'. The term would thus include teachers, baby-sitters, step-parents, foster parents, relatives or others currently caring for the child.

Section 3(5) of the Children Act 1989 gives such persons the right to make decisions on behalf of the child, and is shown below.

> ...a person who (a) does not have parental responsibility for a particular child, but (b) has care of the child may (subject to the provisions of this Act) do what is reasonable in all the circumstances of the case for the purposes of safeguarding or promoting the child's welfare.

Thus staff in an accident and emergency department could obtain the consent of such a person for immediate necessary treatment, such as stitches or injections.

FOSTER PARENTS

Foster parents take care of children without acquiring parental responsibility. The arrangement might result from a private or public agreement. In law, foster parents are regarded as de facto carers. They have no legal rights to hold onto the child but can, like step-parents (see below), apply for a contact or residence order in respect of the child if they have lived with the child for more than 3 years or they have the consent of those who have parental responsibility. A person who has been a local authority foster parent within the past 6 months cannot apply for leave to make an application for a section 8 order unless they have the consent of the local authority, they are a relative of the child, or the child has lived with them for at least 3 years preceding the application (section 9(3)).

As de facto carers, foster parents have the power to make decisions about the care of the child under section 3(5) of the Children Act 1989 (see above).

GRANDPARENTS

If the child has not lived with the grandparents for at least 3 years, the latter are not entitled to apply for a contact order under section 8 of the Children Act 1989 (they could previously apply for access). They can, however, seek the leave of the court to make an application (section 10(1)(a)(ii)).

The grandparents may of course be de facto carers and have the power to make decisions under section 3(5).

STEP-PARENTS

Step-parents who are in de facto care of the child have responsibilities under section 3(5) of the Children Act 1989 in the same way as a teacher or carer (see above). This enables them to make decisions about the care of the child (see Chapter 14). However, there is no additional legal recognition of their relationship with the child.

The step-parent can, however, apply for either a section 8 order or adoption. A section 8 order includes a contact order or a residence order if the step-parent is either a party to the marriage, or has lived with the child for at least 3 years, or has the consent of each of those who have parental responsibility for the child. For adoption the courts may consider whether a contact or residence order is more appropriate before granting an adoption order to a step-parent.

SURROGATE PARENT

Under section 27(1) of the Human Fertilisation and Embryology Act 1990 it is the woman who is carrying or has carried a child as a result of an embryo or sperm and eggs having been placed in her uterus who is to be treated as the mother of the child.

However, section 27(2) states that this principle does not apply if the child is treated by virtue of adoption as not being the child of any person other than the adopter or adopters.

Under section 30 the court can make an order providing for a child to be treated in law as the child of the parties to a marriage if the child has been carried by a woman other than the wife as the result of embryo or sperm and egg donation, or her artificial insemination.

Certain conditions must be satisfied before the court can make an order, including the requirement that the husband and wife must apply for the order within 6 months of the birth of the child. Both husband and wife must have attained the age of 18 years. The court must also be satisfied that no money or other benefit was paid for the arrangement other than reasonably incurred expenses.

Health professionals may never become aware that a child is the result of in-vitro fertilization or similar treatment, unless they become involved in the child's search for information on his or her origins. (This is discussed in Chapter 8.)

GUARDIAN

Whereas in the past the parent was seen as the guardian of the child, the Children Act 1989 has separated the two concepts; the notion of parental guardianship has been abolished by the Act. Guardians are now persons other than parents who are appointed to exercise parental responsibilities. They have the same legal responsibilities as parents. They are not, however, liable for child support as parents are, and they can disclaim their appointment.

Guardians can be appointed in two ways. The first is by private appointment either by the parents with parental responsibility or by the guardians. An unmarried father may not appoint a guardian unless he has acquired parental responsibility. The only formality necessary is that the appointment must be in writing, dated and signed. The appointment can be made by two or more persons.

The second is by court appointment either if there is no parent with parental responsibility or if a deceased parent had a residence order in his or her favour at the time of death.

The guardian has parental responsibility, can object to adoption and can appoint a guardian. The guardian is not liable for the financial responsibility of the child.

Ending of guardianship

The guardian can disclaim his or her appointment within a reasonable time. The appointment can be revoked by the appointing parent or guardian. The guardian may be removed by order of the court on the application of any person who has parental responsibility for the child, or the application of the child concerned with the leave of the court, or in any family proceedings if the court considers the guardianship should be brought to an end, even without an application. The appointment automatically ends with the death of the child or guardian or when the child becomes 18 years of age.

GUARDIAN *AD LITEM*

The guardian *ad litem* is a person with a social work and child care background who is appointed to ensure that the court is fully informed of the relevant facts which relate to the child and that the wishes and feelings of the child are clearly established. The appointment is made from a panel set up by the local authority. A panel manager is appointed who is responsible for arranging the training, and remuneration of the guardian *ad litem*, and general administration. An annual report is prepared on the panel's activities. A panel committee is appointed to assist with liaison between the local authority and the courts.

If a child is separately represented in public family proceedings this will be by a guardian *ad litem* or a solicitor, or both. Under the Children Act 1989 section 41(6) and the Rules of Court, proceedings are specified in which the court must appoint a guardian *ad litem*, unless satisfied that it is not necessary to do so in order to safeguard the interests of the child. Thus there need be no guardian *ad litem* if the child wishes to instruct his or her own solicitor and has the competence to do so. The guardian *ad litem* should be appointed as soon as possible after the commencement or transfer of the proceedings. It is not intended that the guardian *ad litem* should represent the child in the court. This role is undertaken by a solicitor or, if appropriate, a barrister. The functions of a guardian *ad litem* are:

- to safeguard the interests of the child (section 41(2));
- to attend all directions, appointments, and hearings unless excused by the court, and to advise the court on the following matters
  a whether the child is of sufficient understanding for any purpose, including the child's refusal to submit to a medical or psychiatric examination or other assessment that the court has power to require, direct or order;
  b the wishes of the child in respect of any matter relevant to the proceedings, including his or her attendance at court;
  c the appropriate forum for the proceedings;
  d the appropriate timing of the proceedings or any part of them;
  e the options available to it in respect of the child and the suitability of each such option, including what order should be made in determining the application;
  f any other matter concerning which the court seeks his or her advice or concerning which he or she considers that the court should be informed;
- to appoint a solicitor, advise the child as is appropriate having regard to his or her understanding, and instruct the solicitor;
- to file a written report advising on the interests of the child, not less than 7 days before the date fixed for the hearing;
- to make such investigations as may be necessary for him or her to carry out his or her duties, including, in particular, interviewing, inspection of records, and obtaining professional assistance.

Although the local authority pays the guardian *ad litem*, the latter is intended to be independent of the local authority, in order to act in the interests of the child. A decision by the local authority which limited the number of hours which a guardian *ad litem* could spend on a case was quashed by the court because it was essential that the independence of the guardian *ad litem* was not reduced in any way by placing restrictions directly or indirectly on the discharge of his or her statutory duties.

Under section 42 of the Children Act the guardian *ad litem* has a statutory right of access to local authority records at all reasonable times. Access includes examining and taking copies. If the guardian *ad litem* takes a copy of any record which he or she is entitled to examine, that copy or any part of it is admissible in evidence.

What if there is a disagreement between the guardian *ad litem* and the child? There may be a dispute between the guardian *ad litem* and the solicitor representing the child over the competence of the child. The rules enable the solicitor to take direct instructions from the child if, having taken into account the views of the guardian *ad litem* and any court directions, he or she considers that the child has sufficient understanding to issue such instructions.

NEXT FRIEND

The 'next friend' is a person who can sue on behalf of a minor. This must not be a person who is connected with the defendant or interested in the proceedings against the interests of the minor. Preference will be given to the father, mother, guardian, or some other relative or person who has connections with the minor. The court can appoint a next friend for a minor. The person must give written consent to be the next friend and the solicitor must file a certificate stating that he or she knows or believes the person to whom the certificate relates to be a minor and the person so named has no interest in the case or matter in question adverse to that of the minor. The next friend has a duty to continue to act as such unless and until the court substitutes another person to act in that capacity. The next friend is an officer of the court appointed to look after the minor's interests and has the conduct of the proceedings in his or her hands, but he or she is not actually a party to the proceedings and is not, as next friend, entitled to appear in them in person. The next friend will not be ordered to give security for costs. The court can remove the next friend if he or she fails to act as such, or does not conduct the proceedings in a proper manner, and can make a new appointment if the next friend dies.

SOLICITOR

The solicitor is a lawyer who has passed the examinations and entry qualifications of the Law Society. In the past he or she has had no rights of advocacy in the High Courts and above, but now solicitors can obtain these rights. It is still the normal practice to appoint barristers (known as counsel) to represent the client in court, draft pleadings, and advise on legal issues. One of the functions of the guardian *ad litem* is to appoint a solicitor; however, the court can appoint a solicitor when:

- no guardian *ad litem* has been appointed for the child;
- the child has sufficient understanding to instruct a solicitor and wishes to do so; and
- it appears to the court that it would be in the child's best interests for him to be represented by a solicitor.

OFFICIAL SOLICITOR

The official solicitor is appointed to represent children in wardship cases. The Lord Chancellor requires the official solicitor to be appointed in specified proceedings if the child does not have a guardian *ad litem* and the court considers that there are exceptional circumstances which make it desirable in the interests of the welfare of the child for there to be the official solicitor.[2] Such cases include those with a foreign element, and those involving a number of children or a child already represented by the official solicitor in the proceedings. The official solicitor will only be appointed if a case reaches the High Court and the child is without a guardian *ad litem*. The value of the official solicitor is that he or she has great expertise in High Court procedures and child care cases in which wider issues of public policy and complexity are relevant.

If the official solicitor is appointed, the child will be joined as a party in the proceedings and the official solicitor will act as the guardian *ad litem*.

CONCLUSION

Health professionals caring for children should be clear about the distinctions between these various categories of carers and representatives in case they encounter disputes in their work. If there is doubt as to the nature of the relationship between the person accompanying or visiting the child and other persons who seek to represent the child, the health professional would have a duty to ascertain the exact legal standing of these persons. Should a serious dispute over a significant issue emerge between the various persons, the health professional should seek the guidance of his or her NHS trust or employer's solicitor who may need to consult the local authority over obtaining an order from the court. (Disputes over decision-making on behalf of the child are considered in Chapter 14.)

REFERENCES

1 For further details, see: Bainham A, Cretney S: *Children – the Modern Law.* Bristol: Family Law; 1993.
2 Lord Chancellor's Direction: Duties and Functions of the Official Solicitor under the Children Act 1989 [1991] 2 FLR 471 made under section 41(8).

Child health care: the legal framework

SCOPE OF THE CHILDREN ACT 1989

The Children Act 1989[1,2] brought into place a new framework for the law relating to children and although it did not repeal all previous legislation on children, it introduced significant new provisions. Clearly its scope is much wider than is relevant for this book; nevertheless, this chapter aims at setting out the framework of the Act and the basic principles incorporated in it. Reference will be made to the relevant chapters in this book, in which further discussion on the provisions of the Act can be found.

The main principles embodied in the Act are set out below.

- The welfare of the child is the paramount consideration in court proceedings.
- Wherever possible children should be brought up and cared for in their own families.
- Courts should ensure that delay is avoided, and may only make an order if to do so is better than making no order at all.
- Children should be kept informed about what happens to them, and should participate when decisions are made about their future.
- Parents continue to have parental responsibility for their children, even when their children are no longer living with them; they should be kept informed about their children and participate when decisions are made about their children's future.
- Parents with children in need should be helped to bring up their children themselves.
- This help should be provided as a service to the child and their family, and should:
  a be provided in partnership with parents;
  b meet each child's identified needs;
  c be appropriate to the child's race, culture, religion, and language;
  d be open to effective independent representations and complaints procedures; and
  e draw upon effective partnership between the local authority and other agencies, including voluntary agencies.

The main areas covered by the Act are summarized below.

- General principles relating to the welfare of the child (see Chapter 1).
- Parental responsibilities and the appointment of guardians (see Chapter 2).
- Orders with respect to children in family proceedings (see below).
- Local authority support for children and families (see below).
- Care and supervision orders (see below).
- Protection of children (see Chapter 9).

- Community homes (not covered in this book).
- Voluntary homes and voluntary organizations (not covered in this book).
- Registered children's homes (not covered in this book).
- Private arrangements for fostering children (not covered in this book).
- Child minding and day care for young children (not covered in this book).
- Secretary of State's supervisory functions and responsibilities (not covered in this book).
- Miscellaneous and general topics, including the duty to notify the local authority of children accommodated in different establishments, tests to establish paternity, criminal offences, search warrants, and jurisdiction of the courts (wardship jurisdiction is covered in Chapter 9; mental health and the child are covered in Chapter 21).

The Children Act 1989 lays down the basic principles that relate to the care of the child and the considerations that should be taken into account; the nature of parental responsibility and how this is acquired; the powers of the court in family proceedings; the duty of the local authority towards a child in need and the duty to provide care; and supervision and protection when necessary.

As it is not possible to consider in detail all the topics covered in the Children Act, only those areas of direct relevance to the health professional will be covered.[3] Reference can, however, be made to the guidance provided by the Department of Health on the Children Act.[4] The Department of Health has also provided guidance for the NHS.[5] Chapter 2 considers the legal principles relating to parental responsibility laid down by the Children Act 1989. Chapter 9 considers the law and practice relating to child protection and the provisions of Part V of the Act. In the rest of this chapter the other aspects of the Children Act 1989 are considered in brief outline.

FAMILY PROCEEDINGS

Family proceedings include court proceedings under the inherent jurisdiction of the High Court to take care of children and also proceedings in relation to Parts I, II, and IV of the Children Act 1989, the Adoption Act 1976, and legislation relating to matrimonial proceedings. Proceedings under Part V (see Chapter 9) are not family proceedings. A new court at the level of the magistrates court to hear proceedings under the Children Act 1989 has been established. The magistrates are selected from a new panel, known as the Family Panel, and receive special training

Under Part II, orders can be made for children in family proceedings. It is highly probable that the health professional will be caring for children whose parents are divorced or separated and the children will therefore be or have been the subject of such proceedings. The previous orders of custody, care and control, access, committal to care, and supervision, which used to be made under the Matrimonial Proceedings Act 1973, can no longer be made and are replaced by the provisions of Part II. Before making a decree of divorce or nullity absolute, the court now has to consider whether it should exercise any of its powers under the Children Act 1989 with respect to any children of the family. Under Part II the court can make section 8 orders, orders for financial relief (section 15), and Family Assistance orders (section 16).

Section 8 orders
Under section 8 the following may be made: contact order, prohibited steps order, residence order, and specific issue order.

CONTACT ORDER
A contact order requires the person with whom a child lives to allow the child to visit or stay with the person named in the order or for that person and the child otherwise to have contact with each other.

PROHIBITED STEPS ORDER

A prohibited steps order means that no step which could be taken by a parent in meeting his or her parental responsibility for a child, and which is of a kind specified in the order, shall be taken by any person without the consent of the court.

RESIDENCE ORDER

A residence order settles the arrangements as to the person with whom a child is to live.

SPECIFIC ISSUE ORDER

A specific issue order gives directions to determine a specific question which has arisen, or which may arise, in connection with any aspect of parental responsibility for a child.

There are certain restrictions upon the court's powers to make these orders. particularly if the child is in the care of a local authority. The court should not make an order under section 8 which extends beyond the child's being 16 years of age, or make an order after the child is older than 16 years unless the court is satisfied that the circumstances of the case are exceptional. Section 10 covers those persons who are able to apply for a section 8 order. As has been discussed in Chapter 2, this could include a step-parent or a person with whom the child has lived for at least 3 years who is able to apply for a residence or contact order (section 11(7)).

A dispute between parents over the nature of health care for the child is likely to result in an application by one or other parent for a section 8 specific issue order (see Chapter 14).

Financial relief for children (section 15)

Schedule 1 to the Act enacts provisions for the financial relief of the child. The schedule covers the orders which can be made by the court, the rules relating to applications, orders for persons aged over 18 years, the duration of the orders, provisions for lump sums, and the variation of orders for periodical payments. Paragraph 4 sets out the considerations that must be taken into account in deciding whether the court should exercise its powers. These include not only the income or wealth and the financial needs and obligations of each relevant person but also:

- the financial needs of the child;
- the income, earning capacity (if any), property and other financial resources of the child;
- any physical or mental disability of the child; and
- the manner in which the child was being, or was expected to be, educated or trained.

Family assistance orders (section 16)

Section 16 enables the court to make a family assistance order. This will require a probation officer to be made available or a local authority to make an officer of the authority available to 'advise, assist and (where appropriate) befriend any person named in the order.' The persons named could include any parent or guardian, any person with whom the child is living or who has a contact order, or the child itself. The court can only make the family assistance order if it is satisfied that the circumstances of the case are exceptional and it has obtained the consent of every person named in the order other than the child. The order can last for up to 6 months.

The aim of the family assistance order is to provide short-term help to the family in overcoming the problems associated with separation or divorce.

LOCAL AUTHORITY SUPPORT FOR CHILDREN AND FAMILIES

Section 17 places a general duty upon every local authority to 'safeguard and promote the welfare of children within their area who are in need; and so far as is consistent with that duty, to promote the upbringing for such children by their families, by providing a range and level of services appropriate to those children's needs.' Part I of schedule 2 of the Act sets out the duties and powers of the local authority to discharge this general duty of care. The definition of a child in need is:

- a child who is unlikely to achieve or maintain, or to have the opportunity of achieving or maintaining, a reasonable standard of health or development without the provision for them of services by a local authority under Part III;
- a child whose health or development is likely to be significantly impaired, or further impaired, without the provision for them of such services; or
- a child who is disabled.

The definition of disabled is:

- a child who is blind, deaf or dumb or who suffers from mental disorder of any kind or is substantially and permanently handicapped by illness, injury or congenital deformity or such other disability as may be prescribed.

'Development' means physical, intellectual, emotional, social or behavioural development; and 'health' means physical and mental health. Each local authority is expected to provide the services shown below for those children in need.

- Day care for preschool and other children (section 18).
- Review of provision for day care, child minding, and other services (section 19).
- Provision of accommodation for children – general duty (section 20).
- Accommodation for children in police protection or detention or on remand (section 21).

Section 22(3) sets out the general duty of the local authority towards children looked after by them. For any child in its care, the local authority must safeguard and promote the welfare of that child, and make such use of services available for children cared for by their own parents as appears to the local authority to be reasonable in the case of that child.

Before making a decision, the local authority must, so far as is reasonably practicable, ascertain the wishes and feelings of the child, the child's parents, any other person who is not a parent but who has parental responsibility for the child, and anyone else whose wishes and feelings the authority consider to be relevant regarding such a matter.

The local authority is also required under section 22(5) to consider:

- the age and understanding of the child, and such wishes and feelings of the child as they have been able to ascertain;
- such wishes and feelings of any person mentioned in subsection (4)(b)–(d) as they have been able to ascertain; and
- the child's religious persuasion, racial origin, and cultural and linguistic background.

Accommodation

Section 23 sets out the duty of the local authority towards the provision of accommodation and the maintenance of children whom they are looking after.

ADVICE AND ASSISTANCE FOR CERTAIN CHILDREN

If a child is being looked after by a local authority, it shall be the duty of the authority to advise, assist, and befriend the child with a view to promoting his welfare when the child ceases to be looked after by them.

Included in the definition of those children for whom the local authority has this duty are children who have been accommodated by a health authority for a consecutive period of at least 3 months after reaching the age of 16 years. The duty arises when the child is no longer so accommodated. The child must be under 21 years of age for the duty to arise. In certain circumstances the duty applies to those accommodated aged under 16 years (24(2)(d)(i)).

There are provisions (section 25) relating to the keeping of children in accommodation that restricts their liberty which are discussed in Chapter 21 on the care of the mentally disordered child.

CARE AND SUPERVISION

Sections 31–42, listed below, cover the powers and duties available to the local authority towards children suffering or likely to suffer harm and who need to be placed under care or supervision orders.

31   Care and supervision orders.
32   Period within which applications for the order must be disposed of.
33   Effect of care order.
34   Parental contact with children in care.
35   Supervision orders.
36   Education supervision orders.
37   Powers of court in certain family proceedings.
38   Interim orders.
39   Discharge and variation of care orders and supervision orders.
40   Orders pending appeals in cases concerning care or supervision orders.
41   Representation of child and of his interests in certain proceedings by the appointment of a guardian *ad litem* (see Chapter 2).
42   Right of guardian ad litem to have access to local authority records (see Chapter 2).

A care order and supervision order can only be made by the court if it is satisfied that the child is suffering or likely to suffer significant harm as a result of the care given or likely to be given if the order were not made, or the child is beyond parental control. If a care or supervision order is made, the parents will still retain their parental responsibilities and share these with the local social services department.

Schedule 2 sets out further details of the local authority's duties in relation to the children it looks after. Of particular relevance to health professionals is paragraph 12 and the regulations under that paragraph for the local authority to make arrangments in connection with the health and education of such children.

Schedule 3 sets out the provisions on the duties of local authorities in relation to supervision orders and the content of such orders. Thus paragraph 4 enables a supervision order to contain directions for medical or psychiatric examinations, and paragraph 5 enables those for psychiatric or medical treatment. Both paragraphs prohibit such an order unless the local authority is satisfied that, if the child has sufficient understanding to make an informed decision, he or she consents to the inclusion of the examination or treatment, and that satisfactory arrangements have been made, or can be made, for the examination or treatment.

These will not be considered in detail and reference should be made to the Department of Health guidance on the Children Act 1989 and the other works of reference quoted at the beginning of this chapter.

Part V, the provisions relating to the protection of children, are considered in Chapter 9 together with practical advice for health professionals who are involved in an emergency situation.

REFERENCES

1   Bainham A, Cretney S: *Children – the Modern Law*. Bristol: Family Law; 1993.
2   White R, Carr P, Lowe N: *A Guide to the Children Act 1989*. London: Butterworths; 1990.
3   Hendrick J: *Child Care Law for Health Professionals*. Oxford: Radcliffe Medical Press; 1993.

4 Department of Health: *The Children Act, 1989 – Guidance and Regulations.* London: HMSO; 1991. [These are available from HMSO in several volumes covering the following topics. Court orders (volume 1). Family support, day care and educational provision (volume 2). Family placements (volume 3). Residential care (volume 4). Independent schools (volume 5). Children with disabilities (volume 6). Guardians *ad litem* and court processes (volume 7). Private fostering and miscellaneous (volume 8).]

5 Department of Health: *An Introductory guide to the Children Act 1989 for the NHS.* London: HMSO; 1991.

Professional issues and child health care

This chapter is concerned with the various professional groups who undertake the health care of the child. It considers their responsibilities, and some of the future developments that are likely to take place through role expansion and changes in the scope of each profession. Their codes of conduct and the means of enforcement are discussed in Chapter 15.

PROFESSIONS REGISTERED WITH THE UKCC FOR NURSING MIDWIFERY AND HEALTH VISITING

The UKCC as the registration body for nurses, midwives, and health visitors is under a statutory duty under section 2(3) of the Nurses, Midwives and Health Visitors Act 1979, by means of rules, to determine the kind and standard of training to be undertaken before admission on to the register.

The register maintained by the UKCC is divided into 15 parts. Those parts relevant to this book, along with the number admitted on to the register from training in England in 1992, are shown below.[1] Within the brackets are the numbers of practitioners with only one registered qualification; these represent 70.56% of all practitioners.

- Part 1 covers first level nurses trained in general nursing; 15 042, 63.87% (258 105).
- Part 2 covers second level nurses trained in general nursing (England and Wales); 356, 1.51% (103 521).
- Part 8 covers nurses trained in the nursing of sick children; 981, 4.17% (3077).
- Part 10 covers midwives; 1949, 8.28% (1500).
- Part 11 covers health visitors; 682, 2.90% (0: health visitors must be doubly qualified).
- Part 12 covers first level nurses trained in adult nursing; 635, 2.7% (608).
- Part 15 covers first level nurses trained in children's nursing; 69, 0.29% (50).
- Nurses in parts 12 and 15 were trained in adult and children's nursing, respectively, on Project 2000 courses.

The statutory functions of the UKCC for Nursing Midwifery and Health Visiting

The UKCC statutory functions are:

- to establish and improve the standards of training and professional conduct for nurses, midwives, and health visitors;
- to ensure that the standards of training they establish meet any European Community obligations of the UK;

- by rules, to determine the conditions of a person's being admitted to training, and the kind and standard of training to be undertaken with a view to registration;
- by rules, to make provision for the kind and standard of further training available to persons who are already registered;
- to have powers to provide in such manner as it thinks fit advice for nurses, midwives, and health visitors on standards of professional conduct; and
- in the discharge of its function, to have proper regard for the interests of all groups within the professions, including those with minority representation.

Project 2000 programmes

The requirements for the kind and standard of Project 2000 are set out in a Statutory Instrument.[2] The Professional Standards and Development Division of the UKCC has issued requirements for the content of Project 2000 programmes.[3] The Common Foundation programme includes professional, ethical, and moral issues: codes and dilemmas, conflicts, boundaries, and the complementary nature of medical and nursing practice, and patient advocacy. The Branch programme for Children's Nursing includes the following requirements.

- Learning in the Child Branch of project requirements be designed to enable the student to assess, plan, implement, and evaluate the nursing care needs of the child within the family. The nurse of the child be able to address issues of health promotion and sickness, so that each child reaches its full developmental potential.
- Nursing, theoretical frameworks (use of models of nursing with the child and the family), framework of health and illness in children, health promotion, prevention of ill health, development of physical and psychosocial potential of children.
- Priority adapted to meet the maturational needs of children, and provide nursing care in a variety of settings.
- Priority setting, family support systems, setting maturational goals and programmes to develop full potential.
- Continuing care.

This book attempts to cover the legal implications of many of these issues.

Post-registration education and practice (PREP)

The UKCC published in March 1994 the standards it had set in relation to the post-registration education and practice for practitioners.[4] The scheme (UKCC 1994) is summarized below.

- To remain on the register, nurses, midwives, and health visitors will be required to complete a minimum of 5 study days every 3 years, a Notification of Practice form, a Return to Practice programme if they have been out of practice for 5 years or more, and a personal professional profile.
- New standards for specialist post-registration education have been set.

The post-registration education and practice provisions were implemented in April 1995. There are no guarantees that the costs of the minimum 5 days' study leave will be funded by employers and practitioners might find that they are compelled to fund their own continuing education.

Scope of Professional Practice

In June 1992 the UKCC published guidance on the development of the practitioner's role.[5] This guidance suggests that 'practice must, therefore, be sensitive, relevant and responsive to the needs of individual patients and clients and have the capacity to adjust, where and when appropriate, to changing circumstances.' Six principles are put forward to ensure that development takes place safely. These are listed below.

The registered nurse midwife or health visitor must:

- be satisfied that each aspect of practice is directed at meeting the needs and serving the interests of the patient or client;
- endeavour always to achieve, maintain, and develop knowledge, skill, and competence to respond to those needs and interests;
- honestly acknowledge any limits of personal knowledge and skill and take steps to remedy any relevant deficits to meet effectively and appropriately the needs of patients and clients
- ensure that any enlargement or adjustment of the scope of personal professional practice must be achieved without compromising or fragmenting existing aspects of professional practice and care and that the requirements of the Council's Code of Professional Conduct are satisfied throughout the whole area of practice;
- recognize and honour the direct or indirect personal accountability borne for all aspects of professional practice; and
- in serving the interests of patients and clients and the wider interests of society, avoid any inappropriate delegation to others which compromises those interests.

The scope of professional practice and the development of post-registration specialization has increased the number of specialisms within the broad area of paediatric nursing.

Specialization

Although the UKCC has decided that the attainment of a specialist qualification will be recorded on the register, it has not yet set out in what terms the registration will take place: whether in general terms or identifying the exact nature of the specialism studied. As the discussion below shows, the scope for ever-increasing specialisms within paediatric nursing is immense, with the minutest areas of work being concentrated in the hands of one specialist (see especially the work of the extracorporeal membrane oxygenation nurse specialist which is considered below).

PAEDIATRIC INTENSIVE CARE

A report by the British Paediatric Association[6] has highlighted continuing deficiencies in the number of paediatric intensive care beds. The result is that a significant number of critically ill children are still cared for within a predominantly adult intensive care environment or within general paediatric wards. Some children cannot be treated. On the staffing side it has been pointed out[7] that there is a conceptual gap between the educational philosophy of the Project 2000 Child Branch courses which focus on child health, and the knowledge and skills required by registered sick children's nurses in the care of the critically ill child. It is therefore vital that post-registration education responds urgently to bridge this gap. Nurses holding an intensive care qualification, for example ENB 100 (English National Board, Course Number 100) General Intensive Care Nursing, need the facility to gain registration as sick children's nurses, whereas those already holding this qualification require access to specialist intensive care nursing, for example ENB 415 Intensive Care Nursing of Children.

SPECIALIZATION IN NURSING FOR THE SICK CHILD
The development of the paediatric nurse specialist
Sue Jones[8] discusses the current situation in relation to paediatric nurse specialists and identifies:

- neonatal practitioners;
- pain specialists;
- children's emergency nurse practitioners;
- genetic nurse specialists;
- cystic fibrosis specialists;
- continence advisers;

- domiciliary care nurses [Cancer and Leukaemia In Childhood Trust (CLIC) and Macmillan];
- stoma care nurses;
- sickle-cell nurse specialists;
- intravenous therapy nurse specialists;
- nutritional support nurses;
- diabetes nurse specialists;
- asthma nurse specialists; and
- nephrology nurse specialists.

She points out that 'the scope of professional practice[9] has become the vehicle for change in children's nursing. We have moved from few nurses giving intravenous drugs as part of an extended role to the administration of intravenous drugs becoming a basic requirement.'

Many advanced paediatric specialist courses have been developed. One such is on neonatal development. Susan Smith et al.[10] describe how the development of the advanced neonatal nurse practitioners course is set out. All students have two identified mentors.

DEBATE OVER SPECIALIZATION

There is, however, a current debate on the issue of specialization. There are some[11] who would support the need for competent registered nurses who can work more flexibly across care sectors. On the other hand there are those[12] who emphasize the importance in the growth of specialist developments within child care. 'As newer methods of treatment evolve and the care of sick children becomes more complex, it must also be appreciated that children's nurses work in the same settings as their adult nurse equivalents. This is particularly true of the community and as greater numbers of children are cared for at home, the development of paediatric community nursing services becomes more evident.'

It should also be remembered that there will be a multidisciplinary team caring for the sick child, and therefore every paediatric nurse speciality could be mirrored by similar specialisms with the professions supplementary to medicine: child cystic fibrosis physiotherapist, child diabetic dietitian, and so forth.

EXTRACORPOREAL MEMBRANE OXYGENATION NURSE SPECIALIST

The development and the issues which can arise from specialization within intensive care units can be seen from looking in detail at one specific area of specialist practice: the extracorporeal membrane oxygenation nurse specialist within neonatal care.[13]

Extracorporeal membrane oxygenation (ECMO) is a temporary lung or heart–lung support therapy for newborns, children, and adults with acute, life-threatening, reversible respiratory or cardiac failure, who are not responding to maximal ventilatory, medical, and surgical treatment. In neonates it is now considered an effective, life-saving support and has found a place in the intensive care setting. This care is largely managed by the ECMO nurse specialist, known as the ENS. The training provided for the ENS is a course of 40 hours conducted by the ECMO coordinator; it covers technical aspects, protocols, clinical experience, basic respiratory physiology, classes of disease, equipment, insertion and removal procedures, and so on with troubleshooting problems. The duties of the ENS include:

- observation (general);
- taking reports of patients;
- assisting with patient care;
- management of emergency procedures;
- observation of the circuit;
- maintenance of the circuit;
- alterations to blood and gas flow;
- management of haemofiltration; and

- teaching and learning.

The authors state that 'the role of the ECMO nurse specialist is seen as a legitimate part of the nursing function. Indeed there are several advantages in having nurses fill this position, in preference to other personnel.' They maintain that patient care is improved, ward management is facilitated, and there are financial advantages in using this specialist role.[13]

As a nurse the ENS is able to provide sensitively the support, explanations, and information that the family requires.

There are recognized disadvantages to the ECMO procedure. It is expensive, labour intensive and involves a large multidisciplinary team, laboratory services, and blood and blood products. There may be effects on other patients, and the patient receiving ECMO may be affected because of the theatre-like environment necessary to set up the procedure. Staff shortages may restrict other client services, and more than one bed space may be needed, which could decrease occupancy. Questions that should be asked in the future include those given below.

- Who should be the ECMO coordinator?
- Who should train the ECMO nurse specialist?
- Should one nurse be responsible for total bedside care (covering patient and circuit)?
- How should one overcome the necessity for transporting patients on ECMO?

Points to draw from this in relation to the scope include:

- definition of competence;
- course of employment;
- balancing costs and risks;
- role changes between multidisciplinary team;
- leadership issues, control and training;
- who loses out? (costs of what is not being done);
- balance between holistic care and more specialisms;
- protocols;
- review monitoring and amending;
- more can go wrong; and
- parental concerns (it should be noted that the procedure is not a curative but a supportive therapy).

IMPLICATIONS OF SPECIALIZATION

A similar analysis of the issues arising in all the specialisms identified by Sue Jones could be undertaken, which would reveal the need to identify standards and protocols and clarify responsibilities and training.

The result of these developments towards specialization is that the expectations of parents are increased and at the same time the possibility of simple human error increased. Thus the scope for potential litigation or complaints, or both, multiplies.

PROFESSIONS SUPPLEMENTARY TO MEDICINE

Over the past 10 years health professionals traditionally associated with general inpatient care have become increasingly specialized in the provision of child health care both in hospital and in the community. Some specialists within each profession focus exclusively on children, others cover adults and children.

The following professions are controlled by and registered with the Council for Professions Supplementary to Medicine, set up under the 1960 Act: chiropody, dietetics, medical laboratory technician work, occupational therapy, physiotherapy, radiography, and orthoptics. Osteopathy was added in 1993 and chiropractice in 1994.

Each of the professions covered by the Council has a Board which is a body corporate with perpetual succession and a common seal.[14] The Boards have the general function of promoting high standards of professional education and professional conduct among the members of the relevant professions. With the approval of the Council, a Board may appoint committees to carry out, on the Board's behalf, such of its functions as it may determine and are not required to be carried out by an investigating or disciplinary committee. It may also make standing orders for regulating its proceedings (including a quorum or those of a committee). The Board can appoint teaching and other staff in connection with training courses and examinations conducted under arrangements made by it.

Each Board must set up investigation and disciplinary committees. The former has the duty of conducting a preliminary investigation into any case in which it is alleged that a person registered by the Board is liable to have his or her name removed and of deciding whether the case should be referred to the disciplinary committee. The latter has the duty of considering and determining any case referred to it by the investigation committee and any case in which an application is made for the restoration of a person's name to the register.

The Boards may also make regulations for membership of the committees, meetings and quorums all in consultation with the Council for Professions Supplementary to Medicine. The Council can suggest new Boards after an amalgamation. Thus remedial gymnastics lost its separate identity and orthoptics was recognized in 1966.

It is an offence for an individual falsely to claim registered status. The Government has recently stated that it is intending to review the provisions of the Professions Supplementary to Medicine Act 1960.

NONREGISTERED PROFESSIONS

Speech therapists, pharmacists, and psychologists are not covered by the Council for Professions Supplementary to Medicine but have their own professional bodies responsible for training, admission to professional status, and professional conduct.

REFERENCES

1 UKCC: *Statistical Analysis of the Council's Professional Register 1 April 1992 to 31 March 1993*. London: UKCC; 1993.
2 Statutory Instrument 1989 No 1456.
3 UKCC: *PS&D/89/04(B)*. London: UKCC; 17 November 1989.
4 UKCC: *The Future of Professional Practice – The Council's Standards for Education and Practice Following Registration*. London: UKCC; 1994.
5 UKCC: *Scope of Professional Practice*. London: UKCC; 1992.
6 British Paediatric Association: *The Care of the Critically Ill: Report of a Working Party on Paediatric Intensive Care (November)*. London: Critical Care Publications; 1993.
7 Pearce J, Glasper EA, Atkinson B: A response to the British Paediatric Association report of paediatric intensive care. *Br J Nurs* 1995, 2:1095–1096.
8 Jones S: The development of the paediatric nurse specialist. *Br J Nurs* 1995, 4:34–36.
9 UKCC: *Scope of Professional Practice*. London: UKCC; 1992.
10 Smith S, Roch S, Hall M: Neonatal nurse practitioners – developing further education. *Pediatr Nurs* 1994, 6:13–16.
11 Rowden R: Breaking the mould. *Nurs Times* 1993, 89:29–30.
12 Glasper EA: The value of children's nursing in the third millennium. *Br J Nurs* 1995, 4:27–30.
13 Fergusson D, Copnell B: ECMO: the expanded role of the nurse. *Pediatr Nurs* 1993, 5:12–15.
14 *Halsbury's laws of England*, vol 30.

PART 2

THE RIGHTS OF THE CHILD

In this second part of the book we consider the rights of the child. The first chapter considers the duty to provide services for the child and discusses ways in which this duty can be enforced through direct court action on behalf of the child, or through purchasing agreements supplemented by Government controls and monitoring through the Audit Committee and patient charter initiative. The other chapters consider aspects of the rights of the child, including consent, confidentiality, access to records and information, child protection, education of the sick child, financial provisions, and the right to complain.

Child health care: provision and service organization

This chapter examines the question of the duty to provide child health care services and the extent to which the parent or child, or both, can enforce that duty. It also considers the management and administrative context within which child health care services are provided, and discusses the monitoring of the services through the purchasing agreements, the Audit Commission, patient charter standards, and other quality indicators.

STATUTORY DUTIES

What statutory responsibilities are there to provide child health care services?

The responsibilities are set out in the NHS Act 1977 as part of the duties placed upon the Secretary of State to provide health services for the community. These duties are listed below.

The NHS Act 1977
SECTION 1(1)

- It is the Secretary of State's duty to continue the promotion in England and Wales of a comprehensive health service designed to secure improvement:
  a in the physical and mental health of the people of those countries; and
  b in the prevention, diagnosis and treatment of illness, and for the purpose to provide or secure the effective provision of services in accordance with this Act.

SECTION 2

- Without prejudice to the Secretary of State's powers apart from this section, he has power:
  a to provide such services as he considers appropriate for the purpose of discharging any duty imposed upon him by this Act; and
  b to do any other thing whatsoever which is calculated to facilitate, or is conducive or incidental to, the discharge of such a duty.

This section is subject to section 3(3) below. The meaning of the phrase 'without prejudice to the Secretary of State's powers…' means that the examples do not limit the general duty in its scope. Section 3 sets out in more detail the specific provisions which the Secretary of State has a duty to make.

SECTION 3(1)

- It is the Secretary of State's duty to provide throughout England and Wales, *to such extent as he considers necessary to meet all reasonable requirements* [author's italics]:
  a hospital accommodation;
  b other accommodation for the purpose of any service provided under this Act;
  c medical, dental, nursing and ambulance services;
  d such other facilities for the care of expectant and nursing mothers and young children as he considers are appropriate as part of the health service;
  e such facilities for the prevention of illness, the care of persons suffering from illness and the aftercare of persons who have suffered from illness, as he considers are appropriate as part of the health service; and
  f such other services as are required for the diagnosis and treatment of illness.

Other specific powers of the Secretary of State set out in the NHS Act 1977 are shown below.

- Section 5 – school health and dental inspections, treatment and education.
- Section 5(2)(a) – invalid carriages.
- Section 5(2)(b) – accommodation outside Great Britain for those suffering from respiratory tuberculosis.
- Section 5(2)(c) – a microbiological service for which charges can be made.
- Section 5(2)(d) – research into causation, prevention, diagnosis or treatment of illness.

It should be noted that whereas sections 1 and 3 are framed as duties, sections 2 and 5 give the Secretary of State powers. A duty means that there is an obligation upon the Secretary of State to ensure that provision of a service is made. In contrast, he or she has a complete discretion over whether a power should be exercised. However, even when a duty is set down within the section, it is not necessarily absolute. Section 3 shows clearly that it is left to the Secretary of State to determine how this duty is to be performed as can be seen from the words underlined.

The Secretary of State is authorized to arrange for some of the duties to be undertaken by local authorities. Schedule 8 of the NHS Act 1977 enables the local authority to carry out some of the duties placed upon the Secretary of State for Health.

CARE OF MOTHERS AND YOUNG CHILDREN

A local social service authority may make arrangements for the care of expectant and nursing mothers and of children who have not attained the age of 5 years and are not attending primary schools maintained by a local education authority.

PREVENTION, CARE AND AFTERCARE

A local social services authority may make arrangements for the purpose of the prevention of illness, and for the care of persons suffering from illness, and for the aftercare of persons who have been so suffering and, in particular, for the provision for persons whose care is undertaken with a view to preventing them from becoming ill, persons suffering from illness, and persons who have been so suffering, of centres or other facilities for training them or keeping them suitably occupied and the equipment and maintenance of such centres; other ancillary services for the mentally ill. Statutory provisions relating to the education of the sick child can be found in Chapter 10.

The Secretary of State fulfils the responsibilities described in the NHS Act on the previous pages through a range of organizations and persons including health authorities, family health service authorities, and GPs, and local authorities. Health authorities and family health service authorities are to be amalgamated in April 1996 with the formation of new health authorities.

CHRONICALLY SICK AND DISABLED PERSONS LEGISLATION

Provision for disabled people under Chronic Sick and Disabled Persons Act 1970

The statutory duties set out in the Chronic Sick and Disabled Persons Act 1970 are shown below. It is not the intention to consider these duties in detail in this book and reference should be made to the publications available from the Disabled Living Foundation and RADAR (Royal Association for Disability and Rehabilitation).

Section 1 of the 1970 Act states the following.

- It shall be the duty of every local authority having functions under section 29 of the National Assistance Act 1948 to inform themselves of the number of persons to whom that section applies within their area and of the need for the making by the authority of arrangements under that section for such persons.
- Every such authority:
  a shall cause to be published from time to time at such times and in such manner as they consider appropriate general information as to the services provided under arrangements made by the authority under the said section 29 which are for the time being available in their area; and
  b shall ensure that any such person as aforesaid who needs any of those services is informed of any other *service provided by the authority (whether under any such arrangements or not)* which in the opinion of the authority is relevant to his needs *and of any service provided by any other authority or organisation which in the opinion of the authority is so relevant and of which particulars are in the authority's possession.*

The italicized words were introduced by the 1986 Act (see below). Section 2 of the 1970 Act lists the provisions that the local authority has a duty to make when:

- the local authority has the functions under section 29 of the National Assistance Act 1948;
- it is satisfied that the section applies to an individual;
- the person is ordinarily resident in their area; or
- it is necessary in order to meet the needs of that person to make arrangements for all or any of the matters set out below.
  a The provisions of practical assistance for that person in his or her home.
  b The provision for that person of, or assistance to that person in obtaining, wireless, television, library or similar recreational facilities.
  c The provision for that person of lectures, games, outings, or other recreational facilities outside his or her home or assistance to that person in taking advantage of educational facilities available to him or her.
  d The provision for that person of facilities for, or assistance in, travelling to and from his or her home for the purpose of participating in any services provided under arrangements made by the authority, in any services provided otherwise than as aforesaid which are similar to services which could be provided under such arrangements.
  e The provision of assistance for that person in arranging for the carrying out of any works of adaptation in his or her home or the provision of any additional facilities designed to secure his or her greater safety, comfort or convenience.
  f Facilitating the taking of holidays by that person, whether at holiday homes or otherwise, and whether provided under arrangements made by the authority or otherwise.
  g The provision of meals for that person in his or her home or elsewhere.
  h The provision for that person of, or assistance to that person in obtaining, a telephone and any special equipment necessary to enable him or her to use it.

Disabled Persons (Services, Consultation and Representation) Act 1986

One of the major deficiencies of the 1970 Act was the failure to introduce provision for the assessment of persons who were potentially under its jurisdiction. The Disabled Persons (Services, Consultation and Representation) Act 1986 introduced by Tom Clarke MP aimed to meet this and other deficiencies of the 1970 Act. The new Act provided for the improvement of the effectiveness and coordination of services for mentally and physically handicapped people and those who are mentally ill, and established new procedures for the assessment of the needs of disabled people.

However, although it received the royal assent in July 1986, its sections were due to be implemented at dates to be appointed. Resource implications have delayed the coming into force of some of the crucial parts of the Act.

ENFORCEMENT OF STATUTORY DUTIES

Can a parent or child enforce the implementation of these duties in specific cases?

Figure 5.1 illustrates the forms of action that a parent could take if there were a failure to provide a statutory service. If a parent or child were to complain that a service was not being provided, they could either sue the local authority, or the Secretary of State, or the health authority responsible for commissioning that service, or the NHS provider for breach of his or her duty to provide a statutory service. Alternatively, if harm were to have occurred they could sue the same organizations for breach of the duty of care owed in negligence which caused foreseeable harm to the patient. (An action for negligence is discussed in more detail in Chapter 13.)

Several court cases have shown that failure to provide a service or requiring patients to wait for services does not necessarily imply that there has been a breach of statutory duty.[1] Unless the courts can see evidence of irrational or unreasonable priority setting, they will not intervene in the decisions over the allocation of resources. The Health Service Commissioner has taken a similar line in dealing with NHS complaints.[2] The courts therefore failed to find in favour of patients who complained that they had been on the waiting list for hip replacement operations

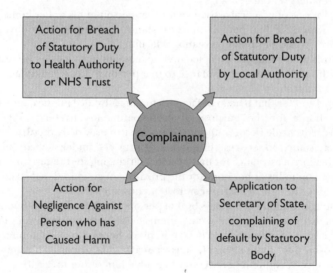

Fig. 5.1 Enforcement of statutory duties.

for too long. There was no evidence that the health authority had acted unreasonably or contrary to the public interest in its allocation of resources.

In a recent case,[3] the father of a boy brought an action against the North West Thames Regional Health Authority when he learnt that the unit at the Westminster Hospital for bone marrow treatment, in which his son was being treated, was to be closed. The father sought a judicial review of the decision.

The court held that there was a failure by the district health authority to consult the community health council according to regulation 19(1) of the NHS (Community Health Council) Regulations[4] over the proposal not to transfer the bone marrow treatment unit at the Westminster Children's Hospital to the Chelsea and Westminster Hospital.

The decision was thus of a limited nature. It did not say that there was no right to close the unit or that the parent had a right to receive care for the child. It was simply that the authority should have followed the correct consultation procedures before closure. The father had no right to be consulted personally. The decision may thus be regarded as a pyrrhic victory for the family, though the child was subsequently treated at a unit in Bristol.

In a commentary on the case,[5] Jean McHale and David Hughes considered that the decision was a hollow victory. The case is contrasted with one involving a school closure,[6] suggesting that applications in NHS cases are in a weaker situation than in school closures.

A news report[7] described an action brought by the father of a 10-year-old girl (known as B) suffering from leukaemia. She had fallen ill at the age of 5 years and Hodgkin's lymphoma was diagnosed. A bone marrow transplant was given in March 1994, her younger sister being the donor. The first course of chemotherapy and the bone marrow transplant failed to work. She was then found to have developed acute myeloid leukaemia and in mid-January 1995 she was given only 6–8 weeks to live. The Cambridge and Huntingdon Health Commission refused to fund a second bone marrow transplant estimated to cost £75 000, on the grounds that:

- she had only a 2.5% chance of putting the disease into remission and making a complete recovery;
- the treatment would cause her considerable discomfort; and
- the treatment would have to be considered experimental and unproven and it could not be justified under Department of Health guidelines on funding for treatment. It was therefore preferable to spend the money on other patients.

Medical experts had advised the parents that her chances of success with the second bone marrow transplant were between 10 and 20%

The judge (Mr Justice Laws) decided that the decision of Cambridge District Health Authority to deny funding for the treatment for the girl had assaulted her right to life. He granted an order for judicial review of the decision not to fund her care but refused an application for an order of mandamus (i.e. an order of the court that the treatment must proceed).

The health authority appealed against this decision and, so great was the urgency, the Court of Appeal met later that same day. It allowed the appeal by the District Health Authority on the grounds that the courts had one function: to rule on the lawfulness of the decision.

The four criticisms made by the High Court judge of the authority's decision were as follows.

1 The relevant director of the authority as the decision-maker had wrongly failed to have regard to the patient's wishes as expressed by her family.

   The Court of Appeal differed. The Director of Public Health of the District Health Authority had taken into account the obvious desire of the father that his daughter be treated when making the decision to turn down the funding request.

2   The director had wrongly used the word 'experimental' to describe the proposed treatment.

> The Court of Appeal held that the treatment did not have a well tried track record of success. It accepted that the proposed treatment had to be regarded as experimental and that the third phase of chemotherapy followed by a possible second bone marrow transplant did not have a 'tried record of success'. It is at the frontier or medical science.

3   The decision could not be justified on the basis that funding the treatment would be an ineffective use of limited resources.

> The Court of Appeal held that difficult and agonizing judgments have to be made as to how a limited budget could best be allocated for the maximum advantage of the maximum number of patients. That was not a judgment for this court. No real evidence was needed to satisfy the court that the authority did not have unlimited resources to purchase and provide all that was needed.

4   The authority failed to consider funding the first £15 000.

> The Court of Appeal stated that it would be flawed to consider that the authority could at least pay the £15 000 towards chemotherapy without committing itself to the further £60 000 needed for the transplant. It would not be reasonable for the authority to embark on expenditure on that basis. Obviously, if one stage were successful, the process would have to go on.

The Court of Appeal was unable to fault the process of reasoning of the authority and allowed its appeal. The Master of the Rolls (Sir Thomas Bingham) stated, 'while I have every sympathy with B, I feel bound to regard this as an attempt – wholly understandable, but nevertheless misguided – to involve the court in a field of activity where it is not fitted to make any decision favourable to the patient.'

There is no doubt that the decision of the Court of Appeal is in keeping with the decisions of the courts cited earlier over the reluctance of the court to interfere with resource allocation decisions within the NHS. Resources are finite, and courts will only intervene if there is evidence of irrational policies or unreasonable actions.

As a result of the publicity attracted by the case, an anonymous donor offered £75 000 to cover the cost of the treatment, and chemotherapy commenced on 13 March 1995. The outcome at the time of writing is that the child has survived further chemotherapy and is now ready for another bone marrow transplant.

In spite of the decision by the Court of Appeal, there is likely to be an increase in litigation as decisions over resource allocation are made more explicit in the internal market. It was reported[8] that the parents of an 11-year-old boy suffering from cystic fibrosis were planning to sue a health authority that had refused to fund experimental treatment for their only child. Doctors had urged the Northumberland Health Authority to authorize the new drug treatment, which costs £7000 per annum. The health authority had refused to do so because it said that the drug, DNase, might not work. The father had stated that: 'We will do anything we can to keep our lad alive and that includes legal action against the authority. It is disgraceful that treatment is being refused because of the cost. The drug would not extend the life expectancy… but it would dramatically improve the quality of his life.' It was subsequently reported that the child's doctor persuaded the health authority to change its mind and the child is now being prescribed the drug.

This is a different situation from that of girl B, with leukaemia, for several reasons. First, DNase is being given to many cystic fibrosis children across the country and, although research is still ongoing, there is evidence from the earlier results that there may be some benefit to some people. The reduction of lung infections may reduce hospital stays and the frequency of intravenous antibiotic therapies. DNase, proprietary name Pulmozyme, works by dissolving the thick mucus in the lungs of patients with cystic fibrosis thus improving lung function. It is administered through a nebulizer. It is based on the findings which have been made since the discovery of the gene responsible for causing cystic fibrosis. Second, there are minimal side effects, and third, the cost is not in the same league as the bone marrow transplant.

Another difficulty is that if health authorities or GP purchasers take the view that only well tried and established treatments should be funded, there will be no place within the NHS for the provision of experimental treatment.

A further problem that is emerging is that different purchasers are taking different views over the funding of expensive treatments. Already there is anecdotal evidence that some GPs are reluctant to take onto their lists, patients with chronic conditions who would make heavy demands upon their time and budgets, and it is clear from the cystic fibrosis case cited above that patients in one area or practice may be refused a treatment that patients in another area or practice are receiving.

One effect of the publicity when treatment is being refused is the rush of offers to the parents of funds to meet the costs, particularly from newspapers who offer funding in exchange for exclusive rights to the story. The effect is to transfer to the private sector the cost of care that the NHS authorities decide not to purchase whatever the clinical benefit to the child. It could be argued, for example, that, if further treatment of the 10-year-old leukaemia patient was not in her best interests, it should not be authorized outside the NHS or inside the NHS, whoever was prepared to pay for it.

In extreme circumstances, a decision to continue treatment funded from private sources which was considered not to be in the best interests of the child could be challenged in the courts (see Chapter 6).

Further disputes over the funding of unusual treatments that often become the subject of extracontractual referrals are likely to increase. The courts have followed a consistent approach: if the health service body as purchaser has acted reasonably in the allocation of resources, then the court will not intervene in its decision-making.

THE GP AS PURCHASER

Over the next few years it is estimated that nearly all the purchasing of secondary care will be in the hands of group fundholding GPs. There has not yet been any case in which the failure of the GP in his or her role as purchaser to buy services for his or her patients has been challenged in the courts. If this were to occur, and it is likely as GP fundholding budgets will be cash limited, there is no reason to suspect that the Court of Appeal would set any principles different from those which they have applied when the health authority has been the purchaser of care. However, the issue raises considerable legal and ethical issues for the GP personally as he or she will be the representative of the patient and the provider of care and also the budget holder; this could generate a conflict of interest or clash of loyalties not easily reconcilable. Community paediatric nurses may become involved in the issues relating to the purchase of secondary services and it is essential that they keep clear records of the advice they give and the reasons for it. They may be called upon to justify their decisions.

THE DUTY TO PROVIDE PRIMARY CARE SERVICES

A GP, under his or her terms and conditions of service, has a duty to provide primary care services to the patients on their list, and to others who are temporary residents or in specified emergency situations. They have the right to ask for any patient to be removed from their list, without giving reasons. Seven days notice of the removal must be given by the FHSA to the patient, who then has the opportunity to seek an alternative doctor. If the patient fails to obtain one, then the FHSA is able to allocate a patient to the list of a GP who will then have to provide services for that patient. Local agreements with the FHSA usually ensure that this allocation will last for up to 3 months, before the GP requests that the patient be moved on. The terms of service of the GP have been amended to allow for the removal of a patient who has threatened or inflicted actual violence on a GP from that doctor's list with immediate effect; the GP must have made a complaint to the police and the violence must have arisen because of a medical or psychiatric condition of the patient.

In such cases of removal of a patient from a GP's list, it would be usual for the whole family to be removed and reallocated (if necessary).

Medical Service Committees

The unreasonable failure of a GP to attend to a patient could lead to a hearing by the Medical Services Committee of the FHSA, which determines whether there has been a breach of the GP's terms and conditions of service set out in the Statutory Instrument. If the GP fails to show that he acted reasonably in making the decision not to visit, he could be faced with, at the minimum, a warning or a withholding of money from fees payable to him. In serious cases the facts are reported to the General Medical Council for consideration through professional conduct proceedings whether the doctor should be struck off from the register. Reforms to the complaints system, including that of complaints against GPs, are at present under consideration and are discussed in Chapter 12.

PLANNING AND STANDARD SETTING OF SERVICE PROVISION

Effective child health services require communication and coordination across a variety of statutory organizations and maximum participation of the voluntary sector. The internal market, in introducing a purchaser–provider split across both health and social services, has facilitated the strategic planning of the services required against the actual resources required. It has also enabled clear standards to be set that can be monitored by purchasers. Reference can be made to publications from the South East Thames Regional Health Authority,[9] which set out the principles and give guidelines in the commissioning of paediatric services. These publications set out the rights of the children and cover various topics, including the principles to be followed, staffing, facilities, treatment, hospitalization, specialist community services, chronic illness and disability, school health, services for teenagers, records and communication, consumers' views, audit and information, and commissioning and contracting issues. They also have an extensive bibliography. They provide a blueprint for standard setting in the commissioning process.

Hospital services

The Department of Health has issued a report setting out guidelines for the care of children and young people in hospital.[10] The areas covered are:

- contracting for hospital services for children;
- delivery of hospital services for children;
- meeting children's special needs;
- other locally provided services for children (comprehensive assessment, mental handicap, child and adolescent psychiatry, respite care, chaplaincy); and
- staffing and training.

The cardinal principles identified by the Department of Health's report are listed below.

- Children are admitted to hospital only if the care they require cannot be as well provided at home, in a day clinic, or on an outpatient basis in hospital.

- Children requiring admission to hospital are provided with a high standard of medical, nursing, and therapeutic care to facilitate a speedy recovery, and minimize complications and mortality.
- Families with children have easy access to hospital facilities for children without needing to travel significantly further than to other similar amenities.
- Children are discharged from hospital as soon as socially and clinically appropriate and full support is provided for subsequent care at home or as an outpatient.
- Good child health care is shared with parents or carers and they are closely involved in the care of their children at all times unless, exceptionally, this is not in the best interests of the child; accommodation is provided for them to remain with their children overnight.
- Accommodation, facilities, and staffing are appropriate to the needs of children and adolescents and separate from those provided for adults; if possible separate accommodation is provided for adolescents.
- Like all other patients, children have a right for their privacy to be respected and to be treated with tact and understanding; they have an equal right to information appropriate to their age, understanding and specific circumstances.

Audit commission review

Major improvements as a result of this guidance issued by the Department of Health were unlikely to have occurred before the Audit Commission published its report.[11] The latter pointed out that children take up 10% of hospital and community health services and that many of the recommendations made in reports in the past over the care of children in hospital are not being implemented; for example the Platt report, which was published in 1959,[12] set out clear principles for the care of children, but these are often neglected.

The Audit Commission in 1993 sought not to rewrite the principles but to investigate why they were not being implemented. They considered six principles relating to the care of children in hospital.

- Child- and family-centred care.
- Specially skilled staff.
- Separate facilities.
- Effective treatments.
- Appropriate hospitalization.
- Strategic commissioning.

The Audit Commission concluded that the root cause of hospitals failing to apply the principles is often a lack of attention of many clinicians, managers, and other staff to these special needs and the needs of children's families, and suggested that the solution is mainly to change attitudes and management practices. Additional conclusions put forward by the Audit Commission are listed below.

- There should be a senior management focus for children's services in every hospital to ensure that the special needs of children and families are recognized in all aspects of care.
- Written policies to make standards clear to all concerned are needed.
- Key indicators which can be monitored must be set.
- Children should receive care from specially skilled staff using facilities specifically designed to meet their needs.
- Experienced medical staff and registered sick children's nurses are essential.
- Improvements in staffing by reallocation or replacing existing staff are needed.
- Separate facilities for children are often more cost-effective because the range of tasks undertaken by staff is more concentrated and there is less duplication of equipment and materials.

- In some areas of care, such as cancer and intensive care of some newborn babies, special skills of staff at large tertiary or regional centres can achieve better outcomes at lower cost than at smaller general hospitals. Mortality rates for low birth weight babies receiving intensive care in large centres can be one-half those at local centres, yet the average cost of providing that care can be as much as 30% less.
- The outcomes of treatments should be monitored routinely. (The Commission uses the example of glue ear and intensive care of newborn babies.) Guidelines are recommended for monitoring outcomes.
- Lack of clear guidance as to when an admission is appropriate and a lack of consideration of the alternatives should be remedied.
- Children are kept in hospital unnecessarily because of administrative delays in arranging discharge or a lack of service which can provide care at home.
- Health authorities set the broad strategy in which services should operate, providing a major catalyst for change. They should ensure that strategies are in place which address the key issues highlighted by the Audit Commission.

Very few of these recommendations can be enforced legally by the parents on behalf of the child. If it can be established that harm has occurred as a result of failures in following what would be considered to be a reasonable standard of care, then it may be possible to bring an action for negligence (see Chapter 13). Otherwise, the parents and child are dependent upon the purchasers of the service using the NHS agreement that they have with the providers to define minimum standards of care and ensure that these are monitored.

To assist in this process, the Audit Commission recommended that indicators should be prepared for measuring the quality of care.

Reference should also be made when considering standards of care to the report of the guidelines on the care of dying children drawn up by the British Paediatric Association, King Edward's Hospital Fund for London, and the National Association of Health Authorities (discussed in Chapter 22).[13]

Philosophy of care in paediatric nursing
The Royal College of Nursing has produced a philosophy of care in paediatric nursing.[14]

THE NEEDS OF THE CHILD AS AN INDIVIDUAL
In working towards the provision of appropriate facilities for sick children, nurses should:

- recognize each child as a unique, developing individual whose best interests must be paramount;
- listen to children, attempt to understand their perspectives, opinions and feelings, and acknowledge their right to privacy;
- consider the physical, psychological, social, cultural and spiritual needs of children and their families; and
- respect the right of children, according to their age and understanding, to appropriate information and informed participation in decisions about their care.

PARTNERSHIP WITH THE FAMILY
Nurses should:

- recognize that good health care is shared with families, who should be closely involved in their child's care at all times, unless, exceptionally, this is not in the best interests of the child;
- promote the active participation of children and their families in care and, by providing teaching and support, assist them to be partners in care; and

- promote the right of the children to have a parent accompany them during hospitalization and treatment.

FACILITIES FOR SICK CHILDREN AND THEIR FAMILIES
The Royal College of Nursing:

- asserts the right of all children in all settings to be nursed by appropriately educated staff and believes that staffing levels and skill mix must reflect the special needs of ill children and their families;
- continually works to identify trends which may threaten the health and well-being of children;
- is working to promote the development of comprehensive, integrated child health services
- promotes the provision of hospital accommodation and facilities appropriate to the needs of children and young people, separate from those provided for adults; and
- advocates the reduction of hospital admissions and inpatient stay by promoting family participation in care, day services, and paediatric community nursing services.

The Royal College of Nursing encourages nurses to pursue these objectives within their own sphere of practice and to promote the educational opportunities necessary to advance the art and science of paediatric nursing.
The Royal College of Nursing has given its support to:

- the UN Convention on the Rights of the Child (1989);
- the Resolution of the European Parliament on a Charter for Children in Hospital (1986);
- the National Association for the Welfare of Children in Hospital (NAWCH, now Action for Sick Children);
- the principles of the Children Act 1989; and
- the Department of Health guidance document 'Welfare of Children and Young People in Hospital' (1991).

The 'child' refers to any individual from birth through childhood and adolescence. The 'family' refers to the child's significant carer(s).

Enforcement of quality standards
Even though these indicators may be included in the NHS agreement (or contract) between purchaser and provider, failure to comply with that identified quality cannot be a source of legal action by either the patient or parent or by the purchaser. This is explained below.

THE PARENT OR CHILD
There may be a successful court action on the parent's or child's part if harm has resulted from failure to implement this standard. The indicators could in such a case be used as evidence of the standard of care which should have been provided but causation, that is, a causal link between the failure to provide the standard and the harm that has occurred would have to have been shown (see further discussion on a negligence action in Chapter 13). A claim that failure to provide the standard prescribed constitutes a breach of statutory duty is, however, unlikely to be successful. As the cases cited at the beginning of this chapter show, the courts recognize a discretion in allocating resources which are not unlimited.

THE PURCHASER
The purchaser is prevented by law in bringing a legal action for breach of contract if the agreement for purchase is with an NHS health service body (e.g. NHS Trust) by section 4 of the NHS and Community Care Act 1990. If a dispute arises between purchaser and provider then the adjudication procedures set up by the Secretary of State under the 1990 Act must be used in the last resort. This does not apply if the purchaser has negotiated for the provision of

services with a provider outside the NHS as here there would be a contract within the meaning understood by the law and either party could sue over any breach by the other side in the civil courts.

Patient charter standards

Of increasing importance in monitoring performance are patient charter standards. These are becoming more sophisticated and are included within the NHS agreement and monitored by the health authorities as commissioners and in turn by the Department of Health. These have become an important means of monitoring performance in implementing the defined standards.

On referral by a GP to a hospital, all patients should now be given a card which records the date of referral and this date will be used to monitor the waiting times for appointments as both inpatients and outpatients.

COMMUNITY PROVISION

Increasing use of day surgery and shorter lengths of stay have meant that more children are being cared for in the community where family care is supported by a wide range of health professionals.

Community child health services need to be closely organized in conjunction with not only the acute services but also primary care services provided by the GP and the primary care team, and also with social services.

Audit Report on community child health and social services

In 1994 the Audit Commission published recommendations on coordinating community child health and social services for children in need.[15] This gives detailed evidence and guidelines for managers and practitioners. Its main conclusions are summarized below.

- Joint assessment of needs and development of a strategy.
- Operational areas of common interest: family support.
- Child protection.
- Support for children with a disability.
- An agenda for health commissioners: surveillance and immunization, child health clinics, GP fundholders, school health, monitoring and evaluation.
- An agenda for providers of community child health: what are the health needs of the population? What priories and criteria are being adopted? What skills are required? What information is required? How should the service be organized?
- An agenda for social services for children: reviewing services and costs, reviewing field social work practice and organization, reviewing residential care.
- Setting a course in social services: improving information systems, field social work, and the role of the field social worker, sharpening procedures for assessments and care planning (clearer guidance and procedures for assessments and care planning are required), making better use of staff through workload management.
- Children looked after: improving the management of services, helping young people leave care at age 16 years and over.

An example of the organization of child health services in practice

The organization of child health care services in Greenwich Health Care Trust is described[16] as attempting to bring all the services for persons aged under 16 years together under one general manager. There are four divisions, each headed by a lead nurse and where necessary a lead consultant and planning and information officer. The divisions cover:

1 severe learning disability;
2 preconception and prebirth;
   preschool;
   school health;
   special education;
   child protection;
3 acute paediatrics;
   special care baby units and neonatal intensive care units; and
4 child mental health.

The last two divisions have a lead consultant. All the divisions report to a general manager.

In some districts paediatric consultants are employed in both community trusts and acute hospital trusts.

An executive letter issued in 1993[17] suggested that medical staff involved in child health care should be transferred from the community to acute trusts. This is not without its critics and one[18] suggests that the Department of Health guidance on child health services undermines the purpose of the internal market.

There will, however, be a constant tension in the newly organized NHS. Provider–purchaser relations must be within an agreed framework for meeting the assessed health needs of the locality and in accordance with an agreed strategy. This strategy prevents a completely open market. Exactly the same can be said of planning for specialist units. These cannot be left to local negotiating between purchasers and providers as, because of the capital investment, they need to be planned on a regional or supraregional basis. This was recommended in the House of Commons' report in 1992.[19] (See Chapter 20 for further discussion of community care and the child and the Department of Health's *Child Health in the Community: A Guide to Good Practice.*)

CONCLUSION

At present the way in which the statutory duties are framed makes it exceedingly difficult for an individual to succeed in an action for enforcement of these statutory duties in his or her favour. The legislation which introduced the internal market did not give the patient a legal right to enforce the duties to provide health care nor to enforce the NHS agreements between purchaser and provider. As developments in medical technology increase, the gap between the availability of resources and the demand for care is likely to increase. This means that more action must be taken to ensure the efficient and effective provision of child health services, to maximize the resources that are allocated, and to ensure that the children and young people receive a service which is in accordance with the principles defined in the reports discussed in this chapter and the charters discussed in Chapter 1.

REFERENCES

1 R *v* Secretary of State for Social Services ex parte Hincks and others. *Solicitors Journal,* 29 June 1979: p436.
2 Health Service Commissioner: *Annual Report 1990/1991.* London: HMSO. [W>599/89–90 on pp90–96 of HC 482.]
3 R *v* North West Thames Regional Health Authority and others, ex parte Daniels (Rhys William). *Times* Law Report, 22 June 1993.

4 Statutory Instrument 1985, No 304.
5 McHale J, Hughes D: Down by law – comment on the Rhys Daniel case. *Health Service Law Journal* 1993, 103:33.
6 R *v* Brent LBC ex parte Gunn. 1985 84 LGR 161
7 *Times,* 10 March 1995: p1.
8 *Times,* 13 March 1995: p3
9 South East Thames Regional Health Authority: *Better Care for Children – Commissioning Paediatric Services.* London: South East Thames Regional Health Authority; 1994.
10 Department of Health: *Welfare of Children and Young People in Hospital.* London: HMSO; 1991.
11 Audit Commission: *Children First: A Study of Hospital Services.* London: HMSO; 1993.
12 Platt Committee: *The Welfare of Children in Hospital.* London: HMSO; 1959.
13 Thornes R: *The Care of Dying Children and Their Families.* Birmingham: Birmingham National Association of Health Authorities; 1988.
14 Royal College of Nursing: *Issues in Nursing and Health, No. 10.* London: RCN; February 1992.
15 Audit Commission: *Seen But Not Heard: Co-ordinating Child Health and Social Services for Children in Need.* London: HMSO; 1993.
16 Green P: Joining Forces. *Health Service Journal* 1995, 103:24–26.
17 EL(93) 28 Medical staffing of child health services
18 Ledwith F: Kid's stuff. *Health Service Journal* 1993, 103:27.
19 Health Committee of House of Commons: *Report on Maternity Services.* London: HMSO, 1992.

Consent to treatment

This chapter considers the issues that surround consent to treatment. The first section will discuss the following issues.

- Why is consent necessary?
- Who can give consent?

The second section will consider:

- the procedure in relation to the giving of consent;
- documentation; and
- what a specific consent can be deemed to cover.

The third section will look at:

- the issue of the circumstances when consent can be dispensed with;
- the information which should be given prior to consent being obtained; and
- the legal consequences of not giving sufficient information.

(Consent in specific situations, such as abortion and sterilization, is considered in Chapter 24 and concerning the dying child is considered in Chapter 22. Consent and the provisions of the Mental Health Act 1983 are discussed in Chapter 21.)

WHY IS CONSENT NECESSARY?

General principles on consent

Every competent adult has a right to give or refuse consent to treatment.[1] If no consent is given, then in the absence of other justification (see below) any touching of the person (with the exception of casual social contact) would constitute in law a trespass to the person. Thus an individual who comes into hospital for an operation should give consent to that operation before a premedication is given. If consent were not given, then the operation would be regarded as a trespass to the person.

If there has been a trespass to the person, then the victim can bring a court action and claim compensation without having to prove that any harm has been suffered. This is known as a court action which is actionable *per se*. In the absence of consent or other justification recognized by law, the fact that an action was undertaken for the benefit of the patient would not be a valid defence.

Consent must be given willingly, that is, without duress or force. It must be given without fraud and the person giving it must be competent to do so. Consent in such circumstances given by an authorized person constitutes a valid defence against an action for trespass to the person.

There is a presumption in law that adult persons have the capacity to decide whether or not they will accept medical treatment, even if a refusal may risk permanent injury to their health or even lead to premature death. However, this presumption of capacity is rebuttable (i.e. it can be refuted). This means that evidence can be brought to show that the person was not capable of giving a valid refusal. In the case of Re T,[1] the woman who was pregnant and under the influence of her mother, a Jehovah's Witness, stated that she would not accept a blood transfusion. This was said at a time when it was not considered a likely and necessary procedure. When a blood transfusion did become a life-saving necessity, the Court held that her earlier refusal was incompetent.

BY WHOM SHOULD CONSENT BE GIVEN?

The child

Specific statutory provisions exist for consent to treatment by those of 16 and 17 years of age. It is therefore necessary to consider the issue of consent separately for those of 16 and above and those below 16 years of age. Both groups will be considered in relation to the rights of the child and also the rights of the parent.

THE CHILD AGED 16 OR 17 YEARS
Statutory right
i. Family Law Reform Act 1969

Section 8 of the Family Law Reform Act 1969 enables a child aged 16 or 17 years to give a valid consent to treatment. The section is set out in full below.

- Section 8(1) The consent of a minor who has attained the age of 16 years, to any surgical, medical or dental treatment, which in the absence of consent, would constitute a trespass to the person, shall be as effective as it would be if he were of full age; and where a minor has by virtue of this section given an effective consent to any treatment it shall not be necessary to obtain any consent for it from his parent or guardian.
- Section 8(2) In the section 'surgical, medical or dental treatment' includes any procedure undertaken for the purposes of diagnosis and this section applies to any procedures (including, in particular, the administration of an anaesthetic) which is ancillary to any treatment as it applies to that treatment.
- Section 8(3) Nothing in the section shall be construed as making ineffective any consent which would have been effective if this section had not been enacted.

Certain points should be noted about the statutory provision for the 16- or 17-year-old to give consent.

- The statutory provision only covers consent to treatment as defined very widely in section 8(2). It thus does not give the 16- or 17-year-old the right to give consent to organ donation or blood, though this may be possible at common law (see below).
- The practitioner can rely upon the consent of the 16- or 17-year-old without requiring additional consent from the parent.
- It is implied that the 16- or 17-year-old has the competence to give a valid consent. The statutory provisions would not validate consent given by a person suffering from learning disabilities who lacked the mental competence to make the decision. There would, however, be a presumption in favour of the 16- or 17-year-old having the capacity to give consent. This presumption could be rebutted by evidence to the contrary.
- The parent is also able to give a valid consent to the treatment of the 16- or 17-year-old. Section 8(3) preserves the validity of any ways of giving consent before the Act came into

force and the parent has the right to give consent on behalf of the child under the age of 18 years (see below).

- There could be a clash between a person aged 16 or 17 years refusing to give consent and the parent wishing the treatment to take place and therefore giving consent on his or her behalf (see below).

ii. Children Act 1989

The Children Act 1989 established that in certain specified proceedings one of the considerations which must be taken into account was 'the ascertainable wishes and feelings of the child concerned (considered in the light of his age and understanding)' (section 1(3)(a)).

In addition specific protection is given in sections 38(6), 43(8), and 44(7) for the child to refuse consent to an examination or other assessment, if the child is of sufficient understanding.

This Act applies to all children whatever their age, though the actual age and maturity will be a major factor in determining the extent to which their views will count. However, as can be seen below, these principles did not prevent the court ordering a girl aged 16 years suffering from anorexia nervosa to undergo treatment in a specialist unit, in spite of her refusal. See the case of Re W which is discussed in full below.

Common law

It does not follow that because consent by the 16- or 17-year-old to treatment and ancillary and diagnostic procedures is only permissible under the Family Law Reform Act 1969, the person cannot therefore give a valid consent to the nonspecified procedures. For example, the statutory provisions would not cover a 16- or 17-year-old giving consent to blood donation or donating an organ, because that is not treatment within the meaning of section 8(2) of the Act. (The donation of the organ would of course be subject to the provisions of the Human Organ Transplants Act 1989.) However, provided the 16- or 17-year-old had the necessary competence to make the decision, consent could be given by the person at common law. Exactly the same principles would apply to areas not covered by the Family Law Reform Act 1969 as apply to the under 16-year-old who is Gillick-competent, which is discussed below.

THE CHILD AGED UNDER 16 YEARS

Unlike the child aged 16 or 17 years, the child aged under 16 years does not have a statutory right to give consent to treatment. Any right to give consent derives from the common law. The courts recognize that in some circumstances this right might exist, and a person who therefore relies on the consent of the under 16-year-old in the specified circumstances would not be committing an act of trespass to the person.

As we have seen the statutory right under the Family Law Reform Act for the minor to give consent to treatment was confined to the 16- or 17-year-old. The doubt as to whether the common law recognized the right of the under 16-year-old to give consent was resolved by the House of Lords in the case brought by Mrs Gillick.

The Gillick case[2]

The facts of the Gillick case were as follows. The Department of Health and Social Security issued a circular to area health authorities containing, *inter alia*, advice to the effect that a doctor consulted at a family planning clinic by a girl under 16 years of age would not be acting unlawfully if he prescribed contraceptives for the girl as long as in doing so he was acting in good faith to protect her against the harmful effect of sexual intercourse. The circular further stated that, although a doctor should proceed on the assumption that advice and treatment on contraception should not be given to a girl aged under 16 years without parental consent and that he should try to persuade the girl to involve her parents in the matter, the principle of confidentiality between doctor and patient applied to a girl under the age of 16 years seeking contraceptives; therefore, in exceptional cases, the doctor could prescribe contraceptives without consulting the girl's parents or obtaining their consent if in the doctor's clinical judgment they should be prescribed. The plaintiff, who had five daughters under the age of 16 years, sought an assurance from her local area health authority that her daughters would not be given advice and treatment on contraception without the plaintiff's prior knowledge and consent while they were aged under 16 years. When the authority refused to give such an assurance, the plaintiff brought an action against the authority and the department seeking:

- as against both the department and the area health authority a declaration that the advice contained in the circular was unlawful, because it amounted to advice to doctors to commit the offence of causing or encouraging unlawful sexual intercourse with a girl of less than 16 years of age, contrary to section 28(1) of the Sexual Offences Act 1956, or the offence of being an accessory to unlawful sexual intercourse with a girl aged under 16 years, contrary to section 6(1) of that Act; and
- as against the area health authority a declaration that a doctor or other professional person employed by it in its family planning service could not give advice and treatment on contraception to any child of the plaintiff below the age of 16 years without the plaintiff's consent, because to do so would be unlawful as being inconsistent with the plaintiff's parental rights.

In the High Court the judge held that a doctor prescribing contraceptives to a girl aged under 16 years in accordance with the advice contained in the Department of Health's circular would not thereby be committing an offence of causing or encouraging unlawful sexual intercourse with the girl, contrary to section 28(1) of the 1956 Act. The judge also held that a parent's interest in his or her child did not amount to a 'right' but was more accurately described as a responsibility or duty, and accordingly giving advice to a girl aged under 16 years on contraception without her parent's consent was not unlawful interference with parental 'rights'. The judge accordingly dismissed the plaintiff's action. The plaintiff appealed to the Court of Appeal.

The Court of Appeal allowed her appeal and granted the declaration sought, on the grounds that a child aged under 16 years could not validly consent to contraceptive treatment without her parents' consent and that therefore the circular was unlawful. The Department of Health appealed to the House of Lords against the granting of the first declaration. The area health authority did not appeal against the granting of the second declaration.

The decision of the House of Lords was as follows.

- (Lord Templeman dissenting) As children become increasingly independent as they grow older and parental authority dwindles correspondingly, the law does not recognize any rule of absolute parental authority until a fixed age. Instead parental rights are recognized by the law only for as long as they are needed for the protection of the child, and such rights yielded to the child's right to make their own decisions when they reach a sufficient understanding and intelligence to be capable of making up their own mind. Accordingly, a girl under the age of 16 years did not, merely by reason of her age, lack legal capacity to consent to contraceptive advice and treatment by a doctor.
- (Lord Brandon dissenting) A doctor who in the exercise of his clinical judgment gave contraceptive advice and treatment to a girl under the age of 16 years without her parents' consent did not commit an offence under section 6(1) or section 28(1) of the 1956 Act, because the bona fide exercise by the doctor of his clinical judgement negated the *mens rea* (see glossary) which was an essential ingredient of those offences.
- (Lord Brandon and Lord Templeman dissenting) It followed that a doctor had a discretion to give contraceptive advice or treatment to a girl under 16 years of age if she had a sufficient

understanding and intelligence to enable her to understand fully what was proposed, that being a question of fact in each case. It also followed that the department's guidance could be followed by a doctor without involving him in any infringement of parental rights or breach of the criminal law. The appeal of the Department of Health would therefore be allowed, the first declaration would be set aside, and the second declaration should be overruled as being erroneous.

The decision was an epoch-making one and has established very clearly that a minor under the age of 16 years may have the capacity to give consent to treatment. It also implies that a minor aged 16 or 17 years may have the capacity to give consent to activities not covered by the Family Law Reform Act 1969. This precedent has been followed in a variety of situations, and has not been confined to consent by a girl to contraceptive advice and treatment.

Its philosophy has been incorporated in the Children Act 1989.

The term 'Gillick-competent' has now come into use and covers those situations in which a child who has no statutory right to give consent can give consent validly at common law. The term also covers the 16- or 17-year-old who gives consent to participation in a research project, organ donation, et cetera which are not included in the statutory right given by the Family Law Reform Act 1969.

Gillick-competent

A new legal phrase has thus been added to the language. Gillick-competent means that a child is considered to have the competence to make a decision in a specific set of circumstances. Clearly the nature of the decision will determine the level of competence required for a valid decision to be made. The courts have thus recognized that the capability of children to make decisions determining their lives is part of the maturing process. The result is a gradual passing of the decision process from parent to child. **Figure 6.1** shows the process in graphic form. The kinds of decisions on treatments and care which are gradually passed from parent to child are indicated below in reverse order of gravity.

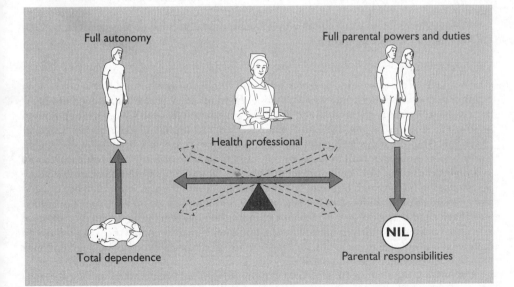

Fig 6.1 Interrelationship between parents, child, and health professionals

- dressing, clothes and shoes
- hairbrushing
- cleaning teeth
- bathing
- nail cutting
- cleaning a wound
- stitching
- medication, external or oral
- X-ray
- medication, intramuscular or intravenous
- dental examination, filling or extraction
- enema
- lumbar puncture
- operation, local or general anaesthetic
- psychotherapy
- behaviour modification
- receiver of transplant from donor
- amputation
- elective or cosmetic surgery
- abortion
- sterilization
- colostomy
- brain surgery
- hormonal implants
- donation of an organ to another

Sometimes researchers find that competence can exist at a very young age. Thus in her research on parents' attitude to self-administration of their asthmatic children, Elizabeth Robinson found that 'maturity is often not age-related. Children as young as 5 years, particularly those with moderate to severe asthma, have demonstrated sufficient maturity to take on self-medication.'[3]

Whether the child is Gillick-competent is a matter to be decided on the actual facts of the situation as the case below illustrates.

Case of Re E (1993)[4]

The hospital authority sought leave of the court to treat a young man with leukaemia in such manner as they considered necessary, including the transfusion of blood and blood products. He was aged 15 years and 9 months and his family were devout Jehovah's Witnesses and refused to consent to transfusions. He had been admitted to hospital 13 days earlier and had deteriorated rapidly. It was a matter of hours, perhaps a few days, before his blood haemoglobin and platelet levels would fall to dangerous levels. On an application by the health authority two nights earlier, he had been made a ward of court. It was argued by his parents that, as he was so close to his sixteenth birthday, an age when his consent to treatment would be required under section 8 of the Family Law Reform Act 1969, and bearing in mind the Gillick case, which says that a child below the age of 16 years can make their own decision on medical treatment when they achieve a sufficient understanding and intelligence to enable them to understand fully what is proposed, it was wrong for the court to interfere and exercise the interventionist jurisdiction vested in a judge in wardship.

The judge for the Family Division held that the lad was intelligent enough to take decisions about his own wellbeing, but that he did not have a full understanding of what refusal to accept blood transfusions would involve. Therefore, his veto was not binding and, as section 8 of the

Family Law Reform Act 1969 did not apply because he was not yet aged 16 years, the wardship proceedings were not an abuse of the process of the court. In deciding whether to give leave to the hospital authority, the welfare of the child was the first and paramount consideration, and had to be decided objectively by the standard of the ordinary mother and father. Yet the court should be very slow to interfere in a decision the child had taken, as the freedom of choice of medical treatment was a fundamental human right in adults, and he was so close to that age. Nevertheless, having given great weight to the religious principles which underlay the family's decision, when viewed objectively the welfare of the child led to only one conclusion, namely that the hospital should be at liberty to treat him with blood transfusions. The wardship was confirmed and the hospital authority was granted leave to give treatment, including blood transfusion, and the consent of the patient and his parents was dispensed with.

The parents in this case were desperate to wait for the boy to become 16 years of age. However, it does not follow that, had he been aged 16 years, a different decision would have been made. As the case of Re W (1992) shows[5] (see below), the court could overrule the refusal of the 16- or 17-year-old minor notwithstanding the Family Law Reform Act 1969 and the Children Act 1989.

In Richardson's ethics cases[6] a similar dilemma is posed for health professionals (Consent to treatment). In the situation envisaged, Max, an American lad, is brought into the Accident and Emergency Department unconscious after a road traffic accident involving the motor cycle on which he was a passenger and of which his brother was the driver. His brother died in the accident. Max, who is aged 15 years, is carrying a card stating that he is a Christian Scientist and rejects all forms of orthodox medical treatment on religious grounds. The staff decide to care for Max with all necessary treatments and after subsequently contacting the parents and also the Christian Scientists discover that their care was in accordance with the wishes of both.

However, one could envisage a situation in which the child's wishes were totally in conflict with the parents', and the child had the full support of a religious group. If such a situation were to occur then the vital legal issues would be as follows.

- Does the child have the capacity to make such a decision?
- Are there any compelling reasons why the child's autonomy should be overruled?
- Is the refusal to consent to treatment a valid refusal according to the principles laid down by the Court of Appeal in Re T?
- If refusal has been given in advance, as in a living will, then other questions arise, such as 'Is this advanced directive valid? Have circumstances changed since that view was expressed?'

This is discussed below.

The situation envisaged by Richardson also highlights how important it is that the health professional understands the significance of certain religious and ethical beliefs. There was clearly a misunderstanding initially about the views of the Christian Scientists. Although it is impracticable to expect all health professionals to have a comprehensive knowledge of different cultures and religious beliefs, their care of the patient must take into account significant cultural and religious differences. This is illustrated in the situation of Ahmed and the sausage which is discussed in Chapter 13.

The Code of Professional Conduct of the practitioner registered with the UKCC states in clause 7: 'Recognise and respect the uniqueness and dignity of each patient and client, and respond to their need for care, irrespective of their ethnic origin, religious beliefs, personal attributes, the nature of their health problems or any other factor.'[7]

Donation of nonregenerative organs

The Gillick principle can also apply to major decisions such as the donation of nonregenerative organs. Therefore the National Organ Donor Register does not stipulate any age limit. Any person who is capable within the law of consenting to treatment is capable of consenting to organ donation. There is no fixed age limit. The new scheme of registering through GPs, however, stipulates for administrative convenience an age limit of 16 years and over for registering with the GP the person's wish to have their name added to the NHS Organ Donor Register by using form FP1. This form enables the person to state whether or not they wish to be placed on the register and, if so, whether the consent applies to some or all of the organs.

PARENTAL CONSENT AND THE 16- OR 17-YEAR-OLD

As we have seen the parent retained the right to give consent on behalf of the 16- or 17-year-old after the Family Law Reform Act came into force. This is one of the effects of section 8(3) (see above). Normally this causes no problems and the practitioner can rely upon the consent of either the 16- or 17-year-old themselves or upon the consent given by the parent or guardian. The possibility of a clash arising is discussed below.

PARENTAL CONSENT AND THE UNDER 16-YEAR-OLD

Parents have a right at common law to give consent on behalf of their child aged under 16 years. This is parallel to the right of the competent child to give consent. It is also a responsibility of the parent under the Children Act 1989. If the parent fails to obtain the necessary treatment for a child, and the child suffers harm, then the parent could face criminal proceedings.

Definition of parent

Chapter 2 considers the different individuals who may have parental responsibilities under the Children Act 1989 and who would be able to give a valid consent to treatment. Even parents who are no longer in daily care of the child do not lose their responsibilities under the legislation.

In addition, the Children Act 1989 section 3(5) enables a person who does not have parental responsibility for a particular child, but does have care of the child, to 'do what is reasonable in all the circumstances of the case for the purposes of safeguarding or promoting the child's welfare' (section 3(5)).

This section would enable a health professional in temporary care of the child to do what is reasonable for the child. However, it would probably only cover immediate and necessary care. If major decisions were required and the situation could await the arrival of the parents, this should be done.

DISPUTE BETWEEN PARENT AND CHILD AND COURT INVOLVEMENT

If, however, there is a dispute between parent or guardian and the child, a difficult situation can arise. It may be possible to reconcile the parent with the child; if not, or in the absence of persons who could give consent and if treatment is essential in a life-saving situation, it may be necessary to obtain the declaration of the court that it is lawful to proceed with the treatment. This occurred in the case of Re W.

The facts of Re W [1992][8]

The child was born in 1976 and was taken into care, at a very early age, when both parents died of cancer. She later suffered from depression and a nervous tic. Symptoms of anorexia nervosa first manifested themselves in June 1990 and by January 1991 she was in need of inpatient treatment in a specialist residential home. While she was there she displayed violence towards the staff and began to injure herself by picking her skin, until she reached a stage when she had to be fed by nasogastric tube and have her arms encased in plaster. Against this background the local authority, deciding that it might become necessary to give her medical treatment against her will, issued an originating summons seeking leave of the court in the exercise of its inherent jurisdiction over children to move the child to a new treatment unit and to give her medical treatment without her consent.

In March 1992 the child reached the age of 16 years and consulted solicitors of her own choice. She wished to remain where she was and vehemently resisted the treatment proposed for her. The issues before the judge were whether, in the light of the provision of section 8 of the Family Law Reform Act 1969 and the fact that the minor was by then 16 years old, he had any jurisdiction to make orders concerning medical treatment which conflicted with her express wishes, and, if so, what treatment should be authorized. The judge held that he had the necessary jurisdiction and authorized the removal of the minor to, and her treatment at, the new treatment unit, subject to arrangements being made for the approval of new foster parents. The child appealed. During the course of the hearing it became clear that unless she submitted to the treatment which she had hitherto refused, she would suffer irreversible harm within a week and, accordingly, the court in an emergency order on 30 June 1992 authorized her treatment at the new unit forthwith.

The Court of Appeal made the following ruling.

- The fact that a child aged 16 years has the right to give consent to treatment under the Family Law Reform Act and common law did not mean that the child's refusal could not be overruled.
- Anorexia nervosa was known to destroy the ability to make an informed choice and treatment should therefore proceed.

The following are some of the principles set out by the Court of Appeal.

- No question of a child consenting to or refusing medical treatment arises unless and until a medical or dental practitioner advises such treatment and is willing to undertake it.
- Regardless of whether the child or anyone else with authority to do so consents to the treatment, that practitioner will be liable to the child in negligence if he or she fails to advise with reasonable skill and care and to have due regard to the best interests of his or her patient.
- This appeal has been concerned with the treatment of anorexia nervosa. It is a peculiarity of this disease that the disease itself creates a wish not to be cured or only to be cured if and when the patient decides to cure himself or herself, which may well be too late. Treatment has to be directed at this state of mind as much as to restoring body weight.
- Section 8 of the Family Law Reform Act 1969 gives children who have attained the age of 16 years a right to consent to surgical, medical, and dental treatment. Such a consent cannot be overridden by those with parental responsibility for the child. It can, however, be overridden by the court. This statutory right does not extend to consent to the donation of blood or organs.
- A child of any age who is Gillick-competent in the context of particular treatment has a right to consent to that treatment which again cannot be overridden by those with parental responsibility, but can be overridden by the court. Unlike the statutory right, this common law right extends to the donation of blood and organs.
- No child of whatever age has power, by refusing consent to treatment, to override a consent to treatment by someone who has parental responsibility for the child and, a fortiori, a consent by the court. Nevertheless, such a refusal is a very important consideration in making clinical judgments and for parents and the court in deciding whether themselves to give consent. Its importance increases with the age and maturity of the child.
- The effect of consent to treatment by the child or someone else with authority to give it is limited to protecting the medical or dental practitioner from claims for damages for trespass to the person.

In their comments on the Re W case and the fact that a Gillick-competent child did not have an unqualified or absolute right to refuse treatment, Korgaonkar and Tribe state that: 'it is most unsatisfactory that uncertainty and doubt remain. Parliament had the opportunity, when drafting the Children Act 1989, to make amends, but failed to grasp it. Children's interests are not best served by lengthy and complicated litigation.'[9]

PARENTAL REFUSAL TO CONSENT

What if the parent refuses to consent to treatment considered essential in the child's interests?

The professionals caring for the child who consider that treatment is essential can either, in an emergency situation carry out the life-saving treatment on the basis of necessity without consent (see below and the case of Re F) or arrange for an application to court under the provisions of the Children Act 1989.

There follows two examples of cases where the courts overruled parents refusal to consent to treatment.

Case of Re S[10]

A girl of 4 years 6 months had been diagnosed as suffering from T-cell leukaemia with a high risk of death. The condition was treatable by intensified chemotherapy which had four phases. The transfusion of blood or blood products was an essential supplement. Her parents were dedicated Jehovah's Witnesses and the family records and instructions had always opposed blood transfusions. A case conference had explored the irreconcilable gulf between the consultant's need to include the transfusion in the range of treatments available and the parents' conscientious objection to consent to the treatment. The local authority had sought leave to invoke the inherent jurisdiction under section 100 of the Children Act 1989 and sought an order permitting a blood transfusion. The following day the parents had issued an application under the Children Act 1989 for a prohibited steps order. The consultant paediatrician had given evidence of the medical need to administer a transfusion in emergency and non-emergency categories. He had been of the opinion that it would have been impossible for him to treat the child intensively without the discretion to administer blood. The consultant had already varied the conventional treatment of her condition to reflect the convictions of her parents. A senior lecturer in paediatric oncology who had shared responsibility for major decisions with the consultant in relation to her treatment had also given evidence on behalf of the local authority. He had stated that either the consultant had the authority to treat her intensively with the discretion to administer blood or there was no medical treatment which held any prospect of cure. The father had been fully supportive of any form of medical or scientific intervention provided it did not breach the veto upon the use of blood. The court allowed both applications of the local authority on the following grounds.

- The welfare of the child remained the paramount consideration. The stark choice was between one medical procedure with no prospect of success and one medical treatment with a prospect of success which was put at 50%.
- The family would recognize that the responsibility for consent was taken away from them and, as a judicial act, this absolved their conscience of responsibility.

Case of Re O (1993)[11]

The child was born prematurely and suffered from respiratory distress syndrome. The parents were Jehovah's Witnesses and did not consent to blood being given. The consultant paediatrician sought the help of the local authority and an application was made to the justices for an emergency protection order. This was granted without formal notice to the parents, although they were aware that such an application would be made. Blood transfusions were administered to the child 3 and 5 days after the hearing. The local authority applied for a care order on the basis that there was an urgent and continuing need for medical treatment, including a blood transfusion to which the parents had refused to give their consent. The matter was transferred to the High Court, who made the following decision.

- The emergency protection order gave the local authority parental responsibility for the child. The effect of sections 44(4)(c) and 2(6) of the Children Act 1989 was that the local authority, the mother, and the father each had parental responsibility and each had the rights and authority which by law a parent had in relation to a child under section 3(1) of the 1989 Act.
- There were substantial limitations to the right provided by section 45(8) of the Children Act 1989 for a parent to apply to the court for the discharge of an emergency protection order. The first limitation was that an application for a discharge could not be heard less than 72 hours after the emergency protection order had been made. Second, no appeal could be made against the making of the emergency protection order.
- The court endeavoured to pay every respect and give great weight to the religious principles which underlay the family's decision and then act as the judicial reasonable parent. After weighing up the various considerations, the court's duty was to give directions that would have the consequence of ensuring that medical advice dictated.
- The gravity of such an application meant that it should be dealt with by a judge of the Family Division. Applications such as these should ordinarily be made under the inherent jurisdiction of the court, but if made under the provision of the Children Act 1989 should be transferred to the Family Division as a matter of urgency; if there were contested issues about the emergency medical treatment, the justice system overrode the views of the parents. The gravity, difficulty, and sometimes complexity of the issues meant that the parents were entitled to look for a decision to the High Court of Justice.

As cases such as those of Re O and Re S are always likely to be emergency problems, it is essential that the hospital trust develops a procedure to enable action to be taken to ensure the welfare of the child. This should be familiar to staff, and should cover weekends and out of office hours, when speedy action is necessary and the unit manager not at work. In an extreme emergency there may not be sufficient time to obtain the decision of the court in carrying out life-saving measures against the wishes of the parents; in such circumstances the health professionals should taken the immediate action necessary to save the life of the child.

OVERRULING PARENTS' CONSENT TO TREATMENT

What if the parents want treatment to take place which is not in the child's best interests? The following case is an example of the parents' consent to a sterilization operation being overruled in the case of a child suffering from Soto's syndrome.

Re D (a Minor) (Wardship: sterilization)[12]

D was born in November 1963 with a condition known as Sotos syndrome, the symptoms of which included accelerated growth during infancy, epilepsy, generalized clumsiness, an unusual facial appearance, and behaviour problems, including emotional instability, certain aggressive tendencies, and some impairment of mental function which could result in dull intelligence or possibly more serious mental retardation. She was sent to an appropriate school but did not do well, partly because she exhibited a number of behavioural problems, including hostility and a certain amount of violence towards other children. Accordingly, in October 1973 she was sent to a school specializing in children who had learning difficulties and associated behavioural problems. The move was a success. She showed a marked improvement in her academic skills, in her social competence and in her behavioural problems. She had an intelligence quotient of about 80, indicating a dull normal intelligence, and she had the understanding of a child of about 9 years of age. A consultant paediatrician confirmed that her clumsiness was likely to lessen and her behaviour to continue to improve. Her mother, however, was convinced that D was seriously retarded mentally and she did not accept that there had been any improvement in the child's behaviour or ability to care for herself. A consultant paediatrician, Dr G, who from an early stage had taken an interest in D's case, thought that her behaviour had deteriorated, that she would always remain substantially handicapped and that she would therefore be unable either to care for or maintain herself or to look after any children she might have. All agreed, however, that she had sufficient intellectual capacity to enable her to marry in due course. When she was a young child her parents had decided that they should apply to have her sterilized when she was about 18 years of age to prevent her from having children who might be abnormal and over the years they discussed the matter several times with Dr G. When D reached puberty at the age of 10 years, the mother's concern increased; she was worried that D might be seduced and possibly give birth to an abnormal child. She consulted Dr G who took the view that there was a real risk that D might give birth to an abnormal child. Accordingly, he agreed that D should be sterilized without waiting for her to grow any older. Arrangements were made for the operation to be carried out in May 1975. Other professional people concerned with D's welfare challenged the social and behavioural reasons for performing such an irreversible and permanent operation on a girl aged 11 years. Dr G, however, refused to defer the operation. Mrs H, an educational psychologist attached to the education department of D's local authority, applied to the court to make D a ward of court and sought an order continuing the wardship to delay the proposed operation or prevent it from being carried out. The court granted Mrs H's application on the following grounds.

- The operation proposed was one that involved the deprivation of a basic human right, that is, the right of a woman to reproduce and therefore if performed on a woman for nontherapeutic reasons without her consent, would be a violation of that right. As D could not given an informed consent, but there was a strong likelihood that she would understand the implications of the operation when she reached the age of 18 years, the case was one in which the court should exercise its protective powers. Her wardship would accordingly be continued.
- A decision to carry out a sterilization operation on a minor for nontherapeutic purposes was not solely within a doctor's clinical judgment. In the circumstances the operation was neither medically indicated nor necessary; it would not be in D's best interests for it to be performed as the evidence showed that D's mental and physical condition and attachments had already improved, that her future prospects were unpredictable and that, although she was as yet unable to understand or appreciate the implications of the operation, it was likely that in later years she would be able to make her own choice.

If harm to a child occurs as the result of the parents' failure to provide a reasonable standard of medical care for the child, even if cultural or ethnic reasons are the cause, the parents could face prosecution. In a recent case parents did not wish their diabetic daughter to be treated with insulin but with a homoeopathic remedy; however, insulin was vital to her treatment. The daughter died and the father was imprisoned, and the mother given a suspended sentence.[13,14]

Disputes between parents and professionals can also arise in the care of neonates; sometimes parents want active treatment when this is not deemed to be in the child's best interests, and sometimes parents want professionals to allow the child to die. (These issues are considered in Chapter 22.)

HOW SHOULD CONSENT BE GIVEN?

There are very few laws relating to the procedure by which consent should be obtained. The following require a written consent in a particular format: the Mental Health Act 1983, the Human Fertilisation and Embryology Act 1990, and the Abortion Act 1967. In other situations, there is no requirement that consent should be given in writing, though good practice would dictate this. Consent can be given by word of mouth or by nonverbal communication (sometimes called implied consent). Implied consent, consent by word of mouth, and consent in writing may all be equally valid, but clearly if there is a dispute over whether consent was actually given there is considerable evidential value in the consent being in writing.

DOCUMENTATION

The NHS Management Executive has given guidance[15] on consent to treatment and has drafted forms which could be used in a variety of circumstances. If the consent is given in writing, it is essential that the forms are correctly completed and the necessary information given to the patient or parent before the form is signed. It must be remembered that the form is only prima facie evidence that consent has been given and this can be rebutted by showing that there was not actual willing consent by a competent person. In research quoted by Priscilla Alderson,[16] a study found that 40% of patients who had signed a consent form had very little idea of what they had consented to. There is no reason to suspect that the figure for parental consent on behalf of children would be significantly higher. She points out (page 94) that 'law cases usually concern parents refusing treatment for their child. A more common problem is parents feeling unable to refuse treatment which turns out to be ineffective or harmful.' There is a clear advocacy role for nurses in this context to ensure that valid consent is given.

WHAT DOES THE CONSENT COVER?

Should the parent (or child) give consent for each individual item of care or can it be assumed that once consent is given it is for a treatment plan? The question is important as some parents may question specific parts of treatment given if it has not been explained to them that this is an essential part of the care.

In the case study on the care of a child with hypospadias[17] (a congenital malformation of the genitalia resulting in the urethral orifice being found on the ventral surface of the penile shaft) Pat Rose states that after a session in the operating theatre to have a fistula repaired, John, a 6-year-old boy, returned to the ward 'with his forearms encased together across his chest in a cylinder of plaster of Paris. This was a complete surprise to the boy, his parents and the nursing staff. The surgeon had done it to ensure that John did not pull out his catheter. The author asks: 'Was it ethically right for the surgeon to decide to encase John's arms in plaster without prior discussion?'

What concerns us here is 'was it lawful?' The parents had signed a consent form which presumably included the phrase 'and any other treatment deemed necessary'. This phrase could be regarded as covering the encasing of the child's arms and presumably it was in the child's best interests according to the principles of Re F (see below). However, it was clearly not an emergency procedure and could have been discussed with the parents and the child before the operation. At the very least there were failures in communication, which can in certain circumstances be regarded as a breach of the duty of care (see below).

To avoid such uncertainties it is preferable if staff are able to discuss with the parent, or the child if competent, or both, the treatment plan and give them an idea of the various procedures likely to be required. Thus the need to take the temperature via the anus, or to give anal suppositiories for pain relief could be spelled out to the parents and child. Does this mean that the parent or child has to give consent to each individual item of care and treatment? The answer is probably that procedures which have a considerable risk should receive specific consent, otherwise it could be assumed that a consent in principle entitles the professionals to carry out treatment and care according to the reasonable standards of the profession. However, good communication between the parents or child and those administering the care is clearly good practice and should cover, in particular, those elements in a treatment plan which may involve a risk or cause concern.

TREATMENT IN THE ABSENCE OF CONSENT

The following are circumstances in which what would otherwise be a trespass to the person is justifiable by common law or statute law.

- Necessity at common law
- Police and Criminal Evidence Act 1984
- Mental Health Act 1983
- Children Act 1989

Necessity

The leading case on the power of the professional to give treatment to a person incapable of giving consent is Re F.

THE FACTS OF RE F[18]

The case was concerned with the sterilization of a mentally disordered woman. This was recommended by her carers and health professionals but no-one in law had the right to give consent on her behalf. An application was made to the court, and the House of Lords declared that it would be lawful for a professional acting in the best interests of the patient and following the Bolam test to give treatment to her without her consent.

There was power at common law for a person to act out of necessity in the care and treatment of a person who was incapable of giving consent.

In an emergency situation a professional could rely upon the principles of the case of Re F in giving treatment to a child who was incapable of giving consent and in which the parents were refusing necessary treatment or not available. Alternatively, if the professionals were deemed to be in the charge of the child, there is power under section 3(5) of the Children Act 1989 for the carer to give consent to treatment (see page 58).

Police and Criminal Proceedings Act 1984

This enables a police constable or private citizen to arrest a person and thus commit an act which would without this lawful justification be regarded as a trespass to the person. Under section 17 a police constable can enter and search premises to save life or limb.

Mental Health Act 1983

The circumstances in which treatment can be given without consent for mental disorder are discussed in Chapter 21.

Children Act 1989

This gives a statutory duty for those with parental responsibility to make decisions on behalf of the child. However, as it has been shown, the wishes and feelings of the child must be taken into account in the light of his age and understanding.

GIVING INFORMATION BEFORE CONSENT IS OBTAINED

The importance of giving full information to the parents or the child before treatment and care proceeds is emphasized above. If there has been a failure to warn the parents or child of the significant risk of substantial harm and that harm occurs, and had the parents or child not given consent had that risk been spelled out, then there could be an action for breach of the duty of care to inform the parent or child. This was established by the House of Lords in the Sidaway case.[19]

To bring an action, the plaintiff would have to show the absence of the significant information, the harm which has arisen, and the fact that had information on these risks been given consent would not have been given.

The research by Priscilla Alderson[20] showed that 'not all the information for consent can possibly be covered in clinics, and this stage can seem too early to discuss consent. However, after a child has been admitted for surgery suddenly it can seem too late to demur. Families need much information before admission to help them to consider decisions and to prepare for surgery. Gaps in information are not routinely filled in after admission, and the clinic is the only chance some families have to talk with the consultant before surgery. However, outpatients clinics are only one stage in the decision making. One of their main purposes is to collect data for discussion at the medical case conference.' She defines informed proxy consent as 'the absence of serious ignorance or misunderstanding about how the treatment is likely to affect the patient'.[16]

CONCLUSION

The area of consent is complex for the health professional and particularly so in the care of the child, when many conflicting views may emerge. The following are examples of guidelines to assist the health professional in the care of the child.

Guidelines for health professionals in child health decision-making situations

- What are the facts of the situation?
- Obtain appropriate advice, knowledge, and instruction.
- Be aware of the legal principles governing the situation.
- Do any procedures or codes of practice apply?
- Ensure that appropriate action is taken to enable the child to be personally represented; this may require an application to court, to an ethics committee, to a social worker and so on
- Identify the interests of each party in the dispute.
- Try to understand the principles that may arise.
- Ensure that your own view is legally justifiable.
- Keep comprehensive records of action taken and advice given, and respective reasons.
- Be prepared to account for your actions and advice.

REFERENCES

1 Re T (Adult: Refusal of Medical Treatment) [1992] 4 All ER 649
2 Gillick v W Norfolk and Wisbech Area Health Authority [1986] 1 AC 112
3 Robinson E: Parents' attitudes to self-medication by their asthmatic children. *Br J Nurs* 1994, 3:651–656.
4 Re E (a minor) (Wardship: Medical Treatment) Family Division [1993] 1 FLR 386
5 Re W (a minor) (Medical Treatment) [1992] 4 All ER 627, [1993] 1 FLR 1
6 Richardson J, Webber I: *Ethical Issues in Child Health Care.* London: Mosby; 1995.

7   UKCC: *Code of Professional Conduct*. London: UKCC; 1992.
8   Re W (a minor) (Medical Treatment) [1992] 4 All ER 627, [1993] 1 FLR 1
9   Korgaonkar G, Tribe D: Children and consent to medical treatment. *Br J Nurs* 1993, 2:383–384.
10 Re S(a minor)(Medical Treatment) Family Division [1993] 1 FLR 376
11 Re O (a minor)(Medical Treatment) [1993] 2 FLR 149
12 Re D(a minor)(Wardship: sterilisation 1976 1 All ER 327
13 *Times*, News Report 6 November 1993
14 Times, Editorial: A right to life: parents cannot condemn their children to die. 8 November 1993.
15 NHS Management Executive: *A Guide to Consent to Examination and Treatment*. London: HMSO;
    1990. [published with DoH circular HC(90)2]
16 Alderson P: *Choosing for Children*. Oxford: Oxford University Press; 1990: p133.
17 Rose P: Care of a child with hypospadias: ethical issues in practice. *Br J Nurs* 1992, 1:393–398.
18 F *v* West Berkshire Health Authority [1989] 2 All ER 545
19 Sidaway v Board of Governors of the Bethlem Royal Hospital and the Maudsley Hospital [1985]
    1 All ER 643
20 Alderson P: *Choosing for Children*. Oxford: Oxford University Press; 1990: p61.

The right to confidentiality

Professionals owe the same duty of care over keeping confidential information about the child as they do over information about the adult patient. The law on maintaining confidentiality is summarized with guidance for professionals in a recent publication by Bryden Darley and others.[1] This chapter explores:

- the nature of this duty;
- the exceptions to it;
- conflict between Gillick-competent child and parent if the child does not want the parent to be aware of information; and
- future developments.

THE NATURE OF THE DUTY OF CONFIDENTIALITY

The duty to ensure that information received from and about the patient is kept confidential is recognized by all health professionals as part of their codes of conduct. It is also recognized by an express or implied term in the contract of employment and this applies also to ancillary, administrative, and clerical staff who might not be members of a professional association and therefore subject to a code of professional practice.

An infringement of the duty could be enforced by the employer through disciplinary proceedings, by the professional body through conduct proceedings, and by the patient through an action for breach of the duty of confidentiality owed to him or her. **Figure 7.1** illustrates the main ways in which the duty of confidentiality can be enforced.

Health professionals should be aware that normally there would be a presumption that the duty of confidentiality exists, and if they were called upon to divulge information which they hold in confidence, they should clearly identify the reasons justifying such disclosure. If they are in doubt over whether confidentiality should be broken, they should seek advice from a senior manager who is not professionally involved with the case. Records should be kept of the reason for the decision whether to disclose.

The duty of confidentiality is set out in the UKCC Code of Professional Conduct.[2] Clause 10 requires the practitioner 'to protect all confidential information concerning patients and clients obtained in the course of professional practice and make disclosures only with consent, where required by the order of a court or where you can justify disclosure in the wider public interest' (see below the advisory paper of the UKCC on confidentiality).

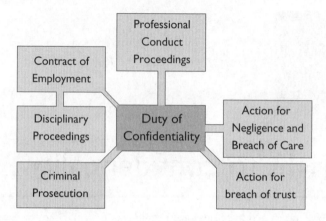

Fig. 7.1 Enforcement of the duty of confidentiality

EXCEPTIONS TO THE DUTY OF CONFIDENTIALITY

The law recognizes certain exceptions to the duty of confidentiality to the child; these are listed below.

- Consent of the parent for the child below the age of Gillick-competence and possibly up to the age of 18 years
- Consent of the child (if of Gillick-competence)
- Disclosure in the interests of the child
- Statutory justification for disclosure
- Disclosure by order of the court
- Disclosure in the public interest

Consent of the parents

A television programme about a children's hospital on a week by week basis takes the general public through the successes and tragedies of the work undertaken and the lives of the patients. One episode concerned the diagnosis of leukaemia in a young boy aged about 3 years and the story of a slightly older girl who had had an operation to pin back her ears. One assumes that their real names were used; in any case there was no attempt to preserve anonymity as the children were often filmed full on and would be recognizable by anyone with more than a fleeting acquaintance. The parents would have given consent to the filming, as of course would the NHS trust where the filming took place. However, they have also given consent to what would, without that consent, have constituted a breach of the duty of confidentiality of information about the child. Presumably the reason must be that the programme was in the interests of the child [this is debatable in view of the filming of the child in distress at receiving injections or the young girl having the bandages being taken off her head ('Don't whinge' says the doctor to her whimpers when the hair was caught in the bandaging)]. Were the children frightened by the presence of the cameras; did this create alarm in a situation which was already terrifying for them? As far as the law is concerned, the parents have the right to give consent to disclosure which, without that consent, would be a breach of the duty to maintain confidentiality. However, is it necessarily in the child's interests?

Similar examples could be given: the child who is being flown overseas for specialist treatment not available in this country; the child who is being used as a donor for a sibling who requires bone marrow; the child whose lack of treatment is being used for political purposes to assert deficiencies in the NHS. Only if it can be shown that the parents have acted contrary to the interests of the child, is an application to the courts likely to succeed. Such an action could take place under the Children Act 1989 (see Chapter 9).

The duty owed to the child is therefore in practice owed to the parents for the child below the Gillick-competence age. If the parents give consent to disclosure, that would normally be a complete defence to any action brought in respect of that disclosure.

Disclosure by the Gillick-competent child

If a child is Gillick-competent, that is, the child has sufficient maturity and understanding, he or she could give consent to a disclosure which, without that consent, would be a breach of confidentiality. The consent could be given either generally or specifically. The onus would be on the person relying on that consent to prove that it was given and that the child was competent. A health professional relying upon that consent to disclosure should ensure that both the fact of the consent and the assessment of the capacity to give that consent were recorded.

The possibility of a conflict between the child and parent is considered below.

Disclosure in the interests of the child

This would cover the giving of information to other health professionals who need that information in order to care for the child. It could also cover the passing of information to the Area Protection Team and the at risk register if the child was considered to be in danger.

Statutory justification

As is the case with adults, there are certain very specific occasions where statute law requires disclosure of information regardless of whether the child or parent gives consent. Legislation includes the following.

- Section 172(4) of the Road Traffic Act 1988.
- Section 18 the Prevention of Terrorism (Temporary Provisions) Act 1989.
- Regulation 3 of the misuse of drugs (notification of supply to addicts) regulations 1973 S1 1973 no. 799.
- Section 11(1) Public Health (Control of Diseases) Act 1984.
- Police and Criminal Evidence Act 1984.
- Abortion regulations 1991 SI 1991 no. 449 paragraph 4.
- NHS (Notification of Births and Deaths) regulations 1982 SI 1982 no. 286.
- Health and Safety at Work Act 1974.
- Reporting of injuries, diseases and dangerous occurrence regulations 1985 SI 1985 no. 2023.

Court order

The court can order disclosure of confidential information at various stages of litigation. In civil cases of litigation arising from personal injury or death, section 33 of the Supreme Court Act 1981 enables disclosure to be made in advance of the writ being issued (see Chapter 13) if the person against whom the order is made is likely to be a party to the proceedings. This would include a situation in which litigation was being contemplated by a person who had been injured or by the relatives of such a person who had died as the result of the negligence of health professionals. Section 34 enables disclosure to be made after the writ has been issued. The disclosure can be ordered against a person who is not likely to be a party to the action but who has in his possession information likely to be of relevance to an issue arising in litigation for personal injury or death. An example would be a case involving a child in a road accident, in which the defendant wishes to obtain information about the child's health to prove that the compensation payable should be reduced on account of the preceding illness or disability of the child.

DURING A COURT CASE

A judge has the right to subpoena a witness who has information relevant to the proceedings together with any documents (subpoena duces tecum, that is, an order to appear and bring with you). The witness cannot refuse to answer questions relevant to the case (relevance is determined by the judge) unless they are protected by legal professional privilege or by the public interest immunity (see below), or the answers would tend to incriminate them in court. If these exceptions do not exist, failure on the witness's part to answer questions deemed relevant by the judge could result in the witness being held in contempt of court.

LEGAL PROFESSIONAL PRIVILEGE

Communications between a client and lawyer in contemplation of court proceedings or in connection with legal advice in relation to court proceedings are privileged from disclosure. It must be established that the prime purpose of the communication was the possibility of legal action. If documents have been brought into existence in such circumstances, their disclosure cannot be ordered by a judge either before litigation commences or once it has begun. The reason for the privilege is to ensure that there can be confidence between client and lawyer in the interests of justice. In the House of Lords decision in the case of Waugh v British Railway Board[3] it was held that if a document had come into existence for two separate purposes (e.g. in the case itself, a fatal accident inquiry report both to enable safety measures to be introduced and to enable the solicitor to advise on any possible litigation which might be brought against the Board), it had to be decided which was the dominant purpose of the report and, if this was covered by legal professional privilege, the document was protected from an order for disclosure. (In this case, the House of Lords decided that the dominant purpose was the safety aspect and it was not therefore privileged from disclosure.)

The ruling was followed in the case of Lask v Gloucester Health Authority.[4] In this case the health authority and solicitors had sworn affidavits that the dominant purpose was for use in litigation but the court on seeing the documents decided that they were not privileged from disclosure.

Health professionals cannot claim a similar privilege in relation to the information which they have obtained in confidence from the child and must be prepared to permit their records and themselves to be subject to the scrutiny of the court. Nor could they avoid the issue by keeping a separate secret file containing confidential information, as this file could itself be made the subject for an order of disclosure and the health professional, if called as a witness, could not refuse to answer any relevant questions.

PUBLIC INTEREST IMMUNITY

Certain documents are privileged from disclosure on the grounds that it would be contrary to the public interest for disclosure to be ordered. Thus if national security was at risk a Minister could issue a notice to that effect. The judge is able to inspect the document and decide if the privilege from disclosure should prevail. For example, it is alleged, in 1987 the Government were aware that 26 babies had died and many others had suffered serious illness as a result of the bacterium, Listeria. This was likely to be found in such foods as soft cheese, cook–chill foods, chickens, and pâté. When parents attempted to bring legal action, the Ministers involved signed public interest immunity certificates to state that Government documents showing its awareness should be kept secret. The judge rejected these arguments and released the documents. Litigation is continuing.

After the Scott enquiry, it is likely that changes will be made to the rules relating to the application of this exception to the rules of disclosure to the court.

Public interest

There are certain exceptional circumstances in which, despite promises of confidentiality to the patient, the professional is entitled to disclose information in the wider public interest.

In two of the very few decided cases on the issue of confidentiality the court held first,[5] that an independent psychiatric report commissioned by the patient could be disclosed to the hospital and the Home Secretary in the public interest against the express wishes of the patient; and second,[6] that an injunction could be granted against a newspaper preventing it publishing the names of two doctors working in the NHS who were suffering from AIDS. The court held that the information obtained from hospital records should be kept confidential and the public interest did not require the publication of the names.

Many codes of conduct of different health professionals recognize this exception to the general rule of confidentiality. For example the UKCC in its advisory paper,[7] section D gives guidelines on 'Deliberate breach of confidentiality in the public interest or that of individual patient or client'. It advises (paragraph 5): 'In all cases where the practitioner deliberately discloses or withholds information in what he/she believes the public interest he/she must be able to justify the decision. These situations can be particularly stressful, especially where vulnerable groups are concerned, as disclosure may mean the involvement of a third party as in the case of children or the mentally handicapped. Practitioners should always take the opportunity to discuss the matter fully with other practitioners (not only or necessarily fellow nurses, midwives and health visitors), and if appropriate consult with a professional organisation before making a decision. There will often be ramifications and these are best explored before a final decision as to whether to withhold or disclose information is made.' The importance of recording the reasons for the disclosure or withholding is emphasized. (The UKCC used bold print.)

This advice would also be pertinent to every other health professional who is the custodian of confidential information.

CONFIDENTIALITY AND WHISTLE-BLOWING

Disclosure in the public interest may also be justified in a so-called whistle-blowing situation, that is, a situation in which an employee is frustrated in attempts to persuade management to give its attention to a situation which is potentially hazardous or dangerous to the safety of patients, staff or others. The NHS Management Executive in its guidance for employees,[8] although requiring NHS trusts to establish a mechanism whereby concerns can be drawn to the attention of senior management, has emphasized that staff must be extremely careful not to breach confidentiality and to take professional advice. Ngwena and Chadwick[9] point out the lack of an independent adjudicatory mechanism in its suggested procedures, but consider that legislation protecting the employee in whistle-blowing situations is unlikely to be supported by the present Government. Individual employers may include in the contracts with employees confidentiality clauses which may preclude an employee making known concerns to outside agencies or individuals. A health professional should always seek advice before breaching such terms but should also be mindful of duties set down in codes of professional conduct to report situations of potential danger to clients or colleagues.

CONFLICT BETWEEN GILLICK-COMPETENT CHILD AND PARENT

Conflict between the Gillick-competent child and the parent when the child does not want the parent to be made aware of information, could occur, for example, if a child tells a therapist that:

- he or she is having a sexual relationship with an adult, such as a parent, teacher, priest, or health professional and does not wish the (other) parent to be told;

- he or she suffering from venereal disease, AIDS, or is HIV positive and does not wish the parent to be told; or
- he or she is on drugs, is an alcoholic, smokes, is pregnant or is having an abortion.

What is the position of the health professional? When would it be justifiable to go against the child's wishes for confidentiality?

If the child is below the age of Gillick-competence and therefore does not have the capability to make such a decision on his or her own account, and the health professional believes that the information is significant and should be reported to the parent in the child's best interests, this would count as a justifiable exception of the duty of confidentiality owed to the child. The health professional should, however, clearly identify and record the reasons for disclosure and the action they have taken.

There may be circumstances in which the health professional should see him- or herself as an advocate for the child and, if no exception to the duty of confidentiality is justified, ensure that every reasonable action is taken to ensure that the child's right to confidentiality is recognized. In addition, the health professional may have a role in enabling the child to be an advocate for him or herself.

If the child is Gillick-competent, there would still have to be a balancing of the interests of the child in making the disclosure against the right of the child to keep the information confidential.

In Jim Richardson's book on ethics,[10] Chapter 10 tells the account of a 15-year-old boy, Alex, who is a haemophiliac. His parents have refused to tell him that he is HIV positive as the result of earlier blood transfusions. He is keeping secret from them the fact that he is having unprotected sex. He confides in a nurse, when he is worried about suffering from venereal disease and the nurse is in possession of both sets of information; the boy does not want his parents told about his sexual activity, and the parents do not want their son told about his HIV status.

What is the legal situation? The right of Alex to know about his HIV status is discussed in Chapter 8. It is not an easily enforceable right, as it is difficult to obtain information if you do not know that the information exists. He should be able to obtain access to his health records, whether they are held in manual or computerized form.

Alex's right to prevent the nurse telling his parents about his sexual activity would depend upon whether any of the exceptions to the duty of confidentiality apply.

If the parents were aware of these activities, they would be able to give Alex the necessary information to protect himself and others. This would be in Alex's interest.

If the parents were told, they would be able to ensure that Alex knew of his HIV status and therefore of the necessity of his taking precautions against spreading the HIV virus. This would be in the public interest.

The advice of the UKCC is applicable in this area. Just as the practitioner is advised to consider many different factors when there is pressure to disclose in the public interest, so should the same issues and steps be followed when considering breaching confidentiality in the interests of the child.

FUTURE DEVELOPMENTS

Department of Health consultation paper on confidentiality

This paper was issued for comments to be returned by December 1994. It discusses the meaning of health information, the obligation in relation to confidentiality, and the use of information in research. In the Appendices are included details of the duty of confidentiality under the Human Fertilisation and Embryology Act 1990 and the amending legislation in 1993, a list of statutes which require disclosure (see above), and a specimen notice for NHS patients.

The document has been criticized[11] and it may well be that the revised edition as a result of consultation may be more focused. One weakness in the document is that it fails to state the legal authority for situations in which it states that disclosure can be made, for example personal health information being passed to social services and in the interests of planning.

Multiprofessional working group

In July 1994 a group of professional associations representing nurses, doctors, dentists, psychologists, midwives, health visitors, professions supplementary to medicine, the Conference of the Royal Colleges, and other interprofessional working groups met with observers from the Data Protection Registrar's Office, the Medical Research Council, and the UKCC. As a result a draft handbook was prepared giving guidance on the use and disclosure of personal health information. It included a Bill to govern the use and disclosure of Personal Health Information.

The Bill makes it clear that: 'Nothing in this Act prevents the disclosure of personal health information with the consent of the person to whom it relates.' A child is defined as an individual who has not attained the age of 16 years.

There has been no statement that the Government is prepared to adopt the suggestions for legislation. However, the feedback from its consultation paper will probably be influenced by the more restrictive approach to disclosure which is shown in the legislation drafted by the multidisciplinary group.

In addition, work has taken place in the Institute of Health Informatics at the University of Wales Aberystwyth[12] on a strategy for security of the clinical record and its transfer in relation to electronic communications of confidential information. It is hoped that these recommendations will also be taken into account by the Department of Health in its final proposals.

REFERENCES

1 Darley B, Griew A, McLoughlin K, Williams J: *How to Keep a Clinical Confidence*. London: HMSO; 1994.
2 UKCC: *Code of Professional Conduct*. London: UKCC; 1992.
3 Waugh *v* British Railway Board 1980 AC 521.
4 Lask *v* Gloucester Health Authority. *Times*, 13 December 1985.
5 W *v* Egdell [1990] 1 A11ER 836.
6 X *v* Y [1988] 2 A11ER 648.
7 UKCC: *Confidentiality: an elaboration of clause 9 of the second edition of the UKCC's Code of Professional Conduct*. London: UKCC; April 1987. [Now clause 10 of the June 1992 edition of the Code of Professional Practice.]
8 NHS Management Executive: *Guidance for staff on relations with the public and the media*. London: Department of Health; 1993.
9 Ngwena C, Chadwick R: Confidentiality and nursing practice: ethics and law. *Nurs Ethics* 1994, 1:136–150.
10 Richardson J, Webber I: *Ethical Issues in Child Health Care*. London: Mosby; 1995.
11 Gibbons B: Draft guidelines are ill-wind for confidentiality. *Pulse* 1995.
12 Griew A: *A strategy for security of the clinical record and its transfer*. Aberystwyth: University of Aberystwyth; 1994.

The right of access to health records and information

To see their health records is an important right for patients, including child patients.[1] In the past the possibility of access has depended upon the agreement of the professionals who have made out the records, and some have been more liberal than others. Ownership of NHS records rests with the Secretary of State. In practice this is delegated to health authorities. The Secretary of State has urged access to be facilitated in advance of possible court orders for disclosure. Such guidance is less significant now that there is a statutory right of access to the records whether held in manual or computerized form. This chapter explores the statutory provisions, especially for access by a child, and discusses some specific situations in which access might be requested. A useful source of reference which covers access provisions and the law relating to confidentiality is by Darley and others.[2]

COMPUTERIZED RECORDS

Patients were given a right of access to personal records held in computerized form under the provisions of the Data Protection Act 1984 and the statutory instrument on access. The provisions came into effect on 11 November 1987.[3]

Access by parents

A parent has a right of access to the records of his or her child, if the child lacks the capacity to exercise their rights to access their own records. A parent would include a person undertaking the responsibilities of a parent. It must be shown that the parent or legal guardian considers it necessary to have access to the data for the purpose of carrying out the duty to take care of the child. The guidance from the Department of Health suggests that health authorities should assume, unless there are grounds to suggest the contrary, that a parent or legal guardian making a request on behalf of a dependent child who lacks capacity is acting in the child's best interests and access should be allowed. The advice of the health professional should be sought by the data user on whether it is known that the child in fact lacks capacity or whether there are reasons to believe that the child would not wish the information to be disclosed. In these circumstances the data user should make further enquiries of the parent or child as appropriate.

Access by the child

If the child has the capacity, he or she can apply for access to his or her personal health data kept in computerized form. The Department of Health recommends[4] that a certificate should be signed in which a responsible adult certifies that the child understands the nature of the application.

Procedure under the Data Protection Access provisions

The application is made to the data user, that is, the person who holds the records. Health authorities and NHS trusts are 'persons' and are therefore capable of holding data. The application would be made to the chief executive of the authority or trust.

The application must be made in writing; it must give sufficient information to identify the person making the application and to locate the information sought; and the required fee must either accompany the application or be sent at a later date.

The application must be processed within 40 days of its receipt, irrespective of whether the fee accompanies the application. If insufficient information accompanies the request, the 40 days runs from when that is provided.

That data user must consult the doctor or dentist who is currently, or was most recently, responsible for the clinical care of the subject to whom the data relates or, if there is more than one such person, the one most suitable to advise on the matters to which the request relates. Failing this, the data user must consult an appropriate health professional.

Refusal of access

Access can be refused if serious harm would be caused to the physical or mental health of the patient, or if access would reveal the identity of a third person who does not wish to be identified. If access is denied, the patient can either apply to the High Court or the County Court for an order of enforcement, or notify the Data Protection Registrar, who has the power to serve an enforcement notice upon the health service body.

The patient has a right to apply to court to request the rectification of inaccurate data. The patient can also seek compensation for harm that has resulted from inaccurate data.

ACCESS TO RECORDS IN MANUAL FORM

On 1 November 1991 patients received the right of access to their health records which were held in manual form.[5] Manual records made before that date are only accessible if they are required to make sense of records kept after that date. This right also applies to the child patient, but there are some specific provisions in relation to health records held about a child.

Right of the child

Section 3(1)(a) of the Access to Health Records Act 1990 gives the right of access to the patient. However, for a record held in England and Wales, if the patient is a child (i.e. someone under 16 years of age), access shall not be given under subsection (2) of section 3 unless the holder of the record is satisfied that the patient is capable of understanding the nature of the application.

No definition of the capability of the child is given in the Act but it is submitted that the Gillick test of competence adapted to the specific conditions of access to records would be applied. (This is discussed in Chapter 6.)

Right of the parent

Under section 3(1)(c) in England and Wales, if the patient is a child, a person having parental responsibility for the patient has a right of access. However, this is qualified by section 4(2), which prevents access unless the holder of the record is satisfied either that the patient has consented to the making of the application, or that the patient is incapable of understanding the nature of the application and the giving of access would be in their best interests.

Access if the patient is incapable of managing their own affairs

Under section 3(1)(e) if a person is incapable of managing their affairs, any person appointed by the court to manage those affairs has a right of access.

Access to the records of a deceased person

Under section 3(1)(f) the personal representatives of the deceased have a right of access to the health records, but this can be prevented by the patient in their lifetime, as under section 4(3) access shall not be given in such circumstances if the record includes a note, made at the patient's request, that they did not wish access to be given on such an application.

There is no reason why this provision should not also apply to a child, providing that they had the mental capacity to make the note refusing access.

General right to prevent access

These qualifications on the right of access to the records by both child and parent exist alongside the power of the holder of the records to exclude access under section 5.

This section enables the holder of the record to refuse access to any part of the health record which, in the opinion of the holder of the record, either would disclose information likely to cause serious harm to the physical or mental health of the patient or of any other individual, or information relating to or provided by an individual, other than the patient, who could be identified from that information; or was made before the commencement of the Act.

Section 5 would thus enable access to be refused to parents if they have not been told of a terminal condition of their child and it is felt that serious physical or mental harm would be caused to them. Serious physical or mental harm is not defined in the Act and there are as yet no decided cases on the interpretation of these words. It is assumed, however, that it must be related to the particular applicant in question and any blanket policy prohibiting access in specified circumstances would not be acceptable as a general rule. For example it would be contrary to the law to have a policy which stated that all patients who were being treated for mental disorder could not have access to their records.

Section 5 also enables access to be refused in such cases in which another individual (who is not a health professional concerned with the patient's treatment), who does not wish to be identified, has reported to the health service concerns about the treatment or care of the child. The anonymity of an informer can thus be protected.

An example of a situation in which anonymity might be required is the case of D v NSPCC[6] in which the House of Lords refused to allow, on grounds of public policy, the disclosure of an informer's name to the parent who considered that the Society had acted negligently in their investigation, which she claimed had caused her severe and continuing shock. The NSPCC refused to disclose the information sought on the grounds that disclosure would be contrary to the public interest as people would be less likely to notify the Society of concerns if disclosure were to be ordered. The House of Lords upheld their views.

In addition, section 5(3) specifically excludes a right of access to part of a record, if the applicant is a person having parental responsibility, appointed by the court to manage the patient's affairs, or the personal representative of a deceased patient, if in the opinion of the holder of the records, that part of the record would disclose either information provided by the patient in the expectation that it would not be disclosed to the applicant; or information obtained as a result of any examination or investigation to which the patient consented in the expectation that the information would not be so disclosed.

Who is the holder of the records?

This is defined in section 1(2) as the GP for records made by the GP or, if there is no GP, the FHSA or, in the case of records made by a health professional in connection with the provision of health services by a health service body, the health service body on whose behalf the record is held. In any other case, the health professional is the holder. (From 1 April 1996 the functions as present carried out by the FHSA will be undertaken by the new health authorities to be appointed from that date.)

ADVICE TO THE HOLDER OF THE RECORDS

The holder is expected to obtain advice from the health professionals who have kept the records or on whose behalf the records have been kept, before they are satisfied as to any matter for the purposes of this Act or form an opinion as to any matter for those purposes. The requirement is, however, only to take advice. It does not require the advice to be followed, though the holder would wish to have clear reasons why he or she decided not to follow the views of the health professional.

The health professional is defined in section 2(1), and section 7(2) clarifies who is the appropriate health professional to provide advice for the purposes of disclosure under section 3.

Value of access

Initially, open access was not universally welcomed within the NHS. However, the many advantages are set out below.

- Openness
- Better communication with patient
- Better standards of record keeping
- Need for professionals to have a good understanding of the relationship between child and parent and the likely wishes of the child
- Correcting incorrect records (under the Data Protection Act there is a right to obtain the correction of any inaccurate records)

SPECIFIC SITUATIONS

What is the legal situation if a child aged 14 years does not wish their records held in manual form to be accessed by their parents? The records may, for example, give details of incest, sexual activity, drugs, drink, or criminal activity.

If this information were given to the health professional 'in the expectation that it would not be disclosed to the applicant, or the information has been obtained as the result of any examination or investigation to which the patient consented in the expectation that it would not be disclosed' (section 5(3)(a) and (b)), access shall not be given.

The following questions must therefore be asked.

- Is the patient a child?
- Does the applicant have parental responsibility for the child?
- Has the child given the information in the expectation that it would not be disclosed to the applicant?

If the answers to all three questions are yes, that part of the records which would be covered by this provision can be withheld from access.

The deceased child

The same provisions apply if the application relates to a child who has died. In addition, section 5(4) prohibits access if the information would not be relevant to any claim that may arise from the patient's death.

ACCESS AT COMMON LAW

The above situations have been concerned with access under statute law. There was, however, a court action[7] to decide whether a patient had a right to obtain access to information kept in his records which predated the implementation of the Access to Health Records Act in November 1991. In this case the applicant, who suffered severe depressional and psychological problems, had fallen in love with his psychiatric social worker, who was in 1966 withdrawn as his social worker. He subsequently asked the two authorities for disclosure of his records as he wished to find out why she was taken off his case, why he had been committed to a mental hospital in 1968, what the basis of his treatment was, and what the final diagnosis of his treatment was.

In July 1991 (i.e. before the implementation of the Access to Health Records Act 1990) the FHSA refused him access to his records on the grounds that they had an absolute right to control access to the records and were acting lawfully in refusing access. The health authority also refused to allow him access when he refused to give an assurance that no litigation was contemplated. He applied for judicial review of these refusals, on the grounds, among others, that he had a right of access to his medical records under the common law or the European Convention on Human Rights, or both. His application was refused on the following grounds. First, that the patient was not entitled to see the conclusions of the doctor; second, that there was no right at common law to access to any records which pre-existed the Access to Health Records Act 1990; and third, that the European Convention did not assist his case as that need only be brought into assistance when the domestic law was unclear, which it was not in this case.

Mr Martin appealed against Judge Popplewell's decision. The Court of Appeal dismissed his appeal.

The implications of this decision are that the patient does not have an absolute right of access to his records at common law.

INFORMAL ACCESS

It must be emphasized that although there is now statutory provision for access to both computerized and manually held records, this does not mean that informal access cannot be permitted without requiring the applicant to go through the formal procedure. It might be that the very fact that there is now a statutory right of access will mean that informal access agreed to by professionals will now be the norm and there will in practice be very few applications under the Acts. The Royal College of Nursing, for example, points out: 'It should be noted that there is nothing within the Act to prevent nurses sharing information with patients. It will be necessary to ensure that they are acting within the UKCC Code of Professional Conduct and, where appropriate, within their employer's policies on access and confidentiality.'[8]

ACCESS AND CONFIDENTIALITY

The fact that access to the relevant records can be refused to the parent does not, however, mean that the information that the child has passed on in confidence cannot be disclosed. Reference must therefore be made to Chapter 7 on the exceptional circumstances in which confidentiality can be breached.

Telling the terminally ill child

It has been noted that, whether the records are in computerized form and therefore come under the Data Protection Act 1984 or whether they are in manual form and come under the Access to Health Records Act 1990, there is not an absolute right of access either by the child or the parent, under the statutes or at common law. Similarly, there is no absolute legal right for parents or for the child to insist upon being given certain information. The patient has a right, and this would apply to the child who is considered to be Gillick-competent and also to the parent, to receive information which should be given according to the reasonable standard of care practised by a professional in those circumstances, that is, the Bolam test is applied.[9]

Difficulties can arise. The parents may wish certain information to be withheld from the child; the child may wish certain information to be withheld from the parent(s).

The problems that can arise are described in a case study by Samantha Heath.[10] James was an 8-year-old boy suffering from acute lymphoblastic leukaemia. His parents were adamant that he should not be told of his possible death and wanted this policy maintained even in the event of James asking a direct question. The writer was faced with the "dilemma of respecting James' parents' wishes", while preserving her own moral code which was to remain honest with James, and to give the explanations he required when asked, "especially as she believed that telling the truth is fundamental to a health-care relationship".

'In the event James outwitted us all. As I went to tell James that I was going home, he asked me to sit on the edge of the bed for a moment. With both parents in the room, he said, 'It's OK now. I know I am going to see Jesus.' He died peacefully at home three days later.'

The author explores the ethical principles which would apply in such a situation. The legal situation is not clear cut and is summarized over the following pages.

Neither parent nor child has an absolute right to obtain information about prognosis, et cetera. Information held on records can be withheld if serious harm would be caused to the applicant or another person, or a third person would be identified. In addition, in giving information to the patient or parent, the doctor does not have an absolute duty to disclose everything. The test used in the Sidaway case recognized that a therapeutic privilege existed with the result that it would be lawful to withhold information in certain circumstances, which any reasonable practitioner following the Bolam test would do.

In going against the parent's wishes and telling the child, the professional, and this would usually be the doctor, can act in the best interests of the child. He or she would, of course, take into account the possible effects on the relationship of the child with the parents in going against their wishes. He or she would also take into account the age and competence of the child.

Edward Purssell[11] in discussing the problem of parents 'not wishing their child to be told', states that 'parents may be hesitant to tell their children about death for any number of reasons, but nurses must not allow this fact to deny the child's right to know about his/her prognosis and treatment.' Unfortunately, this right is not enshrined in any statute and it is a question of the interpretation and application of the Children Act 1989 to the specific circumstances of the case.[12]

In Jim Richardson's book a case is discussed (Chapter 10) in which Alex, a 15-year-old haemophiliac, was known by his parents since he was aged 8 years, to be HIV positive. They initially decided not to tell him about his HIV status and have never been able to tell him since. They have expressly forbidden the nurses and the doctors at the Haemophilia Centre to speak to Alex about the issue. Their reasons are that they wish Alex to enjoy his youth and that to tell him would cast a shadow and blight his life.

What is the legal position? All have to act in the best interests of the child. Under the Children Act 1989 the welfare of the child is of paramount importance. There are, however, diverging views as to what is in the interests of Alex; the parents believe ignorance at this time is best, whereas the health professionals may take a different view, believing that it is important for Alex to know his status.

The consultant in charge of Alex's treatment could decide on the basis of Alex's maturity (i.e. that he is Gillick-competent) that he is capable of understanding and coping with the information and, in spite of the parents' objections, give Alex the full information. Such a course would not be undertaken lightly and every effort would be made to obtain the parents' agreement to this action being taken. One disadvantage is that disclosure by the health professionals might undermine the relationship that Alex has with his parents. The fact that it is discovered that Alex is sexually active having unprotected sex may be a stimulus to ensuring that Alex has the full information despite the wishes of his parents. Any such disclosure must, of course, be accompanied by counselling and all necessary support for him.

If the child wishes information to be withheld from the parents, different considerations arise and these are discussed in Chapter 7.

What if there is a conflict between the nurse and other members of the multidisciplinary team and the doctor? As the doctor is seen as leading the team caring for the child, he or she would in law have the ultimate right of deciding whether or not it was appropriate to give certain information to the child against the wishes of the parents. However, difficulties can arise because many of the team members, especially the nurses, may spend much longer with the child, and therefore form a different view over what should be done. If a conflict arises, it is essential that full information be given to the doctor so that he or she knows the patient's wishes and the reasons why the professionals consider that disclosure is right. The courts see the information which is given to the patient as part of the general duty of care owed to the patient, which includes diagnosis, treatment, information on risks, and every other aspect of care.

Refer to Chapter 7 for the discussion of other provisions relating to disclosure, including preventing disclosure on grounds of legal and professional privilege, and the disclosure of information at the commencement of litigation. Other legal issues relating to the dying child are considered in Chapter 22.

ACCESS TO ADOPTION INFORMATION

Although the effect of an adoption order is to remove all parental responsibilities of the natural parents, there has recently been a recognition that it is sometimes in the interest of the child to have information about the fact that he or she is adopted.

There is, however, no duty in law for the child to be informed that he or she has been adopted. Once they know of that fact, under the Adoption Act 1976 an adopted person aged 18 years and over can obtain a copy of their birth certificate. A 16- or 17-year-old can obtain details if they are intending to marry or are likely to marry within the prohibited degrees. Under the Children Act 1989 an adoption contact register has been established. Part I sets out the names of adopted people over 18 years of age who have obtained copies of their birth certificates and who wish to contact a relative. Part II contains the name and address of any relative who would like to contact an adopted person. Those in Part I can be given information about the relevant relative if such information is listed in Part II.

ACCESS TO INFORMATION UNDER THE HUMAN FERTILISATION AND EMBRYOLOGY ACT 1990

Under section 31 of the Act the Human Fertilisation and Embryology Authority must keep a register containing information about the provision of treatment for any identifiable individual; the keeping or use of the gametes of any identifiable individual or of an embryo taken from an identifiable woman; or whether any identifiable individual was, or may have been, born in consequence of treatment.

A person over the age of 18 years may apply to the Authority to ascertain whether they were or may have been born in consequence of fertility treatment. They must be given a suitable opportunity to receive proper counselling about the implications of compliance with the request. The information that can be given out is specified in Regulations drawn up under the Act. The identity of the donor of the gametes or embryo cannot be given. When a child is under 18 years of age and proposes to marry, they can learn from the Authority whether they and their intended spouse might be related. Again the child must be given a suitable opportunity to receive proper counselling about the implications of compliance with their request.

The identity of the donor is thus kept secret. Only if a legal action is intended to be brought under the Congenital Disabilities (Civil Liability) Act 1976 can the court make an order requiring the Authority to disclose information which will identify the parent.

The Access to Health Records (Control of Access) Regulations 1993 No. 746 which came into effect on 13 April 1993 restricts the right of access to health records to ensure that access shall not be given to any part of a record which may show that an identifiable human being was born as a consequence of treatment under the Human Fertilisation and Embryology Act 1990.

FUTURE DEVELOPMENTS

It was recommended[13] by the Report of the Joint Working Party on Professional and Parent-held records that the use of parent-held personal child health records contributes to high quality child health care through involving parents or carers in the delivery of child health surveillance (see Chapter 23), conveying health promotion information to families and children, empowering parents across the full range of contacts they have with various agencies, and encouraging the professionals to improve communications and reduce duplication of resources. The Department of Health has issued guidance on personal child health records and purchasers are advised to encourage its use by providers.[14] If this advice is followed, it could be that the statutory rights of the parent and child are less significant; however, the issues relating to the right of the child to keep information from parents will continue (see Chapter 7).[15]

REFERENCES

1 Cowley R: *Access to Medical Records and Reports*. Oxford: Association of Health Authorities and Trusts, Radcliffe Medical Press; 1994.
2 Darley B, Griew A, McLoughlin K, Williams J: *How to Keep a Clinical Confidence*. London: HMSO; 1994.
3 Data Protection (Subject Access Modification) (Health) Order, 1987; Statutory Instrument, 1987; No. 1903. [See HC(87)14 HC(87)26 and HC(89)29.]
4 HC(89)29 paragraph 4.
5 NHS Management Executive: *Access to Health Records Act 1990: A Guide for the NHS*. London: National Health Service Management Executive; 1991. [See also RCN Issues in Nursing and Health Leaflet No 16: Access to Health Records: the Nurse's Responsibilities. (Order No. 000 144) London: RCN; 1992.]
6 D v National Society for the Prevention of Cruelty to Children [1978] AC 171.
7 R v Mid Glamorgan Health Services Authority and South Glamorgan Health Authority ex parte Martin [1994] 5 Med LR 383.
8 RCN Issues in Nursing and Health Leaflet No. 16: *Access to Health Records: the Nurse's Responsibilities*. (Order No. 000 144) London: RCN; 1992.
9 Sidaway v Board of Governors of Bethlem Royal Hospital, Royal Maudsley Hospital [1985] 1All ER 643.
10 Heath S: Making decisions in clinical care. *Paediatr Nurs* 1994, 6:20–23.
11 Purssell E: Telling children about their impending death. *Br J Nurs* 1994, 3:119–120.
12 Thornes R: *The Care of Dying Children and Their Families*. Birmingham: Birmingham National Association of Health Authorities; 1988. [See also, Kubler-Ross E: *On Death and Dying*. London: Routledge; 1961. Kubler-Ross E: *On Children and Death*. New York: Macmillan; 1983:pp147–160.]
13 Report of Joint Working party on Professional and Parent held records: British Paediatric Association.
14 Guidance on parent held child health records Executive Letter (93)86 Department of Health.
15 For fuller details of the topics covered in this chapter refer to Cowley R: *Access to Medical Records and Reports: A Practical Guide*. Oxford: Radcliffe Medical Press; 1994.

The right to protection

Chapter 4 covered the general framework for children's rights and protection, and the impact of the Children Act 1989 in particular. In this chapter we consider the situation when a child needs the protection of the law in an emergency situation. The chapter sets out the basic principles of law, looks at the procedure that applies in the case of child abuse, and gives guidance on keeping records, making statements, and giving evidence in court.

The health professional may be involved in the care of the sick child who becomes subject to child protection proceedings. The professional needs to be familiar with the law and legal procedures and also be aware of the possibility that they may be required to give evidence in court proceedings.

This chapter is concerned with Part V of the Children Act 1989 which enables steps to be taken when abuse is suspected or emergency protection may be indicated. Reference should be made to the guidance provided by the Department of Health.[1] Reference could also be made to the South East Thames Regional Health Authority Commissioning guidelines.[2]

THE ROLE OF THE LOCAL AUTHORITY

The local authority has a duty to investigate the situation of a child when directed by the court in family proceedings (section 37(1)) and in the circumstances specified in section 47 of the Act. These include when the child is the subject of an emergency protection order (see below); when the child is in police protection (see below); and when a local authority has reasonable cause to suspect that the child who lives, or is found, in their area is suffering, or is likely to suffer, significant harm.

The authority is required (section 47(1)) to make, or cause to be made, such enquiries as it considers necessary to enable it to decide whether it should take any action to safeguard or promote the child's welfare.

As a result of these investigations, the local authority might decide that:

- no action is required at present (but it should also consider whether a review is necessary at a later date and fix the date for this review) (section 47(7));
- a care assessment order should be sought;
- an emergency protection order should be sought;
- a care or supervision order should be sought; and
- voluntary assistance should be offered under Part III of the Act.

Cooperation with others
The local authority must consult the relevant local education authority, if it appears that there are matters connected with the child's education that should be investigated. It is the duty of any 'person' specified under section 47 of the Act (listed below) to assist the local authority

with its enquiries (in particular, to provide relevant information and advice) if called upon by the authority to do so (section 47(9)), unless it would be unreasonable in all the circumstances of the case (section 47(10)).

- Any local authority
- Any local education authority
- Any local housing authority
- Any health authority
- Any person authorized by the Secretary of State for the purposes of this section. (section 47(11))

Child assessment order

This was a new provision under the Children Act 1989. It can only be sought by the local authority or an authorized person, such as the NSPCC, and it is only available in a situation that is not urgent.

It is available if the court is satisfied that the conditions shown below exist.

- The applicant has reasonable cause to suspect that the child is suffering, or is likely to suffer, significant harm.
- An assessment of the state of the child's health or development, or of the way in which he or she has been treated, is required to determine whether or not the child is suffering, or is likely to suffer, significant harm.
- It is unlikely that an assessment can be carried out without an order being made.

The person making the application must endeavour to ensure that notice of the application for a child assessment order is given to the child's parents, any person other than the parent who has parental responsibility for the child, any other person caring for the child, others who have a contact order, and the child him/herself.

The child assessment order cannot be made if the court is satisfied that there are grounds for making an emergency protection order and that it ought to make the latter rather than an assessment order. The court can treat an application for a child assessment order as an application for an emergency protection order.

The order must specify the date by which the assessment is to begin and have effect for less than 7 days beginning with that date, as is specified in the order. The commencement of the 7 days could therefore be postponed until, for example, the admission of the child to hospital.

The effect of the order is that it becomes the duty of any person who is in a position to produce the child to do so and comply with directions specified by the court relating to the assessment of the child (section 43(6)). It also authorizes any person carrying out the assessment or any part of the assessment, to do so in accordance with the terms of the order (section 43(7)). The child has the right (section 43(8)), if they are of sufficient understanding to make an informed decision, to refuse to submit to a medical or psychiatric examination or other assessment.

DIRECTIONS BY THE COURT

The child can only be kept away from home if directions are specified in the order, if it is necessary for the purposes of the assessment, and for such periods as may be specified in the order (section 43(9)). The court must set out directions about the contact that he or she must be allowed to have with other persons while away from home (section 43(10)).

IMPLICATIONS FOR THE HEALTH PROFESSIONAL

The health professional cannot apply for a child assessment order, but may be caring for a child who is subject to one. He or she should ensure that he or she sees the order, and is fully acquainted with the directions given by the court. He or she should take particular note of persons with whom the child is permitted contact and the right of the child to refuse to submit to a medical or psychiatric examination or other assessment. The right of the child depends upon the child having sufficient understanding to make an informed decision. The health professional may be involved in the assessment of the child's capacity and the reasons for coming to a particular conclusion should be carefully recorded. The health professional may also be involved in the carrying out of the assessment and should refer to the guidance given by the Department of Health.[3] Reference should also be made to the Department of Health Guidance on the Children Act (Volume 1 – Court Orders).

Emergency protection order

It was pointed out that a child assessment order cannot be made if the court is satisfied that there are grounds for making an emergency protection order with respect to the child and an application for a care assessment order may be treated as one for an emergency protection order. The emergency protection order replaces the old safety order.

The provisions for an emergency protection order are set out in section 44 of the Act. The application can be made by any person, a local authority, or an authorized person. The grounds of which the court must be satisfied depend upon who is applying for the order and are listed below.

- In the case of an application by any person, the order for emergency protection may be made by the court if it is satisfied that there is reasonable cause to believe that the child is likely to suffer significant harm if:
  a. he or she is not removed to accommodation provided by or on behalf of the applicant; or
  b. he or she does not remain in the place in which he or she is then being accommodated.
- If the applicant is a local authority, it must show that enquiries are being made under section 47(1)(b) (local authority's duty to investigate), that those enquiries are being frustrated by access to the child being unreasonably refused, and that it has reasonable cause to believe that access to the child is required as a matter of urgency (section 44(1)(b)).
- If the application is made by an authorized person (e.g. the NSPCC), the court can make the order if it is satisfied that the applicant has reasonable cause to suspect that a child is suffering, or is likely to suffer, significant harm; that the applicant is making enquiries about the child's welfare; that those enquiries are being frustrated by access to the child being unreasonably refused to a person authorized to seek access; and that the applicant has reasonable cause to believe that access to the child is required as a matter of urgency (section 44(1)(c)(i), (ii), and (iii)).

The health professional could thus be an applicant for the purposes of section 44 though it is more likely that the local authority or the NSPCC would undertake this role.

The effect of an emergency protection order is threefold as shown below.

- It operates as a direction to any person who is in a position to do so to comply with any request to produce the child to the applicant.
- It authorizes first, the removal of the child at any time to accommodation provided by or on behalf of the applicant and the child's being kept there or second, the prevention of the child's removal from any hospital, or other place, in which he or she was being accommodated immediately before the making of the order.
- It gives the applicant parental responsibility for the child.

Once the emergency protection order has been granted, the applicant's powers to authorize or prevent the removal of the child can only be used to safeguard the welfare of the child. The applicant's parental responsibilities only enable him or her to take such action as is reasonably required to safeguard or promote the welfare of the child. The applicant must also comply with regulations made by the Secretary of State.[4]

In making an emergency protection order the court can give direction on the contact which is or is not allowed between a named person and the child, and the medical or psychiatric examination or other assessment of the child (section 44(6)). However, as with the child assessment order, the child may, if he or she is of sufficient understanding to make an informed decision, refuse to submit to the examination or other assessment (section 44(7)). The court's directions can impose conditions on contact and set out whether there is not to be such examination or assessment (section 44(8)). The court's directions can be given any time while the emergency protection order is in existence and can be varied at any time on the application of the specified persons (section 44(9)). The directions can include a provision that the applicant, in exercising any powers which he or she has by virtue of the order, may be accompanied by a registered medical practitioner, registered nurse or registered health visitor, if he or she so chooses (section 45(12)).

Subject to the directions on contact under section 44(6), the applicant shall allow the child reasonable contact with the following people.

- The child's parents
- Any person who is not a parent of the child but who has parental responsibility for the child
- Any person with whom the child was living immediately before the making of the order
- Any person in whose favour a contact order is in force with respect to the child
- Any person who is allowed to have contact with the child under section 34
- Any person acting on behalf of those persons (section 44(13))

It is an offence for a person intentionally to obstruct any person exercising the power under section 44(4)(b) to remove or prevent the removal of a child (section 44(15)).

ROLE OF THE LOCAL AUTHORITY

If an emergency protection order has been made, regardless of who made the application, the local authority must initiate such enquiries as are necessary to enable it to decide what action it should take to safeguard or promote the child's welfare (section 47(1) and (2)), as stated. As a result of these investigations the local authority may decide that it is necessary to seek a care or supervision order, or it may decide that no action is necessary but a date must be set for this decision to be reviewed (see above and section 47).

DURATION OF AN EMERGENCY PROTECTION ORDER

An emergency protection order lasts for the period specified by the court up to a maximum of 8 days (if the last day of the 8 days is a public holiday, the order can extend to noon on the first later day which is not a public holiday).

The emergency protection order may only be extended once (section 45(6)).

DISCHARGE OF AN EMERGENCY PROTECTION ORDER

The discharge of the emergency protection order can be applied for by:

- the child;
- a parent of the child;
- any person who is not a parent of the child but who has parental responsibility for them; or
- any person with whom the child was living immediately before the making of the order (section 45(8)).

An application for discharge of the order cannot be heard by the court within 72 hours of the making of the order (section 45(9)).

IMPLICATIONS OF THE EMERGENCY PROTECTION ORDER FOR THE HEALTH PROFESSIONAL

If an emergency protection order is being sought or is in place for a child, the health professional should be aware of the legal implications, should ensure that a copy of the court order and its specific directions is obtained, and that the rights of the child given under section 44(7) are protected when appropriate.

The health professional should also be aware of the time limits upon the order and check to ensure that it is still in place. If the court has limited rights of individuals to contact the child, the health professional should ensure that these restrictions are recognized by those on the ward responsible for the child. Anyone seeking to remove the child from the ward should be questioned as to their legal status, and the appropriate action taken. In those rare situations in which it is necessary for the health professional to take action which will lead to an application for an emergency protection order, the health professional should ensure that the necessary grounds are satisfied, that records and evidence are available, and that every effort is taken within the time available to secure the child's welfare by other means. The health authority has a statutory duty to assist in the enquiries by the local authority, in particular by providing relevant information and advice, if called upon to do so, unless this is unreasonable (section 47(9)(10) and (11) and see above). Each professional should therefore take part in the multidisciplinary meetings and case conferences, and share the relevant information, ensuring that records are kept of the information and advice that is given. It may be necessary for the health professional to be involved in subsequent court proceedings.

Removal and accommodation of children by police in cases of emergency

Section 46 enables the child to be taken into police protection. If a constable has reasonable cause to believe that a child would be likely to suffer significant harm, he or she may remove the child to suitable accommodation and keep him or her there, or take such steps as are reasonable to ensure that the child's removal from any hospital, or other place in which he or she is being accommodated, is prevented (section 46(1)).

The child is then referred to as 'having been taken into police protection' (section 46(2)).

As soon as is reasonably practicable after taking the child into police protection, the constable concerned shall:

- inform the local authority within whose area the child was found of the steps which have been, and are proposed to be, taken with respect to the child under this section and the reasons for taking them;
- give details to the authority within whose area the child is ordinarily resident ('the appropriate authority') of the place at which the child is being accommodated;
- inform the child (if he or she appears capable of understanding) of the steps that have been taken with respect to them under this section and of the reasons for taking them; and of the further steps that may be taken for the child under this section;
- take such steps as are reasonably practicable to discover the wishes and feelings of the child
- make sure that the case is inquired into by an officer designated for the purposes of this section by the chief officer of the police concerned; and
- if the child was taken into police protection by being removed to accommodation which is not provided by or on behalf of a local authority, or as a refuge, in compliance with the requirements of section 51 (see below), make sure that the child is moved to accommodation which is so provided (section 46(3)).

In addition to the duties shown above, as soon as is reasonably practicable after taking a child into police protection, the constable concerned shall take such steps as reasonably practicable to inform:

- the child's parents;

- every person who is not a parent but who has parental responsibility for the child; or
- any other person with whom the child was living immediately before being taken into police protection.

of the steps that he or she has taken under this section with respect to the child, the reasons for taking them, and the further steps that may be taken with respect to the child under this section (section 46(4)).

It should be noted that the police do not require the permission of the court to take a child into police protection. Their powers under section 46 are in addition to those in the Police and Criminal Evidence Act 1984 section 17, which enables a police constable to enter and search any premises to save life or limb or prevent serious damage to property.

DURATION OF POLICE PROTECTION

Once an officer has completed any inquiry under section 46(3)(e), that officer conducting it shall release the child from police protection unless he or she considers that there is still reasonable cause for believing that the child would be likely to suffer significant harm if released (section 46(5)).

The section lasts a maximum of 72 hours; no child can be kept in police protection for more than 72 hours (section 46(6)).

While the child is in police protection, the designated officer may apply on behalf of the appropriate authority for an emergency protection order to be made under section 44 with respect to the child (section 46(7)).

Additional provisions for police protection state that while the child is being kept in police protection, neither the constable concerned nor the designated officer shall have parental responsibility for the child but the designated officer shall do what is reasonable in all the circumstances of the case for the purpose of safeguarding or promoting the child's welfare (having regard in particular to the length of the period during which the child will be so protected). The designated officer must also allow specified persons, including the child's parents, to have such contact (if any) with the child as, in the opinion of the designated officer, is reasonable and in the child's best interests.

IMPLICATIONS FOR HEALTH PROFESSIONALS

A child may be brought to hospital under police protection or may be prevented from leaving the hospital; staff should ensure that they are familiar with the grounds and procedure relating to the protection and the time limits. They may be asked to assist in the investigation and assessment and provide advice about the recommended course of action.

ADDITIONAL POWERS IN SUPPORT OF THE PROTECTION OF THE CHILD

In making an emergency protection order the court can:

- include in the order a requirement that a person with information on the child's whereabouts makes this available (section 48(1));
- authorize the applicant to enter premises specified by the order and search for the child;
- authorize the applicant to search for another child on those premises in respect of whom an emergency protection order ought to be made;
- issue a warrant authorizing a constable to assist in the exercise of these powers; and
- direct that the constable in executing the warrant be accompanied by a registered medical practitioner, registered nurse, or registered health visitor (section 48(11)).

The warrant should either name the child, or describe him or her as clearly as possible (section 48(13)).

An ethical or legal situation

In the case 'I don't want to live with Mummy any more', Jim Richardson[5] discusses a situation in which a community child health nurse discovers that one of the children attending her toddlers' group has large bruises on her legs and back; the girl has said that her mother's new boyfriend hit her hard when she was naughty. The nurse promises the person who informed her that it will be kept confidential. However, after a series of unprofessional mishandlings, the child is eventually visited by a social worker, an emergency protection order obtained, and the girl is taken into temporary foster care. Eventually the father is given a residence order.

The case reveals many lessons, listed below.

- The nurse should not have promised that she would keep the information confidential. She could promise that she would recognize the right to anonymity of the informant, but she had a professional duty to take steps to protect the child.
- The necessity for each individual health worker to be familiar with the child protection procedure is brought out very clearly, as it was apparent in this case that the reaction to the information was slow and hesitant.
- Conflict arose between health professionals over how the case should have been handled and a potential 'whistle-blowing' situation arose (see Chapters 7 and 15).
- The nurse had to attend the court and it seems that she had not had full preparation for that.
- Prosecution of the cohabitee was being contemplated and the nurse would have to take on board the possibility of having to give evidence in that type of case as well as in the children proceedings.
- The case also reveals bad communications between the health professionals concerned.

CHILD ABUSE AND NONACCIDENTAL INJURIES

The Area Child Protection Committee

There should exist in each local authority area a forum to ensure cooperation between all the agencies involved in the protection of children at risk. This forum is known as the Area Child Protection Committee (ACPC) and should involve representatives of the medical and nursing services. This representation should be at a senior level, and there should be a designated senior professional for child protection within the hospital.

The ACPC has the tasks of :

- establishing, maintaining, and reviewing interagency guidelines on procedures to be followed in individual cases;
- monitoring the implementation of legal procedures;
- identifying significant issues arising from the handling of cases and reports from inquiries
- scrutinizing arrangements to provide treatment, expert advice, and interagency liaison, and making recommendations to the responsible agencies;
- scrutinizing progress on work to prevent child abuse and making recommendations to the responsible agencies;
- scrutinizing the work related to interagency training and making recommendations to the responsible agencies;
- conducting reviews required under Part 8 of the Guide;[6] and
- publishing an annual report about local child protection matters.

Child protection register

Each local authority must maintain a child protection register:

- to provide a record of all children in the area who are currently the subject of a Child Protection Plan and to ensure that the plans are formally reviewed at least every 6 months;

- to provide a central point of speedy inquiry for professional staff who are worried about a child and want to know whether the child is the subject of a Child Protection Plan; and
- to provide statistical information about current trends in the area.

Access to this register would be permitted to an agreed list of personnel which would include senior medical staff or paediatric social workers in the local hospital departments.

In the incident described above it would have been possible for the senior medical officer on duty to ascertain whether the child was on the register.

The importance of record keeping cannot be exaggerated when a professional suspects that injuries being shown by the child are the result of nonaccidental injury. Kath Butler[7] suggests a simple chart that can be used as a paediatric assessment sheet.

The recognition of the distinction between nonaccidental injury and accidental injury or disease can be extremely difficult as Nigel Speight shows.[8] He provides the following pointers to the diagnosis of nonaccidental injury though he emphasizes that none of them is foolproof.

- There is delay in seeking medical attention.
- The account of the 'accident' is not compatible with the injury observed. Examples include 'I think he got it from lying on his dummy', 'The bruise on his forehead just came up while I was watching', and 'He just brushed against my cigarette, honest'.
- The account may be vague and lacking in detail (vivid, detailed accounts tend to have a 'ring of truth'). The account may vary with each telling, and from person to person.
- The way in which the parents are affected may be abnormal. They may lack normal anxiety for the child's injuries, or be preoccupied with their own concerns and appear suspicious or aggressive, or both.
- The parents' behaviour may be abnormal, for example in disappearing without saying anything or before seeing the consultant.
- The parent–child interaction may be abnormal.
- The child may be failing to thrive, apathetic, frightened or sad; 'frozen watchfulness' is a late and very serious sign. Its absence, however, does not exclude the diagnosis of nonaccidental injury.
- The child may say something!

Speight quotes some cases where admission to the paediatric ward was essential in determining the exact diagnosis. In some cases the outcome was an illness such as neuroblastoma, or idiopathic thrombocytopenic purpura.

In a recent case[9] it was held that in a case of alleged child abuse, in which the medical evidence pointed overwhelmingly to nonaccidental injury, an expert medical witness who advanced an alternative hypothesis that the child's injury had an innocent cause, was under a heavy duty to explain to the court whether that hypothesis was controversial and place before the court and other expert witnesses all material that contradicted the hypothesis. The judge said that it was not for the court to become involved in medical controversy. In the case the judge made an interim care order in respect of the child.

The Department of Health has issued guidance[10] for doctors on the diagnosis of child sexual abuse which may prove of value to other health care professionals. Reference should also be made to the lessons from the Cleveland Inquiry in 1987. A short version extracted from the complete text is available.[11]

PRACTICAL GUIDANCE FOR HEALTH PROFESSIONALS INVOLVED IN CHILD CARE PROCEEDINGS[12]

Working together[6]

The advisory document issued by the Department of Health makes it clear that it is for the local authorities, Social Services Department, and the Police to take the lead in investigating child abuse. Other agencies, such as the NHS, must cooperate fully with them in these investigations. At all times, all the agencies and the individuals employed by them are governed by one overriding principle: the welfare of the child is paramount.

Any health professional involved in child abuse investigations or proceedings will keep this principle firmly in the forefront of his or her mind.

Another important principle, born as a result of the Cleveland Inquiry, is that no professional should endeavour to shoulder the burden of wrestling with an issue arising out of potential child abuse without having the opportunity to share the problem with a senior colleague. This applies to all members of a team from top to bottom. Even the most senior member should not remain unsupported when faced with a difficult issue. All NHS departments should therefore have in place a structure for the sharing between individual professionals of the difficult decisions that may need to be made. The practical golden rule for any NHS professional must be: share the burden. No individual will be praised for wrestling alone with an issue of, for example, confidentiality, when the welfare of a child may be at stake. Quite frankly, it is not worth the risk: the health professional who fails to confide in the manager may find him- or herself subject to scrutiny and criticism.

Looking at the practicalities for an NHS professional involved in a child abuse situation, we need to consider four stages.

- Care
- Investigation
- Preparation of evidence
- Appearance in court

THE CARE
If a child is suspected of being the victim of abuse then the health professional must ensure the recording of a rigorous and comprehensive set of case notes. As they are contemporaneous, they will form the essence of any subsequent investigation whether at a case conference, court hearing or inquiry. If parent-held records are in use, it is for the professional to consider with his or her manager the keeping of a separate record where appropriate and in accordance with his or her employer's policy.

The child's condition and any changes and developments must be noted by the professional involved, together with the details of any conversation with parents in which, for example, advice has been given as to the care of a child, discussions have taken place as to the nature of any injury or its causation, or observations have been made as to the way in which a parent may care for a child whether in a home or hospital situation.

Because these records will be the subsequent source of any evidence which the nurse or any other health professional may be subsequently asked to provide, and for that reason alone, they must be detailed and accurate. Their importance can be spelt out by the fact that as they are contemporaneous they may corroborate the subsequent oral evidence of the professional or any expert evidence that may be produced when issues may be disputed by the parent.

If there is a suspicion that child abuse is taking place, then it is essential that the health professional acts immediately and puts into action the locally agreed reporting procedures. There will no doubt be discussions with the health professional's managers, a GP or a paediatrician may be involved, and there will be continuing liaison with Social Services. The fact that these discussions are taking place should be recorded in the notes, although the content of the notes should be a matter of separate records. In particular, case conference records should not be held on an individual child file.

Health professionals may be in difficulty, particularly those visiting the community or school nurses, when information as to potential abuse may be given by a child or a parent in confidence. The health professional may clearly be anxious to retain a relationship he or she has with that person, particularly with the knowledge that, if he or she betrays that confidence, the confidante may not necessarily cooperate with further investigation. Although this must be a matter for individual professional judgment, the health professional has to take into account his or her special code of conduct. For the practitioner registered with the UKCC, the duty of confidentiality is set out in clause 10 of the Code of Professional Conduct,[13] as described below.

- Each registered nurse, midwife, and health visitor must protect all confidential information concerning patients and clients obtained in the course of professional practice and make disclosures only with consent, if required by the order of a court, or if he or she can justify disclosure in the wider public interest.

The UKCC has expanded the confidentiality clause in an advisory paper[14] which includes guidelines on a deliberate breach of confidentiality in the public interest or that of the individual patient or client.

> *In all cases in which the practitioner deliberately discloses or withholds information in what he or she believes to be the public interest, he or she must be able to justify the decision. These situations can be particularly stressful, especially if vulnerable groups are concerned, as disclosure may mean the involvement of a third party as in the case of children or the mentally handicapped. Practitioners should always take the opportunity to discuss the matter fully with other practitioners (not only or necessarily fellow nurses, midwives, and health visitors), and, if appropriate, consult with a professional organization before making a decision. There will often be ramifications and these are best explored before a final decision as to whether to withhold or disclose information is made.* [Reference should also be made to Chapter 7 on confidentiality.]

Once a decision has been made, the practitioner should write down the reasons either in the appropriate record or in a special note that can be kept on file. The practitioner can then justify the action taken should that subsequently become necessary, and can also, at a later date, review the decision in the light of future developments.

Although individuals must rely on their own interpretation of that duty, they must be aware of the fact that they may reach a judgment that may be contrary to the long-term interests of the child. It is therefore important that they keep the overriding principle of the welfare of the child firmly in the forefront of their mind. In that situation, discussion with a senior manager as to the appropriate course to take must be a prerequisite to deciding upon any further action. A failure to confide in another colleague may lead to the wrong decision being taken. That colleague will be aware of the health professional's own duty in terms of his or her professional code, but may also have a more objective view of the situation.

THE INVESTIGATION

It is the role of the local authority and the Police to take the lead in instituting and carrying out formal investigations. The creation of the ACPC has ensured closer cooperation between these agencies. There should be cooperation at all levels of the Social Services Department and the NHS. Individual health professionals should make sure they are aware of the local guidance produced by the ACPC and DCPC as to how local cooperation will be achieved.

The NHS professional is therefore obliged to cooperate with the Social Services in terms of reaching any decision as to action that should be taken in the interests of the child. There are occasions, of course, when the issues raised by the professional in terms of their professional practice do not entirely coincide with the issues being faced by the Social Services. The Social Services may not fully understand the potential dilemma faced by a professional in terms of the care of the child. By and large, local arrangements for cooperation operate well, and since the creation of the various structures, there has been improved communication between the professional staff. The individual professional problems of the health professional should therefore be understood. However, to ensure that health professionals do not feel isolated, they must feel able to rely on the support of their managers and request access to counselling and maybe even legal advice if they are concerned as to their role.

Case conferences form the essential forum for decision-making in terms of rules as to the subsequent care of the child and the need to instigate court proceedings to achieve an order as described above. Attendance at a case conference should not be taken lightly. The problem for the individual health professional is that case conferences are often called at short notice with little opportunity to prepare information for the conference. Problems of communication can also arise when individual professionals who are directly involved in the case are unable to attend and a member of the team is sent who is not directly aware of all the facts. This should be avoided if at all possible.

Although the case conference is an informal forum for the exchange of views before a decision is made, it is essential that the professional provides accurate and comprehensive information. If mere 'gossip' is exchanged about a particular family, it can only cause subsequent difficulty in the preparation of court proceedings that cannot be backed up by firm evidence. Individual health professionals should make sure that they absorb all the background information that they have about the child or family in question before the meeting so that it is readily available. No-one should ever attend without the case notes! If other colleagues have 'bits and pieces' of information which help to complete the jigsaw, the health professional should make a point of speaking to them to get a full picture. Detailed preparation beforehand will mean that the individual does not feel intimidated by the format of the case conference itself, at which there will be many people. This can particularly arise in that members of the Social Services and Police attend far more of these occasions than an individual may, and also they will be more familiar with the proceedings. If the individual has done his or her homework, then he or she should not feel balked by the whole proceedings. Occasions can arise when the Police or Social Services are misled as to how much information the health professional can give. If the professional is relating information that has been absorbed by another colleague, he or she must make this clear so that sufficient thought can be given to who actually should attend to give evidence in the event of subsequent court proceedings being commenced. Below are listed five quick tips for preparation for a case conference.

- What are the issues?
- Prepare what needs to be said.
- Take the case notes.
- Avoid gossip.
- Provide accurate information from other colleagues.

If health professionals relevant to the case do not all attend the case conferences, it is important that the managers ensure that all personnel potentially involved in the case have some feedback so that they know what decisions have been made should they be subsequently involved. Attenders at the case conference will have a copy of the minutes; if they are not accurate, amendments should be sought to ensure that there are no subsequent misunderstandings.

THE PREPARATION OF EVIDENCE

It will often be the case that an individual nurse is only requested to attend court in a child abuse hearing once, if at all, during the course of his or her career. The golden rule when approached for a formal statement is: 'don't panic'. Just as one would not enter a marathon without training, so health professionals should not contribute evidence for a child abuse hearing without proper preparation of the evidence, including detailed consultation with their managers as to their role, and guidance from their employers' legal advisers as to the proper presentation of a statement. Sometimes, particularly if emergency procedures are being sought, a statement will be required at short notice. However, the advice is to insist that sufficient time is given to allow consultation with a manager and a legal adviser if necessary. Evidence given in haste without proper preparation is not the best evidence!

The importance of note taking has been emphasized; it is essential advice to the individual practitioners that they should not commence writing a statement without access to their original case notes. A statement should not be prepared on the basis of memory alone; any inaccuracy can lead to subsequent problems when the health professional presents him- or herself for cross-examination at a formal court hearing.

The golden rules for formulating a statement
- Consult the notes.
- Give only direct information, avoid that from conversations with other colleagues, Social Services, et cetera.
- Relate the facts from the beginning and keep strictly in chronological order.
- Number the paragraphs individually.
- Avoid giving opinions or forming judgments that cannot be supported by reference to the facts.
- Stick as closely as possible to the facts; this evidence is not from an expert witness.
- Do not comment on medical matters; that is for the paediatrician or GP.
- Try to end the statement with a brief summary of the evidence as seen from a health professional's point of view. Do not stray from this role or be tempted to comment on other issues outside the knowledge of a health professional.

Before the statement is submitted to Social Services, the health professionals must be happy that it is exactly right and it represents exactly what they want it to say. This may require several drafts. A manager should have a look at the evidence, and consider with the health professional the question as to whether legal advice will be helpful.

APPEARANCE AT COURT
Even when formal evidence has been provided, the attendance of the individual health professional will not necessarily be required. Sometimes a decision will be made not to rely on that evidence or, alternatively, the parties to the proceedings will agree that the statement can be produced without the witness having to attend.

However, if the Social Services or the Police have decided that they wish the health professional to give oral evidence, it is usual practice for the health professional to be given sufficient notice that his or her attendance is required. The same rule applies in the preparation of evidence; one should not consider attending court as a witness without proper preparation of the evidence. If the evidence has been prepared and revised properly, even if one is nervous, one will gain confidence from the ability to deliver the evidence well as it is at one's fingertips. Of course, one is nervous, but once one starts to give evidence and concentrate on the questions being asked, there is not time to worry about it.

The waiting outside the court is the worst burden, and one should be prepared with, perhaps, a good book; court timetables are very flexible.

A case involving a child abuse issue will be heard by a Family Court. This can either be a number of lay magistrates sitting together (usually two or three), or a single judge. It is advisable to do some detective work and find out exactly which court one is being asked to attend, its location, and whether there will be a single judge or several magistrates, and so forth.

Family proceedings are slightly less formal than other court proceedings because of their very nature. In particular, only personnel directly related to the case are allowed to be physically present in court; the press and the public are not allowed to attend. Occasionally health professionals are required to give evidence if parents are charged with a criminal offence and the hearing will be held in an open court.

The court procedure is very formal and is governed by rules and regulations as to the giving of evidence. Those rules are a matter for the lawyers and it is not necessary for the health professional to be aware of them, except for the following procedure for giving evidence.

Evidence in chief
The witness is questioned by representatives for the party by whom he or she is being asked to attend.

Cross-examination
The representative for the opposing party is allowed to ask questions on the evidence which the witness has given in chief.

Re-examination
The representative for the first party is allowed to clarify any issues on the evidence given in cross-examination.

Questions by the court
The examination in chief is fairly straightforward and the witness is allowed to refer to the statement which they had previously given to the court and case notes. Before referral to the case notes, the witness should always ask the court's permission to refer to them. At the cross-examination stage, the representative for the opposing party is entitled to clarify and challenge the evidence previously given. The best advice is to take one's time and keep calm in dealing with the cross-examination. One should not be drawn into giving answers to questions to which one really does not know the answer. If one does not know the answer, one should simply say so. One should not feel guilty if one is obliged to make concessions in favour of the opposing party. The role of the health professionals is to give a balanced view as to their judgment of the case to assist the court in coming to a decision. They should not be seen to be taking sides as such. Their paramount concern is the welfare of the child and therefore they must appear to be giving an objective balanced view. If there are facts which can be given that are in the parents' favour, then those facts should be clearly recited and not disguised in any way. One should not be drawn into getting angry with the advocate for the representative for the other side. Accept that the advocate is being paid to test the credibility of the evidence and on that basis that he or she may embark on aggressive questioning. If the questioning is becoming too aggressive, the court will intervene to prevent that happening. One should never allow oneself to feel that one is under personal criticism; an objective view should be maintained as to one's contribution to the case in terms of one's role as a health professional.

No-one should attempt to give evidence in court without prior rehearsal. One should read through the statement on as many occasions as possible before going into court and be fully conversant with the case notes. One might think one knows the notes, but it is only on testing that one finds one does not. One should insist on going through the evidence with either a senior manager who has expertise in this field or one's employer's legal adviser. When one is asked questions about dates and individual facts, one finds that one does not know the case notes as well as one thought. It is very important to get clear in one's mind when events occurred and in what sequence. A handy tip is to use 'post-it notes' to tag onto individual sections of the notes so that references can be found quickly. There is nothing worse that standing in court rummaging through notes to find the appropriate section. For that reason one should make sure the notes are in good order before attending. The original case notes should never be marked with any form of pen or marking device.

Ten tips to successful presentation of evidence
- Revise and rehearse.
- Seek the support of the senior manager and the legal adviser.
- Be fully conversant with your statement.
- Thoroughly revise the case notes.
- Make sure you have essential dates and facts firmly fixed in the forefront of your mind.
- Ensure that you are able to locate specific entries in the records relatively quickly (either with an index or post-it note).
- Take the original notes with you to court.
- Take time in replying.
- Do refer to the notes if you need to be sure of any particular fact, having asked the court's permission before so doing.
- Take your time, keep cool; remain objective and do not answer a question if you do not know the answer.

REFERENCES

1 Department of Health: *The Children Act, 1989: Guidance and Regulations. Volume 1 – Court Orders.* London: HMSO; 1991.
2 South East Thames Regional Health Authority: *A Mandate for Children: A Guide to Commissioning Health Services under the Children Act 1989.* London: South East Thames Regional Health Authority; 1992.
3 Department of Health: *Protecting children: a guide to social workers undertaking a comprehensive assessment.* London: HMSO; 1988.
4 The Emergency Protection Order (Transfer of Responsibilities) Regulations 1991 SI 1991/1414. [See also Department of Health: *The Children Act, 1989: Guidance and Regulations. Volume 1 – Court Orders.* London: HMSO; 1991.]
5 Richardson J. Webber I: Ethical Issues in Child Health Care. London: Mosby; 1995.
6 Home Office, Department of Health, Department of Education and Science Welsh Office Working Together Under the Children Act 1989 A guide to arrangements for interagency co-operation for the protection of children from abuse HMSO 1991
7 Butler K: Nurse-aid management of children. 1: Accidents. *Br J Nurs* 1994, 3:579–582.
8 Speight N: Bruises and burns: accidental or non-accidental. In *Accidents and Emergencies in Childhood.* Edited by Silbert J. London: Royal College of Physicians of London; 1992:pp97–103.
9 Re B (a minor)(Medical Issues: Expert evidence) [1994] 5 Med LR 333.
10 Department of Health: *The Diagnosis of Child Sexual Abuse: Guidance for Doctors.* London: HMSO; 1988.
11 Secretary of State for Social Services: *Report of the Inquiry into Child Abuse in Cleveland 1987.* London: HMSO; 1988
12 I am indebted to Tessa Shellens of Edward Lewis Bevan Ashford who drafted this guidance.
13 UKCC: *Code of Professional Conduct, edn 3.* London: UKCC; 1992.
14 UKCC: *(Advisory Paper) Confidentiality: a Framework to Assist Individual Professional Judgement.* London: UKCC; 1987.

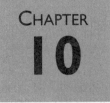

Education of the sick child

The fact that a child is hospitalized does not relieve the authorities of the duty to comply with statutory requirements to provide education. Every effort should be made to ensure that the interruption to the child's schooling is kept to a minimum.[1] At present there are several ways of meeting the educational needs of sick children,[2] including:

- the establishment of hospital special schools;
- hospital teaching units or hospital classes which are not formally classified as hospital schools; and
- home tuition.

HOSPITAL SPECIAL SCHOOLS

The Education (Approval of Special Schools) Regulations 1994 made under the provisions of the Education Act 1993, came into force on 1 April 1994 and allow local education authorities (LEAs) to make statutory proposals to establish, alter or discontinue a special school within a hospital under section 183(2) of the Education Act 1993. All such proposals are subject to the approval of the Secretary of State. Special schools occupying health service premises in hospitals are no longer required to conform to the regulations governing school premises (the Education (School Premises) Regulations 1981 currently under review).

Hospital schools must have governing bodies, the conduct of whose meetings and proceedings is prescribed in the Education (School Government) Regulations 1989. Rules relating to parent governors differ from those for nonhospital schools. Hospital schools are not under the same legal obligations to follow the national curriculum as other special schools, but the Secretary of State hopes that it will be offered whereever possible. The Education (Grant-Maintained Special Schools) Regulations 1994 set out the detailed provisions for hospital special schools to become grant-maintained. These schools, unlike other schools, do not require an affirmative parental ballot before grant-maintained status can be sought.

TEACHING UNITS OR CLASSES WITHIN HOSPITALS

A class in a hospital will not have a governing body, nor funding under Local Management of Schools, nor be eligible to seek grant-maintained special school status. Teaching is to be provided for long-term pupils, that is, those who are, or are likely to be, admitted to hospital for longer than 5 consecutive working days, or chronic sick pupils who are readmitted for periods which in aggregate are likely to exceed that amount.

The teacher(s) will be provided by the LEA and will be expected to work closely with the multidisciplinary team caring for the child and with educational colleagues within the LEA to ensure that the child has every opportunity to keep up with normal school progress. The LEAs are empowered to provide education. They have the freedom to interpret these duties according to the identified needs and resources.

Special groups in hospital

CHILDREN WITH SPECIAL EDUCATIONAL NEEDS

Part III of the Education Act 1993, sections 156–191, covers the provision for children with special educational needs. Section 166 places a duty upon the district health authority or local authority to help the LEA and specifies the action which they should take in certain circumstances.

Some sick children may also have learning difficulties as defined in section 156 of the Education Act 1993. Special provision should be made for those long-term sick children who are also identified as having special educational needs. The LEA should give, or provide on request, a copy of the statement specifying certain special educational or noneducational provision to the hospital school or service. The LEA may have to make an amendment to the statement in order to name the hospital school where a child with special educational needs is likely to be a long-term pupil. The parents have the right to comment on any such amendment in accordance with the provisions set out in Schedule 10 to the Education Act 1993.

CHILDREN AND ADOLESCENTS ON ADULT WARDS

The guidance strongly recommends that children should not be placed on adult wards, unless it is unavoidable. If they are on adult wards, 'information reaching teachers about the child may be haphazard. Administrative, medical and teaching staff need to be alert to this potential difficulty.'

Good communication is essential between hospital staff and the teachers to prevent such children being neglected. It is important to ensure continuity and standards of education for adolescents who may be working for public examinations.

RECURRENT ADMISSIONS

Those children suffering from chronic conditions such as cystic fibrosis, renal and complex cardiac conditions and cancer who may have frequent admissions to hospital should have teaching during each hospital stay if possible. Liaison between the hospital teacher, home tutor, and home school is particularly important to ensure continuity and progress.

PSYCHIATRIC CARE

The admission and treatment of children suffering from psychiatric disorders is considered in Chapter 21. Their condition may make any educational advancements difficult, but it is essential that they have the opportunity and the facilities to learn. The teachers should be seen as being part of the multidisciplinary team caring for the child or young person and should also be involved in planning admissions.

BRAIN-INJURY CHILDREN

Staff caring for brain-injured children must be aware of the changing clinical situation of the child and be flexible in meeting his or her educational needs. 'The hospital teacher needs to be aware of the child's condition and treatment, while remaining professionally and independently responsible for what is taught. Physiotherapists, occupational, speech and play therapists and nursing staff can all help to regain access to the curriculum. Clinical psychologists may need to be involved before the child leaves hospital; links with the Educational Psychology service may be helpful.'

HOME TUITION

As the numbers of children receiving long-term care in hospital have declined and the emphasis is on short-term admissions linked with care in the community; the emphasis in the education of the sick child has passed to home tuition provision. The Education Act 1993 section 298(1), which came into effect 1 September 1994, placed a duty on LEAs to provide suitable education for children out of school for reasons of illness or otherwise. The full subsection is set out below.

- Each LEA shall make arrangements for the provision of suitable full-time or part-time education at school, or otherwise than at school, for those children of compulsory school age who, by reason of illness, exclusion from school or otherwise, may not for any period receive suitable education unless such arrangements are made for them.

This duty applies to children of compulsory school age and the duty is mandatory, that is, the LEA shall make arrangements. In contrast, the duty in relation to those above compulsory school age is permissive. This is set out in section 298(4) and is shown below.

- The LEA may make arrangements for the provision of suitable full-time or part-time education otherwise than at school for those young persons who, by reason of illness, exclusion from school of otherwise, may not for any period receive suitable education unless such arrangements are made for them.

Suitable provision, defined in section 298(7) as 'suitable' education in relation to a child or young person, means 'efficient education suitable to his age, ability and aptitude and to any special educational needs he may have.'

Government guidance was issued in June 1993. Home tuition is not expected to be provided for very short absences from school. Four weeks or more away from school is considered to be the point at which home tuition can be provided. For less than 4 weeks it would normally be expected that the school itself would provide home-work to be done outside school. However, it is a question of discretion and some LEA provide home tuition for 3 weeks away from school if necessary. Any calculation would obviously take into account the length of time that the child has already been in hospital with or without tuition.

The guidance recommends that the LEAs have a written policy on home tuition to cover the organization and staffing of the service, and the timing of provision, and giving a named contact for parents, hospital teachers, and others.

The passing of records between the home school and the hospital, and then to the home tutor is essential to ensure maximum continuity in the teaching. The guidance also recommends that continuity should be further assisted by ensuring that home tutors attend in-service training with other teachers, both hospital and school.

The National Association for the Education of Sick Children has been set up to relieve the educational disadvantages suffered by sick children. It published the results of a survey on the provision by LEAs, the teaching available, home tuition, and the falling number of hospital schools.[3] The Association has a government grant to monitor the effects of implementing the new duty.

SPECIALIZED UNITS FOR PREGNANT SCHOOLGIRLS

One of the biggest disadvantages of pregnancy for a schoolgirl is the loss of educational opportunities. A duty to provide schooling for pregnant schoolgirls is part of the duty to provide education out of school because of sickness or otherwise. Many authorities have arranged home tuition for pregnant schoolgirls, but if demand warrants it some have set up special units. This has the advantage of preventing feelings of isolation for the girls and assists in reducing the stigma. It can also give support and education in parent craft and can involve the assistance of health visitors, welfare workers, and career officers. Such educational assistance can officially begin at 6 months but some will take the girls as early as 4 months. They can stay until 6 weeks after the birth. Attitudes of the schools themselves vary towards the pregnant schoolgirl; some support them in continuing at the school for as long as possible, others encourage them to leave as soon as possible on the grounds of problems with insurance cover.

LIAISON BETWEEN CHILD HEALTH DEPARTMENTS AND THE SCHOOLS

Even if the child is not seriously ill enough to require the support of home tuition, the child suffering from a chronic condition might need to take medication to school. Cooperation should exist between the paediatric health professionals and the schools to ensure that adequate instruction and support is given to the teaching staff. This is further considered in Chapter 20.

CONCLUSION

All those professions involved in the health care of the child should be aware of the importance of meeting the educational needs of the child and ensuring maximum cooperation with the LEA. In an article written before the implementation of the Education Act 1993, Karen Wilson[4] draws attention to the lack of policies and legislation providing guidelines for the provision of education to hospitalized children. It is hoped that the monitoring now being undertaken by the National Association for the Education of Sick Children will ensure that any deficiencies found will be remedied and that the situation will improve.

REFERENCES

1 Department of Health: *Welfare of Children and Young People in Hospital.* London: HMSO; 1991.
2 See DES circular and Welsh Office circular 57/94, which give guidance on the Education Act 1993.
3 Housby Smith N: A new era in education. *Paediatr Nurs* 1994, 6:6,14.
4 Wilson K: Education for the hospitalised child. *Paediatr Nurs* 1993, 5:24–25.

CHAPTER

11

Child health care and financial provisions

For many parents the sickness of a child is not only a time of worry about the child, it is also a time of increasing financial concern. Visiting the child in hospital, taking time off work, and perhaps paying for carers to look after other dependent children all have their financial burdens.

The purpose of this chapter is to indicate to the health professional potential sources of financial support for the family. It is not possible to cover the detail of each of the kinds of assistance that may be available, but the aim is to ensure that the health professional is sensitive to these possible needs of the parents and that the health professional knows how other sources of information could be accessed. For further information about the other conditions and details in relation to the benefits discussed here reference should be made to the local Department of Social Security offices. The Disability Rights Handbook is also a useful source of information and is revised each year.

In the main, the sources of financial assistance are:

- Social Security;
- charitable foundations;
- employers; and
- accommodation in hospital for parents.

SOCIAL SECURITY

Child benefit

Child benefit is payable for every child and is not means tested. A slightly higher amount is paid for the eldest qualifying child in the family and a lesser amount for each child that follows. A qualifying child is one aged under 16 or under 19 years if they are undergoing education of at least 12 hours per week at a school or college. A single parent also receives an additional payment for the first child.

This payment does not increase if the child becomes ill and is admitted to hospital. If, however, the child him- or herself receives income support or severe disability allowance, child benefit ceases to be payable.

Income support

This is a means tested benefit which is payable if a person's assessed income is below a specified amount. Once a person is in receipt of income support, he or she may be entitled to a range of other benefits, such as housing and council tax benefit, free prescriptions, and so on.

To obtain income support, a person is usually required to:

- be in this country;
- be aged 18 years or over (see below for exceptions in which it is payable to a 16- or 17-year-old);
- not be in full-time nonadvanced education;
- not be working 16 hours or more per week;
- not have a partner who is working 16 or more hours per week;
- be available for work; and
- not have capital over £8000.

INCOME SUPPORT AND THE 16- OR 17-YEAR-OLD

Minors aged 16 or 17 years may be able to claim income support if they are suffering from disabilities. In addition, a girl who is pregnant and is incapable of work because of the pregnancy may be eligible for income support.

Certain premiums are also payable in defined circumstances to those on income support. These include a disability premium, a lone parent premium, a family premium, a disabled child premium, a carer premium, and a severe disability premium.

Payments for those with disabilities

In addition to income support and the premiums available in relation to disabilities, the following benefits are also available.

DISABILITY LIVING ALLOWANCE

The disability living allowance includes a care component and a mobility component. It replaces the previous mobility and attendance allowances for those aged under 65 years. The care component of the disability living allowance is payable without any lower age limit, but the mobility component is only payable to children aged 5 years and above. The disability living allowance is payable at three levels: lower, middle, or higher rate depending upon the extent of disability. In a terminal illness the disability living allowance is payable without any qualifying period and applicants are given a high priority. Specific provisions relate to the payment of the disability living allowance for renal dialysis.

The disability living allowance is not means tested and is payable regardless of whether a person is in work.

Stays in hospital

The care component of the disability living allowance is affected by stays in hospital and will stop after the person has been in that accommodation for a total of 28 days. A previous admission that was less than 28 days' duration will be counted together with the current admission.

DISABILITY WORKING ALLOWANCE

The disability working allowance is payable as a supplement to those in work for at least 16 hours per week and who are in receipt of a low wage or who are self-employed. It is payable to those whose disabilities put them at a disadvantage in getting a job. It is tax-free but means-tested.

INVALIDITY BENEFIT AND INCAPACITY BENEFIT

Invalidity benefit includes an invalidity pension and an invalidity allowance. It is payable on the basis of national insurance contributions and is paid after statutory sick pay or sickness pay has ended and a person remains incapable of work.

In April 1995 a new scheme for incapacity benefit was introduced which replaced sickness and invalidity benefit as state provision for those people who, because of their medical condition, cannot be expected to work. Two new tests have been introduced for defining incapacity.

First, there is the 'own-occupation test' in which the GP is asked to provide an opinion about the patient's ability to carry out his or her usual occupation. This will apply until the second test is performed.

Second, there is the 'all-work test' to determine whether the applicant is medically capable of undertaking any work. This test is run by benefits agency assessors and must be undertaken by many of those currently on invalidity benefit. Anyone aged over 58 years who has been claiming invalidity benefit since December 1993 will be exempt from taking the test.

Incapacity benefit is taxable.

SEVERE DISABLEMENT ALLOWANCE

The severe disablement allowance is payable to persons who have been incapable of work for at least 28 weeks but who do not have enough national insurance contributions to qualify for sickness and incapacity benefit. It is not means tested and it is not taxable.

INVALID CARE ALLOWANCE

This is payable to persons aged 16 years or over of working age who regularly spend at least 35 hours a week caring for a severely disabled person. It is now payable to married women as well. It is not means tested and does not depend upon contributions. The person who is being cared for must be in receipt of the disability living allowance care component paid at the middle or higher rate, or receiving a constant attendance allowance. It is not payable if the carer is already receiving as much or more from other benefits such as unemployment benefit, maternity allowance, invalidity benefit, retirement pension, widow's benefits and others. A credit is made for class 1 national insurance contributions for each week a person is receiving invalid care allowance.

Travelling costs to visit hospital or attend outpatients

Those who are on income support or are in receipt of family credit are eligible to obtain assistance with their travelling costs. The hospital procedures for people to recover the costs should be well publicized and health professionals should be familiar with the provisions in order to be able to advise parents about the assistance and how to obtain further information within the hospital. The Department of Health Guidance on the Welfare of Children and Young People in Hospital[1] points out that (paragraph 4.7) 'escorting and visiting children in hospital may impose an additional financial strain on families. Provider hospitals are advised to ensure that the hospital travel costs scheme is publicised within the children's department and that a named member of staff is designated to help advise families on the benefits which may be available to them in these circumstances.'

The guidance also recommends (paragraph 4.8): 'Where a family's financial situation is particularly difficult, parents should be aware of any assistance the hospital social worker can provide. Some bus operators are offering concessionary fares to parents visiting children in hospital on production of passes which are issued by the operator to hospitals. If approached, provider hospitals are asked to co-operate by making arrangements for passes to be completed for parents with children in hospital.'

The research of Gillian Bridge showed that communication between professionals and mothers was not always good: 'Mohammed's mother was spending £3.00 daily on taxis because no-one had told her about mobility and attendance allowances.'[2]

Child Support Act 1991

The Child Support Agency was set up under this Act to enable absent parents to be traced and to ensure that they contributed to the upkeep of their children, thus reducing the support given through the Social Security system. The new system came into force in April 1993 and received considerable opposition from both the absent parent and the parent caring for the child. Amendments were made as a result of the criticism, which took into account some of the specific grievances voiced, such as the failure of the agency to take into account once-and-for-all settlements agreed by the couple at the time of the divorce or separation.[3]

It is possible that health professionals may become aware that bitterness between parents has possibly been increased as a result of the effects of the implementation of the 1991 Act and that this has an impact upon the sick child. There may, for example, be cases of dispute over decisions to be made in relation to the treatment of the child or over visiting. Reference should be made to Chapter 14 where such disputes are considered.

CHARITABLE FOUNDATIONS

There are several trusts which have been established to provide support and assistance to families in difficulties through caring for an ill child. Some may give specific amounts for specified purposes, such as a washing machine to assist with incontinence. Others provide more general help. The full list of such charities and the objects of their trust can be found in the Directory of Grant Making Trusts.[4] This sets out the type of assistance available from each trust. The social worker attached to the children's ward should have access to this information and would know from experience which claims are likely to be successful.

EMPLOYERS

Statutory provision for employment rights

Research across the European Community and other European countries has shown that many countries give a statutory right to certain employees to have leave while children are ill.[5] Thus Austria gives to each employee a statutory right to 1 week of fully paid leave per year to look after a sick family member living in the same household or to look after a child if the person who permanently looks after the child is unable to do so for a pressing reason (e.g. illness). Each employee has a further entitlement to 1 week of fully paid leave per year to look after a sick child below the age of 12 years.

In France from January 1995 each worker is entitled to 3 days per year to care for a sick child (aged under 16 years); this is increased to 5 days if there is a child under 12 months or three or more children in the family. A worker who has a child with a serious illness, accident or handicap is entitled to work part-time for up to 6 months, renewable for a second 6-month period. This leave is unpaid, unless an employee is covered by a collective agreement which provides for payment.

The review by the European Commission network on child care shows that the UK has no statutory provision for the provision of leave to care for sick children or for other family reasons. Nor is parental leave a recognized statutory benefit in the UK, Ireland, or Luxembourg. All other countries within the European Community have provision for parental leave.

A directive covering parental leave and leave for family reasons was drafted in 1983. The latter were defined as 'entitlement to short periods of leave granted for pressing family reasons to workers with family responsibilities'. Four examples were given of such pressing reasons: illness of a spouse, death of a near relative, wedding of a child, illness of a child or a person caring for the child. It was to be left to member states to define cases in which this type of leave should be granted.

This draft directive has not, however, ever been adopted because of the opposition and reservations of some member states.

Contractual rights

Some employers, however, recognize the right to paternity leave or to paid or unpaid absence from work as a result of a family crisis, such as a child in hospital, through the contract of employment. If such a contractual term exists, the employee has an enforceable right to take time off.

Discretionary time off

More frequently, however, the ability of the employee to take time off when an emergency befalls the family or a child is taken into hospital is at the discretion of the employer, that is, there is no term of the contract of employment covering the situation, but the decision is within the gift of the employer. Some employers may give paid time off for the employee to cope with such circumstances; others may grant only unpaid time off, others may expect the employee to take such time out of annual leave entitlement. Some employees may lose out because they fail to make their difficulties in relation to a sick child clear to the employer and may need encouragement to request some assistance from work.

ACCOMMODATION IN HOSPITAL FOR PARENTS

The Department of Health Guidance[6] paragraph 4.9 recommends that as parents or carers are essential for the well-being of the child in hospital, *no charge should be made for their accommodation* [their emphasis]. The question of whether any charges should be made for other services (e.g. meals) is one for determination between the district and the provider hospital; but it is suggested that parents or carers, regardless of whether they stay overnight, should be offered the benefit of any subsidized canteen meals.

CONCLUSION

It is essential that health professionals should be aware of the financial and other help available to the sick child and his or her family. Each hospital should ensure that designated employees receive the appropriate training to be of assistance and that leaflets are drawn up and kept up to date to ensure families are given the necessary information.

REFERENCES

1 Department of Health: *Welfare of Children and Young People in Hospital.* London: HMSO; 1991:p17.
2 Bridge G: A personal reflection on parental participation: how some mothers of babies born with disabilities experience interprofessional care. *J Interprofession Care* 1993, 7:263–267.
3 Wyld N: *When Parents Separate.* London: The Children's Legal Centre; 1994 [for further information on the Child Support Act 1991 and Social Security benefits, see Bainham A, Cretney S: *Children – The Modern Law.* Bristol: Family Law; 1993.
4 Christian Aid Foundation: *Directory of Grant Making Trusts, 1995.* Tonbridge: Christian Aid Foundation; 1995.
5 European Commission: *Leave Arrangements for Workers with Children.* Brussels: EC; January 1994. [See also European Commission: *Network on Child Care and Other Measures to Reconcile Employment and Family Responsibilities.* Brussels: EC; 1994. (and update November 1994).]
6 Department of Health: *Welfare of Children and Young People in Hospital.* London: HMSO; 1991:p18.

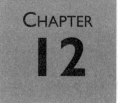
The right to complain

This chapter sets out briefly the means by which complaints about the care of the child can be made. **Figure 12.1** illustrates the parties whom the complainant may address. Complaints may be made in relation to services purchased and provided by the local authority, the services purchased by a health authority and provided by an NHS Trust, and services provided by GPs. The parent has the right to complain on the child's behalf until the child reaches the age of 18 years, but the child, if Gillick-competent, could also complain on his or her own behalf. The complaints system for the NHS is currently under review. A new system is to be implemented on 1 April 1996 and at the time of writing all the details have not yet been published by the Government. Legislation will be required.

LOCAL AUTHORITY

Section 24(14) of the Children Act 1989 requires every local authority to establish a procedure for considering any representation (including any complaint) made to them by a person qualifying for advice and assistance about the discharge of their functions under this part of the Act in relation to the person. The Representation Procedure (Children) Regulations 1991 apply.[1]

If a child has been detained under section 3 of the Mental Health Act 1983 (see Chapter 21) the child or their parent can make a complaint to the local authority under the machinery

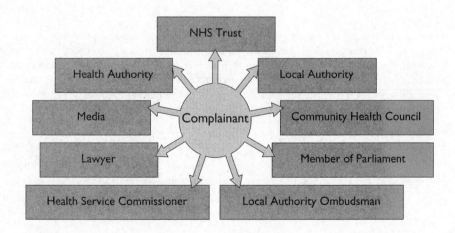

Fig. 12.1 Complaints

established by section 7(b) of the Local Authority Social Services Act 1970, the Local Social Services (Complaints Procedure) Order[2] about the provision of after care services under section 117. If not satisfied the child or parent could complain to the Commissioner for Local Government.

COMPLAINT RELATING TO THE PROVISION OF HOSPITAL AND COMMUNITY NHS SERVICES

The Hospital Complaints Procedure Act 1985 required each hospital to set up a complaints procedure with an officer designated to hear complaints. The Government required this procedure to be established also for the provision of community health services.

If the complainant of a nonclinical complaint remains dissatisfied, he or she can complain to the Health Service Commissioner. In the case of a person who has been detained under the Mental Health Act 1983, the dissatisfied complainant can also apply to the Mental Health Act Commission.

FHSA COMPLAINTS

At present complaints relating to the independent practitioners who have a contract of services with the FHSA, (GPs, dentists, pharmacists) are dealt with by the FHSA, informally if possible initially and then through FHSA service committees which hold a hearing into the complaint. It is recommended that these FHSA committees should be chaired by a lawyer. They must have an equal number of (at least two) lay people and relevant professionals. There can be an appeal against the FHSA committee decision to the Secretary of State. From 1 April 1996, the function of the FHSA will be carried out by new health authorities. Service committees will not be used for complaints.

Can a parent make a complaint without the consent of the child

If the child is under the age of 18 years the parent can make a complaint without the child's consent, though clearly, if the child is Gillick-competent, his or her cooperation should be sought and the complaint only pursued against the wishes of the child if there were substantial justification. Once the minor comes of age, then the decision whether to pursue the complaint is that of the minor.[3]

WILSON REPORT

The present system for dealing with complaints relating to health services is seen to be confusing, bureaucratic, slow, and inefficient. An expert committee was therefore set up by the Government under the Chairmanship of Professor Alan Wilson to review NHS complaints procedures.[4] The report examined the current situation and set objectives for any effective complaints system. The principles it laid down for any effective complaints system, which have been accepted by the Department of Health, are set out below.[5]

- Responsiveness
- Quality enhancement
- Cost effectiveness
- Accessibility
- Impartiality
- Simplicity
- Speed
- Confidentiality
- Accountability

The report recommended that these principles should be incorporated into an NHS complaints system, and the areas covered are listed below.

- There should be a common system for all NHS complaints.
- The complaints procedure should not be concerned with disciplining staff.
- Staff should be empowered to deal with complaints informally.
- There should be training of staff.
- Support should be provided for complainants and respondents.
- The degree of investigation should relate to the complainant's required degree of response.
- Conciliation should be made more widely available.
- Time limits should be set.
- Deadlines should be set for the acknowledgement of complaints (2 working days), the response to the complaint (3 weeks), and further action and response (2 weeks).
- Confidentiality should be preserved and complaints filed separately.
- There should be a system for recording and monitoring complaints.
- Impartial lay people should take part in the system.
- Key aspects of the system should be set by the Department of Health but detailed implementation and operation should be left to individual organizations.
- Procedures should be threefold:
  1. immediate first line response;
  2. investigation and conciliation; and
  3. action by FHSA officer or chief executive officer for trusts; a panel should be set up to consider those complaints that cannot be resolved in the earlier stages.
- There should be training in communication skills.
- Oral and written complaints should be treated with the same sensitivity.
- Community service staff should have particular training in responding to complaints.
- Purchasers should specify complaints requirements in their contracts with providers outside the NHS.
- Complaints about policy decisions should be referred to the Health Service Commissioner if they cannot be resolved locally by the purchasers.
- If more than one organization is involved, it should be the organization receiving the complaint that ensures a full response is sent.
- There should be close liaison with local authorities, and the Government should consider further integration of NHS and local authority complaints procedures for community care.
- There should be a screening officer for stage 2 procedures.
- The jurisdiction of the Health Service Commissioner should be extended to GPs and the operation of the FHSA committees.
- There should be recommendations as to how complaints procedures should be implemented.

NEW COMPLAINTS PROCEDURE

This came into effect on 1 April 1996 and implemented the majority of the recommendations contained in the Wilson report. At the time of writing, the Government has only just published its initial views on the outcome of its considerations on the Wilson report. It has reached agreement on the overall framework for the new complaints procedure and has largely endorsed the recommendations of the review committee.

- It has accepted the principles that should guide the handling of the complaints system as set out in the Wilson report and listed above.
- It accepts that there will be three elements to the new arrangements, although the expectation is that the majority of complaints should be capable of being resolved locally

by the organization concerned. If that fails, there will be a second stage review followed, if necessary, by access to the Ombudsman.

First stage
The complaint should be dealt with speedily and often an oral response will suffice. If investigation or conciliation is required, an initial response should be made within 2 working days and a final response within 4 weeks. Chief executives should personally approve and sign the response to all formal complaints. In family health services, practices will be expected and encouraged to set up their own practice-based complaints procedure.

Independent review
If the complainant remains dissatisfied, they will have access to an independent review and, as necessary, further consideration by an independent panel. This will be organized by a nonexecutive director of the trust or health authority to whom the complaint was made.

All panels will have an independent lay chairman. The nonexecutive director will also be a member.

For nonclinical complaints, the panel will consist of: a nonexecutive director of the relevant health authority or, if appropriate, a GP fundholder.

For family health service complaints, the panel will include the convening health authority nonexecutive director and an independent lay person.

For clinical complaints, the panel will be advised by two independent clinical assessors.

Health Service Commissioner (Ombudsman)
The final option for unresolved complaints will be recourse to the Ombudsman. Legislation will be introduced to widen the Ombudsman's jurisdiction to cover clinical complaints and those about family practitioners. Disciplinary matters will still not be included in his or her jurisdiction.

Time limits
A time limit is to be introduced of 6 months from the event that gave rise to the complaint, or 6 months from the complainant becoming aware of it, up to a maximum of 12 months from the event. There will be discretion in allowing longer periods of time.

Patients' charter
From 1 April 1996 a new standard on complaints will be introduced in the Patients' charter.

Further guidance
Guidance is to be issued on the outstanding details.

Complaints within the family health services
As can be seen they are to be brought within the common complaints system.

CONCLUSION

It remains to be seen if the new system to be implemented on 1 April 1996 will succeed in following the principles recommended by the Wilson report. Monitoring will be through the Patients' charter standards and it is likely that league tables will be published. It is in the interests of all health professionals to ensure that any complaints by parents and children over the provision of health services are resolved as speedily as possible and informally, thus not requiring the complainant to make use of the formal procedure. Health professionals should recognize that it takes courage to make a complaint and many clients, especially the parents of children with a chronic condition, are reluctant to voice their concerns. Staff advocacy is essential to ensure any shortcomings in the service are rectified.

REFERENCES

1 The Representation Procedure (Children) Regulations 1991. SI 1991/894.
2 The Local Social Services (Complaints Procedure) Order SI 1990. No. 2244.
3 R*v* Secretary of State for Health ex parte Barratt [1994] 5 Med LR 235.
4 Department of Health: *Being Heard. The Report of a Review Committee on NHS Complaints Procedures.* London: HMSO; 1994.
5 Department of Health: Welsh Office letter, dated 23 March 1995. In *Acting on Complaints.* London: HMSO; 1995. [2273 1P 45K.]

PART 3

PROFESSIONAL AND PARENTAL LIABILITY

In this part of the book we consider issues of liability for harm to the child arising from the actions of the health professional or the parent. Also considered are the laws relating to liability towards the employer and the professional body concerned with maintaining standards of professional practice. The vast area of health and safety laws is discussed. Areas such as complementary medicine, research and teaching, and substance abuse are also considered.

Child health care and negligence

This chapter covers the legal issues which arise in the professional care of the child, and liability in the tort of negligence. For convenience this large area will be subdivided into first, the law – plaintiff's case: duty, breach, causation, and harm – and types of liability; second, the defences that are available; third, the procedure and the assessment of compensation (known as 'quantum'); and fourth, specific examples.

THE LAW: A PLAINTIFF'S CASE

This first section looks at the present law relating to liability for negligence in causing harm to children. It sets out the basic principles of law, and the different types of liability.

All professionals owe a duty of care to their patients and if it can be established that they are in breach of this duty and, as a reasonably foreseeable result of that breach of duty, have caused harm, then they or their employer may be liable for that harm. Each of these elements will be considered in detail in relation to decided cases involving child care or with specific examples taken from paediatrics.

The duty of care

It is axiomatic that a duty of care is owed to the patient by the professional. The extent, however, of that duty may be uncertain. Is, for example, a nurse responsible if he or she is allocated to patient A and fails to intervene to prevent harm to patient B for whom he or she is not directly caring? Is a physiotherapist responsible if he or she notices that a nurse is giving liquids to a child who has at the head of the bed 'nil by mouth'?

The existence of the duty of care was spelled out in the case of Donoghue *v* Stevenson[1] in which it was said by Lord Atkin, in now famous words:

> '...*acts or omissions which any moral code would censure cannot in a practical world be treated so as to give a right to every person injured by them to demand relief. In this way rules of law arise which limit the range of complainants and the extent of their remedy. The rule that you are to love your neighbour becomes in law: You must not injure your neighbour, and the lawyers' question: Who is my neighbour? receives a restricted reply. You must take reasonable care to avoid acts or omissions which you can reasonably foresee would be likely to injure your neighbour. Who then, in law, is my neighbour? The answer seems to be persons who are so closely and directly affected by my act that I ought reasonably to have them in contemplation as being so affected when I am directing my mind to the acts or omissions which are called in question.*'

This statement may cause difficulties: one being that in practice a person does not direct their mind to the possibility of harm being caused to another person. Had they done so, perhaps the harm would not have arisen. However, despite many refinements and applications to very different situations since 1932, it has virtually withstood the test of time and is basically unchanged.

Sometimes the concept of proximity is used to define whether a duty of care exists; sometimes the concept of proximity is used to define whether the harm that has occurred was a reasonably foreseeable consequence of the defendant's acts or omissions, or whether there was a breach of the duty of care. However the concept is applied, it is used to restrict the liability of a person for harm that has occurred.

The extent and nature of the duty of care has been considered in subsequent cases, including the following which are relevant to health service professionals who care for children.

HOME OFFICE V DORSET YACHT COMPANY LTD[2]

In this case a party of borstal trainees were working on Brownsea Island in Poole harbour under the supervision and control of three borstal officers. During the night seven of them escaped and went aboard a yacht which they found nearby. They set this first yacht in motion and collided with a second yacht, the respondent's yacht, which was moored in the vicinity. Then they boarded the second yacht. Much damage was done to this yacht by the collision and some by the subsequent conduct of these trainees. The owners of the second yacht sued the Home Office for the amount of this damage. The issue came before the House of Lords on a preliminary point of law: did the Home Office owe a duty of care to the yacht owners (assuming that the facts could be established)? The House of Lords held by a majority that a duty of care was owed and allowed the case to go for a full trial of the facts. Lord Reid stated that he could see 'no good ground in public policy for giving immunity to a Government department' from being responsible for the liability caused by the carelessness of the officers as they would have known that the trainees were capable of damage of the kind which occurred.

The implications of this decision are clear. If, for example, a paediatric nurse failed to supervise a child patient adequately with the result that the child went into the ward kitchen and caused an accident, scalding a ward orderly who was making tea, the employers of the nurse could be held liable for the negligence which foreseeably led to the injury. He or she had a duty of care to control the child and therefore to those who might be harmed as a result of the unsupervised actions of the child.

The following case of an injury caused by an unsupervised child is of great relevance to those working in paediatric departments.

CARMARTHENSHIRE COUNTY COUNCIL V LEWIS[3]

A lorry driver was killed when, in swerving to avoid a child (approaching his fourth birthday) who ran on to the road, the lorry struck a lamp post. It was admitted that the lorry driver himself had not been at fault. The child attended a nursery school which was maintained by the county council, the local education authority and which was near to this road. A teacher, Miss Morgan, was about to take this child and a girl out for a walk, but found that a third child had cut himself, and spent 10 minutes looking after that child. During this period, the child who was to be involved in the accident left the classroom. He went across the playground, through the gate, down a lane and 100 yards along the road in question to the point where the accident occurred. The widow of the driver brought an action alleging that her husband's death was due to the council's or their servant's negligence. The trial judge found for the widow, the Court of Appeal dismissed the appeal by the council, and the House of Lords, in a majority judgment upheld the decision in favour of the widow.

Lord Reid in discussing the nature of the duty owed to others said (in answer to the argument that if such a duty was held to exist, it would put an impossible burden on harassed mothers who would have to keep a constant watch on their own children): 'I do not think so. There is no absolute duty, there is only a duty not to be negligent, and a mother is not negligent unless she fails to do something which a prudent or reasonable mother in her position would have been able to do, and would have done. Even a housewife who has young children cannot be in two places at once, and no one would suggest that she must neglect her duties, or that a young child must always be cooped up. But I think that all but the most careless mothers do take many precautions for their children's safety, and the same precautions serve to protect others. I cannot see how any person in charge of a child could be held to have been negligent in a question with a third party injured in a road accident unless he or she had failed to take reasonable and practicable precautions for the safety of the child.'

Professionals caring for children could substitute themselves for the mothers in the passage quoted from Lord Reid's statement and note that the duty of care can extend to third parties whom it can be reasonably foreseen could be injured as a result of the actions of a child.

Later cases have restricted an extension of this duty of care.[4]

Standard of care and breach of duty

In determining whether there has been a breach of the duty of care, it must first be decided what is the standard of care. In reaching a decision on what is the expected standard in any given situation, the courts have applied what has come to be known as the Bolam test. In the case of Bolam v Friern Hospital Management Committee,[5] Judge McNair stated, 'The test is the standard of the ordinary skilled man exercising and professing to have that special skill.'

In the Bolam case a patient was given electroconvulsive therapy without relaxant drugs or anaesthetic. He fell off the table and sustained pelvic and other fractures. The judge, in applying the above test to the facts, decided that there was no negligence involved. The case concerned events that took place in the 1950s. Were the same facts to apply today, a different decision would be made because of the change in standards since then.

This test set out in the Bolam case was followed by the House of Lords in the case of Maynard v West Midlands Health Authority[6] in which Lord Scarman said (quoting an earlier case[7]): 'The true test for establishing negligence in diagnosis or treatment on the part of the doctor is whether he has been proved to be guilty of such failure as no doctor of ordinary skill would be guilty of if acting with ordinary care.'

In a recent case it was held by the Court of Appeal[7] that the phrase 'a responsible body of medical opinion' used in the Bolam case could refer to a small number of medical practitioners. In the case, the plaintiff brought an action alleging negligence by a consultant orthopaedic surgeon and a consultant neurosurgeon. She argued that the Bolam test was not designed to enable a small number of medical practitioners, intent on carrying out otherwise unjustified exploratory surgery, to assert that their practices were reasonable because they were accepted by more than one doctor. She argued that a small number of surgeons could not be a 'substantial' body. Her argument failed. The court held that the issue could not be determined by counting heads. It was open to the judge to find as a fact that a small number of specialists constituted a responsible body and that that body would have considered the surgeon's decision justified or, more succinctly, that the plaintiff had failed to discharge the burden of proof that the surgeon had been negligent.

Several implications, listed below, flow from the use of the Bolam test.

* Standards change as knowledge and skill develop and therefore the standards which the court will be applying are those practised by reasonable professionals at the time of the incidence of the alleged negligence.
* If there is a dispute over the appropriate standard between the plaintiff and the defendant(s) and expert evidence is given that shows a conflict in the standards which should have applied, 'It is not enough to show that there is a body of competent professional opinion which considers that theirs was a wrong decision, if there also exists a body of professional opinion, equally competent, which supports the decision as reasonable in the circumstances.

It is not enough to show that subsequent events show that the operation need never have been performed, if at the time the decision to operate was taken it was reasonable in the sense that a responsible body of medical opinion would have accepted it as proper.'[6]

- Standards cannot simply be the local ones, if these are lower than it would have been reasonable to expect.
- The law does not recognize a concept of team liability (see Chapter 14).
- The standard is tested against the roles held by professionals and not by the people in them. This means that if a nurse is carrying out work normally performed by a doctor, the patient is entitled to the standard of care which a doctor should exercise in that position rather than that of a nurse.
- Evidence from experts from a responsible body is essential to define standards.
- The reasonable standard is based on what is reasonably foreseeable. In a recent case in Australia[9] it was held that a nursing sister was under a duty to warn an enrolled nurse of the real risk that a patient might drop to the floor. In this case the enrolled nurse, who worked part-time in a nursing home, injured her back when assisting an awkward 67-year-old patient to walk with the sister in charge. The patient had suddenly bent her knees and dropped to a kneeling position, causing an injury to the plaintiff's back. The plaintiff alleged that the sister was negligent in that she did not warn her of the patient's propensity to drop or slump. This was accepted by the court: a risk which was not far-fetched was real and therefore foreseeable.
- The standards may also take into account cultural difference of the patients.
- Although there may be no cause for action against a health authority for breach of a statutory duty, there may be an action for negligence if harm has occurred as a result of failure in implementing the duty. Thus, in a case in which Nasima Begum, an 11-year-old girl, died in June 1994 after waiting nearly 1 hour for an ambulance to take her to the Royal London Hospital in Whitechapel, the parents have now declared their intention to sue the Secretary of State for negligence.[10]

STANDARDS AND THE CARE OF THE CHILD

Unfortunately, the standard of care to which the child is entitled is likely to be the subject of great controversy; in an editorial Sally Nethercott argues that sick children deserve a better quality of care.[11] Her comments come after the publication of the Royal College of Nursing review of guidelines following the Allitt enquiry (see Chapter 16). However, every incident of harm that arises should lead to an evaluation of the standards that should be maintained. This is further discussed in relation to kidnapping and bogus professionals (see page 161).

There is also the issue as to whether the sick child is entitled to receive more and more expensive high technology treatment as in the case of Laura Davies. This 3-year-old girl underwent several operations performed abroad, because the facilities were not available here, before she died. George Castledine[12] questions whether children should always get the treatment they need and suggests that nurses must push for more open and broader discussions on issues surrounding the allocation and distribution of scarce resources. There are, however, two separate issues: the entitlement to treatment and the standard of the treatment that is provided. The first question has been answered by the courts negatively in that they have emphasized that there is no absolute right to receive treatment within the NHS. This is discussed in Chapter 5. In contrast, once treatment has commenced the standard of care that must be provided is determined in accordance with the Bolam test set out above. These two issues of resource allocation before care commences and the standard of care when it is given must be kept separate.

WAS THERE A BREACH OF THIS STANDARD?

Once standards which should have been followed are ascertained, the question then is to determine whether what the defendants did was in accordance with that standard. This is a question of fact, and proof of the facts will depend upon the evidence which is available through witnesses and documentation.

There are, unfortunately, numerous examples of failures to follow the recognized standard in child care. These are discussed in detail below (Specific situations).

Causation

Even though the person claiming compensation is able to establish that there has been a breach of the duty of care, an action for negligence will not succeed unless it can be shown that there was a causal link between the harm which has occurred and the breach of duty. There must be a factual link, and it must also be established that the harm which arose was a reasonably foreseeable consequence of the breach that occurred. The burden is upon the person bringing the action (the plaintiff) to show on a balance of probabilities that this causal link is proved.

A case concerned with oxygen therapy in a premature baby is one of the leading cases decided by the House of Lords on the issue of causation.

WILSHER V ESSEX AREA HEALTH AUTHORITY[13]

The facts were as follows. The plaintiff was an infant child who was born prematurely suffering from various illnesses, including oxygen deficiency. His prospects of survival were considered to be poor and he was placed in the 24-hour special care baby unit at the hospital in which he was born. The unit was staffed by a medical team consisting of two consultants, a senior registrar, several junior doctors and trained nurses. While the plaintiff was in the unit, a junior and inexperienced doctor monitoring the oxygen in the plaintiff's blood stream mistakenly inserted a catheter into a vein rather than an artery, and then asked the senior registrar to check what he had done. The registrar failed to see the mistake and some hours later, when replacing the catheter, did exactly the same thing himself. In both instances the catheter monitor failed to register correctly the amount of oxygen in the plaintiff's blood, with the result that the plaintiff was given excess oxygen. The plaintiff subsequently brought an action against the health authority claiming damages and alleging that the excess oxygen in his bloodstream had caused an incurable condition of the retina resulting in near blindness. The trial judge awarded the plaintiff £116 199. The defendants' appeal to the Court of Appeal failed and the defendants then appealed to the House of Lords.

The House of Lords found in favour of the defendants on the grounds that the plaintiff had not established that it was the excess oxygen which caused the blindness. It was emphasized that the onus of proving causation was on the plaintiff and that in the case before the House the plaintiff had not shown that of many possible causes it was the excess oxygen which had caused his condition. The House of Lords therefore ordered a retrial on the issue of causation. Lord Bridge of Harwich said by way of sympathy with the plaintiff's family: 'To have to order a retrial is a highly unsatisfactory result and one cannot help feeling the profoundest sympathy for Martin and his family that the outcome is once again in doubt and this litigation may have to drag on. Many may feel that such a result serves only to highlight the shortcomings of a system in which the victim of some grievous misfortune will recover substantial compensation or none at all according to the unpredictable hazards of the forensic process. But, whether we like it or not, the law, which only Parliament can change, requires proof of fault causing damage as the basis of liability in tort. We should do society nothing but disservice if we made the forensic process still more unpredictable and hazardous by distorting the law to accommodate the exigencies of what may seem hard cases.'

There is no report that the retrial ever took place, and it is assumed, therefore, that an agreement was reached outside the court.

The case, the statements in the Court of Appeal, negligence by senior staff, and direct liability of the hospital are discussed further below.

In a recent case[14] a child suffering from rhesus incompatibility with her mother was born suffering from neonatal jaundice. The jaundice worsened and an exchange transfusion was carried out. The child suffered brain damage which she alleged was caused by kernicterus. The health authority admitted liability in failing to carry out an exchange transfusion earlier but held that causation was only established in two out of the four essential elements of the child's disability: choreoathetosis and deafness. The court held that on the evidence causation was established. The plaintiff was awarded a sum totalling £847 639 (which included the sum of £110 000 for pain and suffering and the sum of £630 000 for future care).

In contrast, causation was not established in a case[15] in which, shortly after her birth, a baby became ill. The GP and midwives visited the baby but only arranged for the baby to be seen by a consultant on the third day. She was later diagnosed as having scleroedema from her shoulders to her buttocks and mental disabilities. The mother alleged that the doctor and midwives had failed to diagnose and treat hypoglycaemia. The defendants admitted negligence in failing to have the baby admitted to hospital sooner, but denied that their negligence was causative of the baby's mental disabilities. The court held that the defendants were not negligent in failing to diagnose hypoglycaemia because readings from dextro-sticks, a video of the baby, and the absence of signs of spasticity indicated that there was no hypoglycaemia. There was no evidence that the baby ever went into a coma, suffered convulsions, or had apnoea. Nor was there anything in the literature to suggest that hypoglycaemia could cause brain damage. It was therefore impossible to say that hypoglycaemia had caused the baby's condition.

Harm

The plaintiff must show, in bringing an action for negligence, that harm has occurred. This is in contrast to an action for trespass to the person, for which harm need not be established. A trespass to the person exists if, without any justification recognized in law, there is a touching or threat of touching. This kind of legal action is known as 'actionable per se'. In contrast, in an action for negligence the plaintiff must be able to show that harm has resulted from the actions or omissions of the defendant or his employees. In a recent case in which a hypodermic needle was found in a baby after discharge from hospital, the parents failed to obtain legal aid on the baby's behalf to sue the NHS trust because it did not appear that the baby had suffered any harm (see Foreign bodies in children, page 137).

All four elements – duty, breach, causation, and harm – must be established before a claim for compensation for the harm that has arisen will succeed.

WHAT IF THE CHILD DIES?

There is no payment to the child's parents or to the estate of the child of any sum in respect of loss of future earnings. (It may sometimes be possible for the parents of a child of working age to establish that they were dependent upon his or her earnings.) Loss of expectation of life has been abolished as a loss for which compensation can be paid.

There is payable a sum for bereavement which is expected to include funeral expenses, an amount currently fixed at £7500.

PAYMENT FOR NERVOUS SHOCK AMOUNTING TO AN ILLNESS

Sums have been awarded if a child has died and the circumstances have led to considerable distress to the parent(s) amounting to a physical or mental illness.

In one such case[16] a baby was born on 23 July 1989 and was found to suffer from cerebral palsy. She died on 19 November 1989. Both parents claimed compensation for post-traumatic stress disorder in addition to the cost of the care of the baby. Liability for the harm was established and the mother obtained £8500 general damages and the father £7500. The symptoms suffered by both parents included abnormal grief reaction. In addition the mother suffered feelings of guilt, inability to sleep in the dark, and a complete loss of interest in sexual relations.

In another case[17] decided in 1989 the parents of a baby who died 2 days after the birth were awarded a total of £300 000. The defendants had admitted liability; the child's death had been caused by medical negligence. The defendants also accepted that the psychiatric illness from which the parents suffered, and which contributed to the breakdown of their marriage, was caused by the death of their son.

If a child survives after the negligent act or omission and subsequently dies, damages are payable for all the costs of care up to the death subject to deductions for Social Security payments.

HARM FROM SEXUAL ABUSE

Recent cases have shown that if an individual can establish that he or she was abused as a child, then he or she may be able to claim compensation. This might not be practicable if the perpetrator was a member of the family and has no assets or insurance cover to compensate the victim; however, as Korgaonkar and Tribe have shown,[18] it might be possible to recover from an employer, such as a local authority, if an employee was at fault. Once the victim reaches the age of 18 years, time will start to run against him or her and the action must be brought within 3 years (see below defence of limitation).

DIFFERENT KINDS OF LIABILITY

In this section personal liability, vicarious liability, team liability, liability for nonemployees such as parents and visitors, and the direct liability of the employer will be considered.

Personal liability

Each person who owes a duty of care to another person and who is in breach of that duty of care and thereby causes harm, is personally liable for that harm. In principle, therefore, individual professionals who are negligent during their work can be sued and are liable to pay compensation for the harm which has occurred as a result. However, an employed person would be covered by the vicarious liability (see below) of the employer. It is the practice, therefore, for the employer to pay the compensation to the person harmed or the personal representatives.

This principle of vicarious liability does not apply to the self-employed person who has no employer to pay out the compensation (though he or she may be liable vicariously for any employees which he or she employs). The self-employed person must therefore ensure that he or she obtains the necessary insurance cover to meet any claims based on his or her personal liability.

Vicarious liability

An employer is vicariously liable, that is indirectly liable, for the negligence and any other wrongful acts of any employee acting in the course of employment.

NEGLIGENCE AND OTHER WRONGFUL ACTS

The four elements of negligence, that is duty, breach, causation, and harm, must be established against the employee in order to hold the employer vicariously liable. In addition, the employer can use against the plaintiff any defence which would have been open to the employee had the employee been sued personally (see below for defences).

Other wrongful acts could include criminal acts such as theft, and civil wrongs such as trespass and defamation. The employer is only liable, however, if such acts were committed in the course of employment (see below).

EMPLOYEE

It must be established that the negligent person was an employee. This is normally easy but certain situations, in which independent self-employed persons or agents or bank persons are used, can create difficulties. In addition, if a person is seconded from one employer to another, it is not always clear which employer is responsible vicariously for the negligent acts of that person. Reference must be made to the agreement by which this individual is working within a particular workplace to determine whether that individual has the status of an employee and if so who is the relevant employer in relation to the negligent act. The courts have used the criteria set out below to decide whether someone has employee status. A contract of service exists if:

- the servants agree that in consideration of a wage or other remuneration they will provide their own work and skill in the performance of some service for that other;
- they agree expressly or impliedly, that in the performance of that service they will be subject to the other's control in a sufficient degree to make that other master; and
- the other provisions of the contract are consistent with its being a contract of service.

IN THE COURSE OF EMPLOYMENT

It is only if the plaintiff can establish that the negligent acts or omissions were performed in the course of employment that the employer will be held vicariously liable. There are many decided cases in which the employer has argued vigorously that the negligent person was not acting in the course of employment at the time of the negligence and therefore there is no vicarious liability. As a result the courts have laid down guidelines to determine what is meant by the course of employment, as listed below.

It will be seen that the definition of the course of employment is wider than the job description of any individual employee and can include acts which are expressly forbidden by the employer and which could lead to summary dismissal. This may be considered unjust to the employer but it is important to note that the concept of vicarious liability is based on the interest of the public in ensuring that persons obtain compensation from an organization or an individual who will probably be insured. The employer may not be in any way to blame. For example, an employer may have provided a suitable environment in which a child could be cared for and have ensured that staff were trained for their work, and a staff nurse could, out of sheer carelessness, give the wrong dose of drug to a child, thus causing the death of the child. It would be the employer who would have to pay compensation to the parents, not the staff nurse.

The course of employment is:

- an act authorized by the employer;
- an act not authorized but performed for the purposes of the employer's business; or that is incidental to the employment; or that is for the protection of the employer's business;
- an act is prohibited by the employer with the prohibition not taking the conduct outside the sphere of employment; or
- the employer is under a duty to the person who has suffered loss from the employee's fraud or dishonesty.

Team liability

The Court of Appeal has held in the Wilsher case[19] that the law does not recognize a concept of team liability. Each individual professional is personally responsible for his or her own actions and the team itself does not have responsibility. If tasks are delegated to junior members of a team, the person delegating would not be vicariously liable for any harm caused by the junior member, but may be responsible in his or her own right if he or she has delegated inappropriately (i.e. the experience or knowledge of the person to whom the activity was delegated, did not justify the delegation) or the level of supervision provided was inadequate.

Liability for nonemployees
PARENTS AND VISITORS TO THE HOSPITAL
Parents
Is the hospital vicariously liable for any harm that results from the actions or omissions of the parents? The answer is probably no, but it would depend upon the circumstances.

If the parent is assisting in the care of his or her child in hospital and there is no fault on the part of the hospital, then it is unlikely that the hospital would be responsible for the parent. However, if a nurse asks a parent to undertake an activity on his or her behalf, perhaps in relation to a child who is not the child of that person, then there could be vicarious liability. The parent would have acted like a volunteer, a quasi-employee, and it would be reasonable to hold the hospital liable for the negligence of this individual and therefore to be responsible for meeting any claim which had been brought by the parents of the child who had been harmed. Much would depend upon the appropriateness of asking the parent to undertake the activity. There could be direct and vicarious liability on the part of the employers. (The liability of the parent is considered in the next chapter.)

Visitors
What is the situation regarding liability for other acts of visitors if these have not been requested? For example in Jim Richardson's case,[20] 'Ahmed and the Sausage', the situation is described in which the mother of another child on the ward gives Ahmed a sausage, in ignorance that this was strictly contrary to Ahmed's parents' instructions. No physical harm has befallen Ahmed, but what if a visitor gave food or drink to a child who was due for surgery and had a notice 'Nil by mouth' prominently displayed at the head of the bed? Would the hospital be liable if the child choked in theatre as a result of being given food or drink by a visitor to another patient?

The answer is that in the absence of any special circumstances it is unlikely that the hospital would be seen as vicariously liable for the actions of a visitor. However, if there were failures on the part of the staff, for example in not providing adequate supervision of the child due to go to theatre, or in failing to display a clear enough notice, the hospital could be vicariously liable for the deficiencies of its own staff. It also may be liable if a member of staff has asked another visitor to undertake activities which lead to harm being caused. In addition, it might be directly liable if it has failed to provide a safe environment for patients in the hospital.

The direct liability of the employer
Even if the employer is vicariously liable for the negligence of an employee acting in the course of employment, the employer may also be directly liable for the harm which has occurred. Thus the employer may have given inadequate resources for work to be performed, or may have failed to train staff adequately, or may not have taken care to ensure that the premises and equipment were safe. In addition, the employer may have failed to set up a safe system of work. Sometimes these failures could be attributed to individual employees; at other times they are a direct failure of the organization itself, in which case there would be direct liability for any harm which results from these failures.

In the early case of Cassidy v Ministry of Health,[21] Lord Denning stated, "In my opinion, authorities who run a hospital, be they local authorities, government bodies, or any other corporation, are in law under the self-same duty as the humblest doctor. Whenever they accept a patient for treatment, they must use reasonable care and skill to cure him of his ailment. The hospital authorities cannot, of course, do it by themselves. They have no ears to listen through the stethoscope, and no hands to hold the knife. They must do it by the staff which they employ, and, if their staff are negligent in giving treatment they are just as liable for that negligence as is anyone else who employs others to do his duties for him... It is no answer for them to say that their staff are professional men and women who do not tolerate any interference by their lay masters in the way they do their work... The reason why the employers are liable in such cases is not because they can control the way in which the work is done – they often have not sufficient knowledge to do so – but because they employ the staff and have chosen them for the task and have in their hands the ultimate sanction for good conduct – the power of dismissal... I decline to enter into the question whether any of the surgeons were employed only under a contract for services, as distinct from a contract of service. The evidence is meagre enough in all conscience on that point, but the liability of the hospital authorities should not, and does not, depend on nice considerations of that sort. The plaintiff knew nothing of the terms on which they employ their staff. All he knew was that he was treated in the hospital by people whom the hospital authorities appointed, and the hospital authorities must be answerable for the way in which he was treated."

Initially Lord Denning would appear to be setting out the basic concept of vicarious liability and the responsibility of any employer for harm caused by his employees. However, at the very end of the quoted passage where he dismisses the significance of the nature of the contract between the health authority and the professionals it is clear that he is considering a wider concept, that is, the direct liability of the organization for what is undertaken on its behalf.

In spite of these words, the distinction has been kept between vicarious liability and direct liability, and until 1990 doctors and dentists, even when employed in the NHS, were expected to meet claims attributed to their negligence, from the protection provided by the medical defence unions. In 1989 a new scheme[22] was agreed between doctors, dentists, their professional defence organizations, and the health authorities that the health authority or NHS trust would accept vicarious liability for any harm which they caused. It could, therefore, be said that in the context of the NHS the distinction between vicarious and direct liability has lost its significance as the NHS trust would be liable to pay the compensation under one or both of those headings and it does not matter which. However, doubts still remain.

ARE INDEPENDENT HEALTH PROFESSIONALS COVERED BY THE NHS TRUST WHEN THEY WORK ON ITS PREMISES?

Is any distinction to be drawn between liability for agency or bank staff, clinical supervisors employed by a college who supervise students on NHS trust premises, and others who may work on the premises and are not recognized as being employees? Is the trust directly or vicariously, or in both ways, liable for them all?

More recently Sir Nicolas Browne-Wilkinson stated in the Court of Appeal in the Wilsher case,[23] 'I agree with the comments of Mustill LJ as to the confusion which has been caused in this case both by the pleading and by the argument below which blurred the distinction between the vicarious liability of the health authority for the negligence of its doctors and the direct liability of the health authority for negligently failing to provide skilled treatment of the kind that it was offering to the public. In my judgment, a health authority which so conducts its hospital that it fails to provide doctors of sufficient skill and experience to give the treatment offered at the hospital may be directly liable in negligence to the patient. Although we were told in argument that no case has ever been decided on this ground and that it is not the practice to formulate claims in this way, I can see no reason why, in principle, the health authority should not be so liable if its organisation is at fault.'

There is a logic now that the NHS trust is responsible for the compensation payable for the negligence of its professional staff while acting in the course of employment; this requires the NHS trust to be directly responsible for harm which occurs.

INDEMNITY

It is an implied term in every contract of employment that the employee will act with all reasonable care and skill and obey the reasonable instructions of the employer. If the employee has acted negligently, he or she is in breach of that implied term. In theory, therefore, the employer has a right of indemnity against the negligent employee and can recover from this employee compensation which the employer has had to pay out for the employee's negligence. The House of Lords confirmed in 1957 that this right of indemnity exists and this has not been overruled.[24]

There was concern that some NHS trusts might seek to enforce this right to be indemnified by the negligent employee in a case involving midwives, and this concern led to the Minister of Health writing to the Royal College of Midwives emphasizing the concept of vicarious liability and the expectation that the NHS trust would not pursue any right to indemnity.[25] However, as claims in respect of negligence increase, with a potential drain of revenue resources, it is by no means clear that there will not be future cases in which the employer's right to be indemnified by the negligent employee is not exercised.

PARENTAL LIABILITY FOR THE CHILD

This is considered in the next chapter.

DEFENCES

Here are some unacceptable defences which would not prevent the employer being liable if harm were to be caused.

- I was too busy.
- No-one had taught me that procedure.
- I thought that someone else was looking after him.
- The procedure was being carried out by a recently qualified nurse.
- We had no funds to get the equipment repaired.
- As a result of a cost-reduction exercise, we had centralized our cleaning services and no longer checked on the sterility of incubators.
- We did our best.

The following are acceptable defences.

- The facts are disputed and the plaintiff's facts are wrong.
- The elements of negligence are not present, that is, there was no duty of care owed, or no breach of duty occurred, or there was no causation or harm.
- The plaintiff was contributorily negligent.
- The time within which the law requires the action to be brought has passed.
- Liability has been excluded.
- The plaintiff has voluntarily assumed the risk of being harmed.

The facts are disputed

The defendant may assert that the facts are not as the plaintiff alleges and that there was no breach of duty, causation or harm.

Many cases never develop beyond the issue of what are the facts. Once there is agreement on the facts, there may well be a settlement: either an acceptance of liability by the NHS trust or an agreement by the plaintiff that there was no breach. As the plaintiff has to prove on a balance of probabilities that there has been negligence by the defendants or their servants which has led to harm, many cases will fail simply because the witnesses giving evidence for the plaintiff fail to 'come up to proof'. This means that the statements they originally made on which the plaintiff may have based his or her case are contradicted or in some way not supported by the oral evidence of the witness in court.

From the defendant's point of view, comprehensive records are vital to resist any claim by the plaintiff and to establish that there was no breach of the duty of care. This is considered further in Chapter 16.

In many cases, the outcome revolves entirely upon the facts and what can be proved.

The elements of negligence are not present

The plaintiff cannot establish that each of the elements of negligence are present. Expert witnesses may, in giving evidence, not agree that there was a breach of the duty of care as measured by the Bolam test; causation in particular may be difficult to establish.

Contributory negligence

This can be a total or partial defence to an action of negligence. It is based on the principle that plaintiffs also have a duty of care to themselves and if their injuries are partly caused by their own fault, the defendant's liability should be reduced proportionally. This is enacted in section 1(1) of the Law Reform (Contributory Negligence) Act 1945: 'Where any person suffers damage as the result partly of the fault of any other person, a claim in respect to that damage shall not be defeated by reasons of the fault of the person suffering the damage, but the damages recoverable in respect thereof shall be reduced *to such extent as the court thinks just and equitable having regard to the claimant's share in the responsibility for the damage.'* [Author's emphasis.]

The emphasized wording make it clear how the court is to assess the percentage of fault attributable to the plaintiff. It is entirely a question of the facts of the case.

Examples of contributory negligence in clinical care include failure to obey the instructions of the professionals, failure to take the recommended medication, failure to return to seek advice when suggested warning signs had been pointed out, and failure to keep to the recommended diet. In all these examples, it must be shown that the harm that occurred relates in some way to these failures by the patient. If these failures existed but have no bearing on the harm which the patient suffered, then they should be discounted for the purpose of deciding if there was any contributory negligence.

CONTRIBUTORY NEGLIGENCE AND CHILDREN

How does this concept of contributory negligence relate to actions brought by a child? The courts recognize that a child could be expected to take less care of itself than an adult. The following case provides an example.

Gough v Thorne[26]

On 13 June 1962 a group of children were crossing the New Kings Road, Chelsea, London. They were Malcolm Gough, who was 17 years old; his brother John who was 10 years old; and his sister Elizabeth, the plaintiff, who was aged 13 years 6 months. They were coming from the Wandsworth Bridge Road, crossing the New Kings Road, and going to a swimming pool on the other side. They waited on the pavement for some little time to see if it was safe to cross. Then a lorry approached, coming up the Wandsworth Bridge Road and turning left into New Kings Road. The lorry driver was virtually halfway across the road towards the bollards when he stopped, about 5 feet from the bollards. He put his right hand out to warn the traffic that was coming up the road. He saw the children waiting; he beckoned to them to cross, and they did. They had got across just beyond the lorry when a 'bubble' car, driven by the defendant, came through the approximately 5-foot gap between the front of the lorry and the bollard, just missed the eldest boy, struck the young 10-year-old boy, and ran into and seriously injured the plaintiff, Elizabeth, aged 13 years 6 months. The judge held that the 'bubble' car was going too fast in the circumstances, and that the driver did not keep a proper lookout because he ought to have seen the lorry driver's signal and he did not see it. On the issue of contributory negligence, the trial judge found that Elizabeth was one-third to blame for the accident.

Lord Denning in the Court of Appeal disagreed: 'I am afraid that I cannot agree with the judge. A very young child cannot be guilty of contributory negligence. An older child may be; but it depends on the circumstances. A judge should only find a child guilty of contributory negligence if he or she is of such an age as reasonably to be expected to take precautions for his or her own safety: and then he or she is only to be found guilty if blame should be attached to him or her. A child has not the road sense or the experience of his or her elders. He or she is not to be found guilty unless he or she is blameworthy.'

Lord Salmon expressed the situation in the following words: "The question as to whether the plaintiff can be said to have been guilty of contributory negligence depends on whether any ordinary child of 13½ could be expected to have done any more that this child did. I say 'any ordinary child', I do not mean a paragon of prudence; nor do I mean a scatter-brained child; but the ordinary girl of 13½."

Application to the health care of the child

It is extremely unlikely that a defence of contributory negligence can therefore be sustained in an action for negligence brought by a child, except in cases in which the child is an older child and has knowingly been partly liable for the harm that has occurred. The standard of care given by professionals in health care must therefore take into account the reduced responsibility of the child for his or her own health. For example in administering medication, there should be adequate supervision to ensure that it is taken, and other treatments which in the care of the adult could be left to be performed by the patient him- or herself must be supervised by the professional. The same principle applies in health and safety and risk management, and this is discussed in Chapter 16.

Limitation of time

Any action for negligence must be brought within 3 years of the plaintiff knowing that harm has occurred as a result of fault by the defendant. An action begins with the issuing of the writ. The definition of knowledge is given in the Limitation Act 1980 (section 14). It means that the plaintiff must know:

- that the injury was significant;
- that the injury was attributable in whole or in part to the alleged wrongful act or omission;
- the identity of the defendant; and
- the identity of any other person who caused the act or omission, if that person was not the defendant (e.g. the employee, if the employer is the defendant being sued for vicarious liability).

The fact that the plaintiff does not know that the act was wrong as a matter of law does not prevent knowledge, for the purposes of the limitation of time, arising. However, it is not necessary for the plaintiff to have actual knowledge of the facts. If it would be reasonable for the plaintiff to have acquired this knowledge from facts observable or ascertainable by them, or from facts ascertainable by them with help from experts which it would have been reasonable for them to have consulted, they would be deemed to have constructive knowledge such that time will then start to run against them.

There is an exception to the 3-year time limit from the date of the knowledge (actual or constructive) of the injury and wrong; that is, those under a disability. The rule is that if a person is under a disability, the action may be brought at any time within 3 years from the date when he or she ceased to be under a disability or died, whichever occurred first (section 28(1) Limitation Act 1980). This phrase 'under a disability' covers minors and those of unsound mind.

MINORS

Time does not run against a minor until the minor is 18 years of age. This, of course, has profound implications in a childbirth case. Time might run against the mother immediately, if she has the requisite knowledge, but will not run against the child until his or her eighteenth birthday.

In a case in which a child, born on 3 February 1959,[27] was not diagnosed with congenital dislocation of the hip until she was 3 years old, the writ was not issued until 11 November 1988. The defendants argued that her action was time barred because she had visited a doctor when she was 8 years old who said that she would have to have a series of operations and that it was unfortunate that it had not been diagnosed when she was younger. The judge held that the action was not statute barred because she did not have actual or constructive knowledge of the negligence until she applied for a job in 1984 and was seen by a doctor as a result of which she consulted solicitors in January 1985.

In another case an adult brought an action relating to negligence when she was a child;[28] the plaintiff was born on 18 March 1959 jaundiced and with rhesus incompatibility. Following an exchange transfusion, an infection set in. She alleged that because of the negligence of the health authority, she had developed septic arthritis. She also claimed that the defendants were negligent in the performance of a series of leg operations carried out on her when she was aged 16 and 17 years in 1975 and 1976. The writ was issued in July 1989 and amended in November 1989 to add the alleged negligence at birth. Initially the defendants obtained an order that the issue of limitation be tried first. However, the plaintiff's appeal succeeded and the judge said that both the limitation point and the issue on liability would be decided at the trial. The defendant's appeal to the Court of Appeal was dismissed. It held that as the limitation issue was concerned with the plaintiff's actual or constructive knowledge of the negligence and was therefore dependent upon the expert medical evidence, and the issue on liability was similarly dependent upon expert medical evidence, the limitation issue could not readily be separated from issues of causation and negligence, and therefore the limitation defence should not be dealt with separately and summarily.

THOSE OF UNSOUND MIND

Time does not run against persons of unsound mind until the disability ends or the person dies. In some cases, the disability may not end before death, when time starts to run. Thus, if a minor was brain damaged at birth, and it was alleged that this resulted from negligence, could, as long as they are still alive, always have an action brought in their name. It is never 'statute barred'; the limitation of time does not apply.

In a recent case it was held by the trial judge that there is an inherent power of the court to override the rule that there is no limitation of time in such cases (see below). This was not accepted by the Court of Appeal.

The implications of the rules about limitation of time can be seen in the case of Bull v Wakeham. In this case Stuart, one of twins, was born on 21 March 1970. The mother alleged that he was brain damaged because of failures in the care provided. The mother commenced an action on her own behalf and also as next friend in the name of the child which was heard on 9 April 1987 (17 years after the birth). The writ was issued on 23 April 1979.

The mother's claim

The judge found that she knew all the facts relevant to her own claim as soon as they occurred on 21 March 1970, therefore that was the date from which the 3-year period ordained by section 11(4) of the Limitation Act 1980 ran. The judge refused to exercise his discretion to exclude the time limits under section 33 of the 1980 Act (see below). Her action was therefore held to be statute barred.

The child's claim

Time did not run against the child until he ceased to be a minor. This would be at 18 years. However, as a brain damaged person, time would not run against him until his disability ceased. Stuart's claim was therefore not out of time, and could be heard and was upheld.

From this case, it would be apparent to health professionals caring for children that records of childbirth must be kept for at least 25 years after a birth and even longer if the child is mentally disordered (for further details, consult 'The Legal Aspects of Midwifery'[29]). Records of children who were not under a disability should be kept for at least 6 years after they reach the age of 18 years. The implications for record keeping are discussed below.

In a recent case the trial judge held that the statutory rules on the fact that there is no time limitation if the plaintiff was under a disability could be overruled by the inherent powers of the court. In this case[30] a child was born on 31 October 1963. On about 1 September 1964 he underwent an internal operation and at was alleged that he had developed respiratory difficulties which led to hypoxia and cardiac arrest. This resulted in lasting brain damage and he was therefore a person under a disability. The writ was issued on 13 July 1992, that is, 28 years after the date of the alleged negligence. The defendants sought to strike out the claim as being an abuse of the process of the court because of the delay. The judge held that the plaintiff's action would be struck out as an abuse of process for the following reason.

The terms of the Limitation Act 1980 section 28 were permissive. They did not bestow an absolute right on a plaintiff under a disability to institute proceedings in all circumstances and were subject to the inherent jurisdiction of the court to strike out proceedings. In the case the defendant was prejudiced by the long delay in that the plaintiff relied upon the maxim res ipsa loquitur (see page 133), with the consequence that the principal disadvantage of the unavailability of evidence fell on the defendant.

In the appeal against this decision[31] it was held that the appeal would be allowed because the writ was issued within the time permitted by Parliament and there was no evidence of an abuse of the process: the delay did not need any explanation.

In commenting on the case Margaret Puxton QC stated, 'There is no reason why claims should not be brought 60, 70, or even 80 years after the accident happened in brain damage cases – indeed it is surprising that we have not seem more of these very late claims.' The implications for potential defendants are, of course, enormous.[32]

Judge's discretion

Under section 33 of the Limitation Act 1980 the judge has the right to exclude the time limit if he considers it equitable to do so having regard to the degree to which the ordinary limitation rules prejudice the plaintiff and any exercise of the power would prejudice the defendant. As has been seen in the Bull v Wakeham case, the judge refused to exercise his power to exclude the time limit in the mother's favour. He said it would not be equitable to allow her action to proceed bearing in mind the prejudice to the authority.

Exclusion of liability

A person may attempt to exclude his or her liability for causing loss or damage. They might, for example, refer to a notice or ticket or to some other document or spoken word. Is this exclusion valid? The answer depends upon whether the harm which has occurred is personal injury and death, or loss or damage, or both, of property. The Unfair Contract Terms Act 1977 states that, in business situations, a person cannot by reference to a contract term or notice given to persons either individually or generally, exclude his liability for death or personal injury. Business includes a profession and the activities of any Government department or local or public authority. However, if there is loss or damage to property an exclusion notice might be effective.

The significance for the professional caring for the child is that liability for negligence cannot be excluded in advance. Thus an NHS trust cannot successfully avoid an action for negligence by saying in advance to its patients and the parents: 'We have inadequate resources to care for you, and if you come it is on the understanding that we exclude ourselves from liability.' Similarly, if a mother wishes to have a particular form of delivery which is considered hazardous, the midwife could not say: 'Well, provided I am excluded from liability, I will deliver you in the manner you wish.'

Damage to property may be excluded provided that it is reasonable to do so. The requirement of reasonableness is satisfied if it would be fair and reasonable to allow reliance upon the term, having regard to all the circumstances obtaining when the liability arose or (but for the notice) would have arisen. It is for the person who is relying upon the exemption notice and is claiming that the term satisfies the requirement of reasonableness to show that it does.

This may be of importance in the care of a patient's property. If a notice is placed in a paediatric clinic, to the effect that the NHS trust is not responsible for loss or damage to property however caused, this may be effective in relieving the NHS trust of liability even if one of their employees is at fault. It would be for the trust to prove that it was reasonable for it to rely upon the notice excluding liability. Clearly, however, in relation to the property of a child in applying the requirement of reasonableness, it would be more difficult for the defendant to rely on the exclusion clause.

Voluntary assumption of risk

Another defence on which a defendant may sometimes rely is that, even though duty, breach, causation, and harm can be shown, the plaintiff voluntarily agreed to waive the right to bring an action for negligence. This is known as 'volente non fit injuria', that is, 'to the willing there is no wrong'.

A parent may, for example, want a procedure to be carried out that might be contrary to the policy of the hospital, and agree to sign a document stating that he or she voluntarily took on the risks involved and would not hold the professionals in any way responsible should harm occur to the child involved. In the case of the unborn child and an action under the Congenital Disabilities Act, if the parent voluntarily assumes the risk of being injured through negligence, and the child is harmed by that negligence, then this could be used as a defence (see page 145). However, it is unlikely that this would succeed in an action brought in the name of the child for postnatal harm, when the parent had consented to that risk. The parent's consent is unlikely to be an effective defence.

A health professional caring for children would be wise not to rely upon this as a defence.

THE PROCEDURE AND ASSESSMENT OF COMPENSATION

Procedure in relation to claims brought by a child
THE PROCEDURE

In Jim Richardson's book[33] a case is described of an overdose given by mistake to a child. This will be used as an example of the procedure that would be followed.

If harm to a patient arises, such as an overdose of medication, and it is suspected that the harm arose as a result of the fault of a named or unknown individual, the child can sue in his or her own name through the guardian who is known as a next friend (see Chapter 2), to obtain compensation. Should the minor sue as a plaintiff without a next friend, the proceedings may be set aside and the plaintiff's solicitors may be ordered to pay all the defendant's costs of the action. The defendant could agree to the action proceeding without a next friend.

When minors reach 18 years of age they can choose whether the proceedings are to continue or not. If they choose to continue them, the proceedings will then be conducted in their own names and they will then be liable for the costs of them from that point on.[34]

Legal aid

Advice would be obtained from a solicitor and from experts in the field and, if appropriate, legal aid sought to bring a case.

The child is entitled to have legal aid in his or her own right. The application must be made on behalf of the minor by the person who is acting, or intends to act, as the next friend or guardian *ad litem*. The charge in favour of the Legal Aid Fund upon any money or property recovered is not affected by infancy.[35]

A writ would then be issued and, within 4 months of its being issued, it must be served upon the defendant. The time limits within which the writ has to be issued are discussed above.

WHO IS THE DEFENDANT?

In the case of an employee working for a trust, the defendant would be the trust on the basis of its vicarious liability for the negligence of the employees of the trust while working in the course of employment. Although personal negligence may be alleged against the employee, it is accepted that the employer would defend the case on the basis of its vicarious liability.

It may be that the defendant accepts that an employee was negligent and that it is vicariously liable, in which case the amount of compensation (known as 'quantum') would be agreed with the solicitor of the plaintiff. If agreement cannot be reached, there could be a court case over the amount of compensation, liability being admitted. (In such cases, the defendant would probably pay into court a sum of money representing what the plaintiff has been offered and refused. The amount is kept secret from the judge and if he or she eventually awards a sum of this amount or less than this sum, then the plaintiff would have to pay the defendant's costs from the date of payment in. The rationale for this is that, if the plaintiff had accepted the defendant's offer, the costs of the court hearing could have been avoided.)

An example can be seen in a recent case in which a couple who had a baby 6 years after the husband had a vasectomy won a claim in the High Court for damages against the surgeon for failing to warn that the procedure might not be effective.[36] The doctor had admitted failing to give warnings of the risk. The judge awarded the couple £500 for anxiety and distress over the unexpected birth of their son. (They already had two children.) He dismissed their claim for damages of £69 000 for the child's upkeep, an extension to their home and loss of earnings. He ruled that they would not have taken further precautions even if they had been warned. The couple had rejected an out of court settlement offer of £10 000 and their £500 could be clawed back by the Legal Aid Fund.

Sometimes both liability and quantum are contested; sometimes there is agreement over quantum but not an acceptance of liability, and the court hearing will therefore centre on whether the defendant's employee(s) were negligent and whether this negligence caused foreseeable harm.

After the service of the writ, a statement of claim is sent to the defendant and this sets out the main points of the case against the defendant and their employee(s). The defendant responds to this with a defence setting out the points of his or her defence to the claim. These documents are known as part of the pleadings and are usually drafted by barristers. There follows further documents requesting answers to certain questions and a request for the disclosure of relevant documents.

DOCUMENTARY EVIDENCE

What would be relevant documents in a case involving a drugs overdose? Some of the documents for which disclosure would be ordered are listed below.

- Patient records
- Patient medication charts
- Duty rotas

- Procedures and protocols
- Professional guidelines that staff followed
- Policy on the prescribing and administration of medication, including a policy on PRN drugs (as required medication)
- Records relating to oversight by the pharmacy department
- Instructions from manufacturers of the drugs

Eventually, and this could be several years after the date of the events complained of, the case would be set down for hearing. This would take place in the County Court if less than £50 000 was claimed and in the Queen's Bench Division of the High Court for sums over £50 000.

The usual procedure followed in court is shown below.

- Opening speeches
- Plaintiff's witnesses:
  examined in chief
  cross-examined
  re-examined
- Defendant's witnesses:
  examined in chief
  cross-examined
  re-examined
- Closing speeches
  decision by the judge (it may be reserved, i.e. given at a later time)

After the opening speeches, the barrister for the plaintiff would bring each witness in turn into the witness box and examine him or her in chief on the statement previously made. This would be done without leading questions being asked and would be aimed at eliciting the evidence which that witness could bring. After the examination in chief, there then comes the cross-examination for the other side. Here leading questions can be asked designed to show that the witness is contradicting him or herself and is unreliable. Alternatively, the cross-examination could aim at strengthening the case for the other party.

The order shown above might be varied if the plaintiff is able to establish what is known as a 'res ipsa loquitur' situation (i.e. 'the thing speaks for itself').[37] This is discussed below (Burden of proof).

TWO KINDS OF WITNESSES
Witnesses of fact
Some witnesses are called to give evidence of the facts which are in contention. Thus if the prescribing and administration of drugs are at issue, witnesses of fact could include the ward sister, other trained staff present, student nurses, support staff, doctors, the pharmacists and other professionals involved in the care of the patient who may have relevant information, and hospital managers. Many of these would be called as witnesses by the defence. However, other professionals could be called by the plaintiff to show the extent of the harm and pain and suffering of the child, and others, such as a district nurse or GP, could give evidence as to the condition of the child before admission. The relatives could give additional evidence of the child's condition and deterioration.

Witnesses of fact are extremely dependent upon the clarity and comprehensive nature of the records which they made at the time. Given the delays before a civil case comes to court, it can be many years before the witnesses are first cross-examined on those events, and therefore the records play a major role in the way the hearing proceeds. If a child is the plaintiff and the action does not commence until the child is over the age of 18 years, it is clear how great the reliance will be on what has been recorded.

Practitioners should be aware of the guidance issued by the UKCC on record keeping. (See further discussion on record keeping in Chapter 16.) However, the fact that information is contained in records does not mean that it is true, and the judge will determine, in the light of the way the witness stands up to cross-examination, the weight which can be attached to his or her records.

Expert witnesses

Other witnesses are called to give evidence, not because they were present at the time, but because they are recognized as leading figures in their professional field and could therefore give evidence of the standard of care which could have been expected by the patient, and advise upon protocols and professionally accepted procedures. They may also be able to give evidence on causation. Such expert witnesses could include nursing advisers of other trusts, professional bodies, National Boards, nurse tutors, doctors, pharmacists, and pharmaceutical manufacturers. These experts would have advised the plaintiff's solicitor before the case commenced over whether there was a *prima facie* cause of action. Once it was clear that the plaintiff contemplated legal proceedings, the defendants would seek expert advice on whether the case should be settled or defended.

BURDEN OF PROOF

The burden of proof is upon the plaintiff to establish the facts of negligence and the existence of liability on a balance of probabilities. This means that if the plaintiff fails to establish the facts through his witnesses and documentation, the court must find in favour of the defendant.

Sometimes, however, the plaintiff (the person seeking compensation) could rely upon the legal device known as 'res ipsa loquitur', that is, 'the thing speaks for itself'. This means that if an incident occurs, such as leaving a swab in a patient, or amputating the wrong limb, the plaintiff can say to the defendant, 'Prove that these events occurred without negligence on your part.' To establish that it is a res ipsa loquitur situation the plaintiff must be able to show three things, namely that:

- the management of the incident was under the control of the defendants;
- something has occurred which with reasonable care being taken would not have occurred; and
- the defendants have not offered any explanation for what happened.

It must also be established that harm has occurred as a result of the breach of the duty of care, that is, causation (see above).

An example of res ipsa loquitur being pleaded in a case was that of Saunders v Leeds Western Health Authority.[38] In this case it was held that the plaintiff was able to rely upon the maxim res ipsa loquitur in establishing negligence against a medical authority when the heart of a fit child arrested under anaesthetic. The plaintiff was a fit child aged 4 years when she underwent an arthroplasty operation under general anaesthetic and she suffered a cardiac arrest and brain damage as a result The defendants disputed that it was a res ipsa loquitur situation relying on the fact that her regular pulse had abruptly stopped and it was possible that a paradoxical air embolism had caused the arrest without negligence on their part. The court held that the defendant's evidence was honest but mistaken. The explanation they put forward would be rejected because it required a chain of occurrence of which there were only three cases in the literature and these involved neurosurgery patients under different circumstances.

Assessment of compensation

An example will be given from a decided case of the types of headings considered by the courts as attracting compensation. The following award was made in the case[39] of a boy aged 17 years suffering from dyskinetic athetoid cerebral palsy due to negligence at birth. The mother had been in hospital for 2 days when the plaintiff was delivered by emergency caesarian section on 23 September 1975. The baby had suffered tachycardia, profound bradycardia, and severe hypoxia, and was moribund. His dyskinetic athetoid cerebral palsy caused constant varying muscle spasms and distortion of movement which disrupted his torso, limbs and face, caused physical impairment, and distorted speech. He could attempt to take hold of objects, undress and dress himself with minimal supervision, feed himself using utensils, attend to his bodily functions, wash and bathe with minimal supervision, walk only a few steps at a time, shave with a cordless electric razor, and had to have objects close by to grab hold of to steady himself. The health authority admitted liability on 27 May 1992. A sum of £674 500.32 was awarded made up as follows:

pain, suffering and loss of amenity	90 000.00
interest on general damages	8 028.00
past parental care	35 262.40
additional household costs	7 000.00
travel (already occurred)	2 304.52
special needs	9 781.92
special damages	54 348.44
less deductible benefits	(30 633.73)
less interest on interim payments	(1 628.67)
pre-trial loss	22 086.04
interest on special damages	9 022.14
future loss and expenses	159 816.98
future care	189 013.44
physiotherapy	11 312.00
travel	18 700.00
accommodation (capital)	52 876.22
accommodation (annual cost)	18 812.54
holidays	14 000.00
lost earning capacity	107 930.16
Total	**701 597.52**
***Less* future benefits**	**(27 097.20)**
Total awarded	**£674 500.32**

COMMENT

It will be noted that the biggest heads of damage are pain, suffering and loss of amenity; future loss and expenses, future care, and lost earning capacity. The courts must also take into account the benefit obtained from Social Security payments both before the trial and in the future, and these are deducted from the award.

It will also be noted that the parents' contribution to the child's care in terms of their own personal care before the court hearing is also quantified. The sum awarded to the child for future care may cover the value of care provided by the parents, but it also leaves the child free to purchase care from persons of his choice.

STRUCTURED SETTLEMENTS[40]

Structured settlements permit damages to be paid by annual instalments for the duration of the loss and enjoy a tax regime which may reduce the cost. The Inland Revenue approved of such schemes in 1987.[41] The scheme consists of a lump sum payment to the plaintiff to cover immediate capital needs and the rest is used to purchase an annuity from a life office. Periodic payments are then made by the life office to the defendant who then makes them to the plaintiff. The settlement must be agreed by both parties. In the health service, if the defendant is a health authority, there are self-funded structured settlements, in which the health authority is able to make a periodic payment to the plaintiff rather than purchase an annuity from a life office. The court must approve the figure for compensation if the plaintiff is a minor. One of the advantages to the plaintiff is in the taxation. The plaintiff does not pay tax on the income received through a structured settlement, and therefore obtains more money than he or she would otherwise have received. As the plaintiff is only entitled to receive sufficient to compensate him or her for the loss which he or she has suffered, a discount is therefore agreed between plaintiff and defendant which is about 10% of the amount structured. The Department of Health currently administers the structured settlement schemes on behalf of health authorities and approval must be obtained from both the Department of Health and the Treasury.

SPECIFIC SITUATIONS

In the final section of this chapter on negligence we look at particular areas of concern to those who work with children. There are, of course, numerous examples of claims for compensation arising from the care of children. One of the most comprehensive sources of information about litigation in paediatrics is the chapter by Campbell.[42]

The topics which are to be considered here are:

- claims resulting from high technology in child health care;
- claims resulting from failures in communication;
- pain relief in children;
- foreign bodies in children;
- errors in drug administration; and
- simple human error.

Claims resulting from high technology in child health care

Campbell shows how the increase in developments in medical technology has increased the potential for litigation. He suggests a possible classification of cases which result from such developments.

- Progress in medical treatment [an example is retinopathy of prematurity (formerly known as retrolental fibroplasia); the Wilsher case decision has made such cases more difficult to win].
- New or quasi-experimental treatments.
- Unproved treatments.
- Iatrogenesis imperfecta, in which investigations and treatments are initiated not because of symptoms or signs of illness but because of false-positive laboratory tests.

He cites examples of litigation in intensive care and assisted ventilation – litigation because of failure to provide intensive monitoring or treatment. 'Some [cases] will result from actual or perceived delays in the recognition that intensive therapy, particularly assisted ventilation, is necessary and some will result from complications that arise during treatment, for example accidental ventilator disconnection.'

Campbell shows that catheterization of the umbilical artery or vein is also fraught with potential difficulties. He emphasizes that the need to use these vessels should be clearly indicated and recorded in the clinical notes and that there should also be some evidence that the risks were appreciated by the staff and that the procedure was discontinued immediately it was no longer necessary.

Claims resulting from failures in communication

'Practical procedures that result in serious complications frequently end in litigation, especially when there has been some failure in communication with the parents.'[43] Campbell cites a case in which a child lost part of a forearm and hand when ischaemic gangrene resulted from thromboembolic complications of an inadequately supervised radial artery catheter inserted for blood gas monitoring. He suggests that the condition of the child may not have justified the risks involved in this particular monitoring. However, no instructions on the care of the catheter were given to nurses or written in the notes and it was clear that early warning signs of ischaemia such as 'blanching of fingers' were ignored. 'Thus although in other respects the care of the infant was exemplary, it was not possible to defend what happened as a regrettable yet, in some circumstances, unavoidable complication of intensive care.'

Another example he gives is of a case in which a child died from the familial disease of severe combined immunodeficiency and the family had received no genetic counselling. Failures in communication within the general practice led to this previous history not being recorded and a second child later died after many infections.

Another case which shows both failures in infection control and in communications is given by Campbell. He cites the case of an 8-day-old infant who was discharged from a newborn unit without the knowledge of the GP and without any arrangements for hospital follow-up even though she had had a persistent mild fever and an inflamed heel thought to be caused by the repeated heel stabs necessary for measuring serum bilirubin. She had had rhesus haemolytic disease which had been successfully treated by an exchange transfusion on the second day of life. She was brought back to hospital 10 days after discharge with extensive osteitis involving both ankles. She was left with considerable disability and was awarded damages in excess of £100 000.

The case highlights:

- failure to identify the infection pre-discharge;
- failure in communications with general practitioners; and
- possibly failure to advise the parents over signs to look for and action to be taken.

The work of the Central Public Health Laboratory Service on infection control and its identification of failures to recognize and record significant facts relating to infections illustrate the low standards of practice and the potential vulnerability to litigation.

Pain relief in children

The assessment and treatment of pain is a good example of changing standards of care, when higher expectations by the child and parents are justified. Sue Price[44] describes the progress which has been made in assessing and measuring pain. 'Over the last decade there has been an increasing amount of research on pain in infants and children. This research has not only extended our knowledge of children's pain experiences but also identified a number of indicators of pain in children, such as changes in physiological signs or behaviour.' She concludes that it is no longer acceptable for children's pain to be undertreated.

Karen Wilson states that, 'Much of the research into paediatric pain suggests that the prescription of analgesics by doctors and their administration by nurses is inadequate, yet little seems to be done to overcome these problems.'[45]

Foreign bodies in children

A hypodermic needle was alleged to have been found in a baby 2 weeks after his discharge from special care baby unit. The incident took place after discharge from the Treliske Hospital in Truro.[46] The management stated that an independent investigation into the incident would be set up, led by child health experts. From the few facts available it appears that the baby was admitted to the special care baby unit and received blood, lumbar puncture and swab tests. The mother claimed that the needle must have travelled from the baby's stomach round to his back. Legal Aid was refused to the child on the grounds that there was insufficient evidence of injury. The preliminary report of the independent inquiry has confirmed the fact that there was a needle and has highlighted mistakes made by staff who failed to notice the needle in an X-ray.[47] The paediatric registrar who studied the X-ray failed to show it to a qualified radiologist who might have picked up the mistake.

Errors in drug administration

An example is given in Jim Richardson's book of a drugs error. He describes the case where a 7-year-old boy was given chlorpheniamine instead of chloral hydrate as a preoperative drug. The mistake arose because of pressures on the ward and the need to give a baby the chlorpheniamine intravenously. When the error was spotted, the nurse ensured that both the paediatrician and the anaesthetist were advised of the mistake. She failed, however, to inform either the ward sister or the senior nurse manager. Nor did she complete an incident report; therefore the nurses on the next shift were not aware of the mistake.

In applying the law to these facts it is clear that a duty was owed to the patient; it is also clear that there was a breach of this duty. However, in the event, the mistake did not appear to cause the boy any harm as the anaesthetist said that the boy had received much the same sort of drug as he would have given him for the operation. Even though the parents were initially very concerned, they would be unable to bring a civil action for compensation as there was no evidence that the boy suffered harm. However, the nurse could still face disciplinary proceedings by her employers and she was given a written warning. She could also face professional conduct proceedings by the UKCC. It is pointed out in the situation discussion that she had a duty to obey the policies of her employer.

The fact that she was very much under pressure would not have been an acceptable defence in a civil case (had harm been established); however, it should go to mitigate the sanctions operated by the employer, as the employer has a direct duty to ensure that the patient will be safe by employing adequate competent staff. However, there would be a duty upon employees to notify the employer of the situation and there is no evidence that the nurse concerned brought the situation to the notice of her managers.

The authors quote an article by Arndt[48] which suggests that it is constructive to focus on the event and the circumstances which surrounded it rather than on the person who made the mistake. This may be useful in taking management action to ensure that such an event does not reoccur; however, the courts would focus on both in determining whether there was liability in the civil law, and the disciplinary and the professional conduct proceedings would have to focus on the person as well. It should also be remembered that had the child died, there would also be an inquest and possible criminal proceedings to be faced. It is also important to be alert to the possibility that an 'Allitt' situation could exist (see Chapter 16).

Simple human error

There are claims for unsightly scars from intravenous infusions which have 'tissued' and caused ischaemic necrosis of surrounding tissue. This is a relatively common problem with the use of pressure pumps. There are many other cases of negligence brought because of harm arising from simple human error. Constant vigilance in maintaining reasonable standards of care is essential.

CONCLUSION

There is no doubt that parental expectations in relation to child health care are high, and as a consequence litigation is increasing. In addition, there are emotional factors when harm occurs to a child which can lead to the initiation of a civil action even when liability is strongly contested. The Government is exploring the possibilities of alternative dispute resolution through some form of arbitration, which may speed up the hearing of such claims. However, at present there is no suggestion that the UK will accept the system of no-fault liability which exists in New Zealand, Sweden, and Finland where fault does not have to be established but simply that a medical accident that would not normally take place has occurred.

REFERENCES

1 Donoghue (or M'Alister) v Stevenson House of Lords [1932] All ER Rep 1.
2 House of Lords [1970] 2 All ER 294.
3 House of Lords [1955] 1 All ER 565.
4 Hill v Chief Constable of West Yorkshire House of Lords [1988] 2 All ER 238 and Calveley v Chief Constable of the Merseyside Police [1989] 1 All ER 1025.
5 Bolam v Friern Hospital Management Committee [1957] 2 All ER 118.
6 [1985] 1 All ER 635.
7 Hunter v Hanley 1955 SLT 213.
8 Defreitas v O'Brien (and another Times Law Report 16 February 1995).
9 De Koning v Cheb Management Party Ltd [1994] 5 Med L R 250.
10 Times News Report 3 March 1995.
11 Nethercott S: Sick children deserve a better quality of care. Br J Nurs 1994, 3:379–380.
12 Castledine G: [Comment]. Br J Nurs 1993, 2:1077–1078.
13 [1986] 3 All ER 801.
14 Fairhurst v St Helens & Knowsley Health Authority [1994] 5 Med LR 422.
15 Marsden v Bateman [1993] 4 Med LR 181 Current Law 1994, 262: pages.
16 Re W 1993. Association for the Victims of Medical Accidents Medical and Legal Journal 1993, [Annual Report].
17 Tredget and Tredget v Bexley Health Authority [1994] 5 Med L R 178.
18 Korgaonkar G, Tribe D: Child sexual abuse and the right to compensation. Br J Nurs 1993, 2:286–287.
19 Wilsher v Essex Area Health Authority [1986] 3 All ER 801 Court of Appeal.
20 Richardson J, Webber I: Ethical Issues in Child Health Care. London: Mosby; 1995.
21 Court of Appeal [1951] 1 All ER 574.
22 HM(89)34.
23 [1986] 3 All ER 801.
24 Lister v Romford Ice and Cold Storage Co. Ltd [1957] 1 All ER 125.
25 Dimond BC: Reliable or liable? Indemnity and insurance. Mod Midwife 1994, 4:6–7.
26 Court of Appeal [1966] 3 All ER 398.
27 Colegrove v Smyth and others [1994] Med LR 111.
28 Fletcher v Sheffield Health Authority [1994] 5 Med LR 156.
29 Dimond BC: The Legal Aspects of Midwifery. Cheshire: Books for Midwives Press; 1994.
30 Headford v Bristol and District Health Authority [1994] 5 Med LR 406 QBD.
31 Headford v Bristol and District Health Authority [1995] 6 Med LR 1 CA.
32 Margaret Puxon Comment on Headford v Bristol & District Health Authority [1995] 6 Med LR 5.
33 Richardson J, et al.: Ethical issues in child health care. London: Mosby; 1995.
34 Halsbury's Laws of England, vol 5(2), edn 4. London: Butterworths; 1993.
35 Law Society v Rushman [1955] 2 All ER 544.
36 Damages after vasectomy fails. Times News Report 17 March 1995.
37 Dimond BC: The Legal Aspects of Nursing, edn 2. Hemel Hempstead: Prentice Hall; 1995.
38 Saunders v Leeds Western Health Authority and Robinson 1984 [but reported (1993)] 4 Med LR 355.
39 Nash v Southmead Health Authority [1994]5 Med L R 74.

40 See also Law Commission Report No 224 Structured Settlements and Interim and provisional damages. (September 1994).

41 Hay K: Structured settlements in the NHS Health Care. *Risk Report* 1995, 1:20–21.

42 Campbell AGM: The Paediatrician and Medical Negligence. In *Medical Negligence*. Edited by Powers M, Harris N. London: Butterworths; 1994.

43 Campbell AGM: The Paediatrician and Medical Negligence. In *Medical Negligence*. Edited by Powers M, Harris N. London: Butterworths; 1994:p709.

44 Sue Price: Assessing children's pain. *Br J Nurs* 1994, 3:1046–1048.

45 Wilson K: Management of paediatric pain. *Br J Nurs* 1993, 2:524–526.

46 Laurance J: Baby had needle in body for two weeks. *Times* 24 January 1995.

47 *Times* News Report 2 February 1995.

48 Arndt M: Nurses' medication errors. *J Advanc Nurs* 1994, 19:519–526.

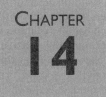

Parental liability and involvement

It has long been recognized that family-centred care should be actively encouraged in the care of the sick child. The considerable advantages have been analysed by Philip Darbyshire.[1] However, the involvement of the parents in the care of the sick child, whether in hospital or the community, can give rise to legal issues.

These include:

- the duty of care of the professional to prevent harm to the parent;
- liability of parent for the negligence of the child;
- liability of practitioner in relation to supervision and delegation from professional to parents;
- controlling the activity of parents in relation to their children;
- disputes between parents; and
- Congenital Disabilities (Civil Liabilities) Act 1976.

THE DUTY OF CARE OF THE PROFESSIONAL TO PREVENT HARM TO THE PARENT

Are parents also patients? Does the professional have a duty of care to the parent as well as to the child? For example, parental stress in paediatric intensive care has been discussed by Colin Way.[2] He points out that one of the principal causes of parental stress is role conflict between parents and the professional staff, especially in the definition of parental participation in care. Such a conflict could have legal implications. It has recently been recognized[3] that a local authority in its duty of care to a social worker had a responsibility not to cause the employee unnecessary stress. There is no reason why the same principles could not apply in the context of the relationship between hospital and parent, even though there is not an employer–employee relationship. A duty of care could be seen to be owed by the staff to ensure that parental stress is not increased by conflicts and uncertainties over the parent–nurse role and relationship. Should a parent seek to sue for compensation for such stress, he or she would have the burden of proving that the stress caused by the professional staff is over and above that which has been caused by the condition of the child.

In addition, as Philip Darbyshire points out,[4] parents had to perform the most delicate of social balancing acts. They had to be obviously and demonstrably caring, but not overly so lest they be thought neurotic. They had to show great interest yet not appear to be nosey or a nuisance. They had to be keen to participate yet not take nurses' valued work away from them. They were to do whatever they would do at home yet also fit in with the hospital's policies and practices.

Situations which raise considerable concern are shown in the research of Gillian Bridge.[5] Her investigation led her to write, 'What I found was disturbing; indicative of the need for more research and above all for the voices of mothers to be heard by professionals.'

The duty of care of the child health care professional may extend to a duty towards the parents if it is reasonably foreseeable that harm would arise from actions or omissions of the professionals. Thus, if negligent advice were given to the parents which would cause loss to them, or if the negligent actions of staff would cause unnecessary suffering to the parents, a duty of care may be seen to exist. Reference should be made to the discussion on when a duty of care arises in Chapter 13, pages 115–117.

LIABILITY OF PARENT FOR THE NEGLIGENCE OF THE CHILD

In what circumstances could a parent be held liable for the actions of his or her child? The basic principle is that it is only if the parent is at fault him- or herself that he or she could become liable for the actions of the child.[6] Thus if the parent fails to supervise the child properly and the child causes a road accident by running in front of a vehicle, the parent could be liable to any injured person, because they are at fault through inadequate supervision (see the case of Carmarthen CC v. Lewis [1955] 1 All ER 565 which is discussed in Chapter 13, page 116). In the context of a paediatric ward it is essential to determine whether the parent or the health care practitioner is supervising the child at any given time.

LIABILITY IN RELATION TO SUPERVISION AND DELEGATION FROM PROFESSIONAL TO THE PARENTS

Clearly any system of care which involves cooperation and the involvement of the parents must be well planned, and the activities which are appropriate for delegation and the extent of any supervision necessary clearly identified. In the Care-by-Parent project set up in Cardiff[7] it was noted that 'The role of the nurse with responsibility for care-by-parent is to teach, supervise and support the parents. In the initial stages, this requires a great deal of nursing time: to teach the correct way of doing things and recording findings is time consuming and may need to be repeated several times. A learner nurse may find a job simple after many hours of teaching and instruction, but the parent lacks this and, usually also, the nurse's knowledge base… Care-by-parent can be achieved in any ward setting, but only with commitment from the whole multidisciplinary team.' In the scheme reported there was a full-time post of care-by-parent sister.

What, however, is the legal situation if the care-by-parent sister assumes that the parent has understood a particular instruction but in fact the parent has not and, through ignorance and negligence, causes harm to the child? Is the sister at fault, with the consequence that the NHS trust becomes vicariously liable for her actions or is the parent responsible?

It is clear that if the hospital is introducing a care-by-parent scheme, it still retains a duty of care in the laws of negligence for the safety of the child. The sister would have to follow the reasonable standard of the responsible nurse working in those circumstances with those particular patients (i.e. the Bolam test) in deciding what activities could be delegated to the parents, what training was necessary, and the level of supervision that was required. The sister would also have to show that she ensured that the parents had understood the instructions and were capable of performing the activities competently. Records are clearly essential here and it may also be useful to have some instructions in writing. This could be of assistance to the parents and it would also establish the kinds of instruction given.

CONTROLLING THE ACTIVITY OF PARENTS IN RELATION TO THEIR CHILDREN

Unfortunately, even though it is recognized that 'a cardinal principle of hospital services for children is complete ease of access to the child by his or her parents… The care provided by a hospital has to centre firmly on the recognition of the **child as a member of a family**',[8] there may be occasions when the hospital has to exercise some restraint over the parents. It may be that they are bringing into the hospital food or drink that is inappropriate for the sick child, that they are accompanied by other young children who are creating a disturbance on the ward, or that they are failing to cooperate with the ward regime or necessary restrictions placed upon the sick child. Problems can range from the parent refusing to accept nonsmoking instructions to the parent not observing control of infection regimes.

What powers, if any, does the hospital have over the parents? Parents, although their presence is usually essential for the improvement in the child's health, are on the hospital premises as visitors. They can therefore be expected to obey reasonable instructions as the condition of their entry onto the premises. In extreme circumstances there could be grounds for evicting the parents from the premises. Because of the disadvantages to the child, staff would be reluctant to take this option, but it is important that the staff know that this is available to them if it is necessary for the care of the child or of other patients.

Special provisions exist when there are reasonable grounds for suspecting child abuse (see Chapter 9). For further discussion on liability and rights of the occupier see Chapter 16.

DISPUTES BETWEEN PARENTS

Disputes can arise between separated and divorced parents which may involve practitioners caring for the child.[9]

Situation
The parents are divorced; the mother cares for the child and the father has access. The father visits the child in hospital and sees the child's medical records from which he notes the address and telephone number of the mother, which she had kept secret from him. He then at a later date harasses the mother. She complains to the ward sister about the information being given to the father. What is the legal position?

Parental divorce or separation and even orders by the court do not end parental responsibility. This is the effect of the Children Act 1989. There is in law no reason why the father could not have informal access to the records of a young child (below the age of Gillick-competence). However, if information such as the address and the telephone number is given to staff on the understanding that it will be kept confidential, it would be an abuse to pass this information to an unauthorized person.

Although a divorce has taken place, both parents still retain parental responsibilities and can make decisions on behalf of the child, unless prevented by an enactment (see Children Act 1989 section 2 (5) and (7), below).

SEPARATED PARENTS AND DISPUTES OVER CHILD HEALTH CARE

Situation
The mother has care of the children and has decided that she will not agree to the children receiving the triple vaccine because she fears the risk of a reaction. The father is caring for the children for a few days and brings them to the clinic for the vaccines to be given. The health visitor notes in the records that despite encouragement, the mother has persistently refused to permit the vaccinations to be given. What is the legal position? Can the health visitor take advantage of the father bringing the children to the clinic and giving his consent for the children to be vaccinated?

Under the Children Act 1989 section 2(1) both parents retain parental responsibility for their children. Under section 2(7) if more than one person has parental responsibility for a child each of them may act alone and without the other (or others) in meeting that responsibility; but this does not apply where an enactment requires the consent of more than one person in a manner affecting the child. Even if one parent has a residence order in his or her favour, the other still retains parental responsibilities and can exercise these to the full. It also follows that one parent does not have the right of veto over the other's actions. The fact that the father has parental responsibility does not entitle him to act in any way which would be incompatible with any order made with respect to the child under the Act. The Law Commission[10] gave this example: if a child has to live with one parent and go to a school nearby, it would be incompatible for the other parent to arrange for him to have his hair done in a way which will exclude him from the school. It would not, however, be incompatible for that parent to take him to a particular sporting occasion over the weekend, no matter how much the parent with whom the child lived might disapprove.

APPLYING THE LAW TO THE FACTS OF THE SITUATION ABOVE

Separated parents both retain parental responsibilities. There is no requirement for both parents to give consent to vaccinations. The father can therefore give a valid consent to the vaccination of the children. The health visitor could rely on this consent and would not be liable to an action for trespass to the person. In law, therefore, the health visitor could proceed with the vaccinations. She might, however, decide that, as this would be contrary to the wishes of the mother, she would rather not go against those wishes and instead could ask the parents to agree together on the action to be taken. If necessary, she could seek the intervention of the court.

Some assistance to the legal position might be obtained from disputes between separated parents over education and access to school reports and parent–teacher meetings. Some information must be given to parents as a statutory duty, such as the updated curricular report. There is a lot of other nonstatutory information given out by schools, and Bainham suggests that the legal position on how far such information should be sent to divorced or separated nonresidential parents is not entirely clear. As divorced parents do not lose their parental responsibility, this would suggest that schools should treat them on the basis of complete equality with residential parents and send all information to them. This would be in keeping with the spirit of the Act but not necessarily the letter, as parental responsibility does not carry with it a right of consultation or notification about matters affecting the child. On the other hand, many 'absent' parents are not actively involved with their children and to duplicate all information might result in unnecessary expense. Bainham suggests[11] that the most practical solution might be for schools only to send out the duplicate information if so requested. He points out that in any unresolved disagreement, an application can be made to the court for a specific issue of prohibited steps order (see below) to obtain a ruling on an educational issue.

The same principles will apply in disputes involving health care. Such disputes might occur in relation to:

- accessing records and information;
- telling the child about a depressing prognosis or diagnosis;
- complaining on behalf of the child;
- giving consent or withholding consent or taking the discharge of the child;
- visiting the child in hospital;
- caring for the child, giving them food, treatments, baths, etc;
- dressing or clothing the child;
- giving the child gifts; or
- taking the child out of hospital temporarily.

PROHIBITED STEPS ORDER

If one parent wishes to prevent the other taking action which he or she does not consider is in the interests of the child, he or she may seek a prohibited steps order. This can be ordered under section 8 of the Children Act 1989 and means that no step which could be taken by a parent in meeting his or her parental responsibility for a child, and which is of a kind specified in the order, shall be taken without the consent of the court. Thus if one parent feared that the other was likely to agree to a mentally impaired daughter being sterilized, that parent could obtain a prohibited steps order preventing consent being given without the consent of the court.

If the child is considered to be of Gillick-competence and disagreed with actions that the parents were intending, he or she could seek the leave of the court to obtain a prohibited steps order. The child would have to apply to the High Court.[12] The court must be satisfied that the child has sufficient understanding to make the proposed application (section 10(8)). (See Chapters 4 and 9 for further discussion of the orders under the Children Act 1989.)

SELECTIVE TREATMENT OF NEONATES

There may be disputes between parents and professionals over the care of neonates. This topic is discussed in Chapter 22 where the issues relating to the dying child and the rights of the child are considered in the light of recent court cases.

CONGENITAL DISABILITIES (CIVIL LIABILITIES) ACT 1976

The Congenital Disabilities (Civil Liberties) Act gives rights to the child, once born, who has been harmed as a result of a prebirth incident of negligence. Until the fetus is born it has no right to bring an action.[13]

The main features of the Act are shown below.

- An action is given to the child, if it is born alive, for harm caused by negligent actions to the father or mother, which resulted in the child being born disabled.
- The mother is only liable if she was negligent while driving a car.
- Liability to the child can be excluded to the same extent and is subject to the same restrictions as liability in the parent's own case.
- If the disability arises from an event preconception, then the defendant is not liable if both parents knew of the risk of the child being born disabled. However, if the father is the defendant, this does not apply if he knew of the risk but the mother did not.
- The mother is not liable to the child, unless she was driving a motor vehicle and is in breach of her duty of care to the unborn child and as a consequence the child is born disabled.
- The Human Fertilisation and Embryology Act 1990 added new sections to cover the possibility of a child suing for negligence over fertility treatment. A person involved in such litigation would be able to obtain information from the Register kept by the Human Fertilisation and Embryology Authority.

Professional liability and congenital disabilities

The Act states that: 'The defendant is not answerable to the child... when responsible in a professional capacity for treating or advising the parent, if he took reasonable care having due regard to the then received professional opinion applicable to the particular case; but this does not mean that he is answerable only because he departed from received opinion.'

This means that if the professional takes reasonable care when acting in a professional capacity for treating or advising the parent of the child born disabled, he or she should not be deemed negligent. The statute uses the test of the 'then received professional opinion to that particular class of case' which is similar to the Bolam test discussed in Chapter 13, page 117. However, as in the Bolam case itself and Maynard's case (see Chapter 13, page 118, Standard of care and breach of duty), the fact that a professional departs from the received opinion is not in itself evidence of negligence: nevertheless, records would have to show clearly the reasons why the professional acted in the way she or he did.

Liability of the mother

As can be seen from the main features of the Act, the only situation in which a child can bring action against the mother under the Act is if the child was injured while she was driving a car negligently. In such a case, of course, the mother would be insured and the insurance company would be responsible for paying out the compensation. The Act does not encourage litigation between child and mother.

Common law and civil liability to the unborn child

At common law (i.e. judge-made law) the child, if born alive, can bring an action in respect of prebirth neglience or illegal activities. This is illustrated in the case of B v Islington Health Authority[14] in which it was held that children with disabilities caused by the alleged negligent medical treatment before they were born had a cause for action against the health authorities. This case was brought over injuries suffered before the 1976 Act came into force. It is now uncertain to what extent the common law exists alongside the statutory position, and whether the Act has precluded the possibility of anyone using the common law to bring an action for congenital disabilities which the Act precludes.

CONCLUSION

Health professionals should welcome and encourage the involvement of parents in the care of the sick child. They should also, however, be aware of some of the risks that could arise and ensure that agreed procedures are laid down and followed to prevent reasonably foreseeable harm arising as a result of parental involvement in the care. They should also be trained in how to deal with disputes that may arise between parents and which could affect the child.

REFERENCES

1 Darbyshire P: Family-centred care within contemporary British paediatric nursing. *Br J Nurs* 1995, 4:31–33. [See also, Cleary J: *Caring for Children in Hospital: Parents and Nurses in Partnership*. London: Scutari Press; 1992. See also, While A (Ed): *Caring for Children Towards Partnerships with Families*. London: Edward Arnold.]

2 Way C: Parental stress in paediatric intensive care. *Br J Nurs* 1993, 2:572–577.

3 Walker *v* Northumberland County Council. *Times* Law Report 24 November 1994 Queens Bench Division.

4 Darbyshire P: Family-centred care within contemporary British paediatric nursing. *Br J Nurs* 1995, 4:31–33.

5 Bridge G: A personal reflection on parental participation: how some mothers of babies born with disabilities experience interprofessional care. *J Interprofession Care* 1993, 7:263–267.

6 Donaldson *v* McNiven [1952] 2 All ER 691

7 Cleary J: *Caring for Children in Hospital: Parents and Nurses in Partnership*. London: Scutari Press; 1992:106

8 Health Policy and Public Health Directorate – The Scottish Office Home Health Department: *At Home in Hospital*. Edinburgh: HMSO; 1993:p22.

9 White R, Carr P, Lowe N: *A Guide to the Children Act 1989*. London: Butterworths; 1990.

10 Law Commission 1988 No 172 Report on Guardianship and custody para 2.11

11 Bainham A, Cretney S: *Children – the Modern Law*. Bristol: Family Law; 1993.

12 Wyld N: *When parents separate*. London: Children's Legal Centre; 1994.

13 Dimond BC: *The Legal Aspects of Midwifery*. Hale, Cheshire: Books for Midwives Press; 1994.

14 B *v* Islington Health Authority 1991 1 All ER 325

Employment and professional issues

The purpose of this chapter is to explore the relationship of health professionals with their employers and with their professional bodies in terms of the accountability that the registered professional employee owes to the employer and the registration body. It is not the intention in a work of this kind to give full details of all laws relating to the contract of employment or the details of professional registration and accountability. The aim is to set out the framework so that the health professional can refer for further information to the relevant works listed under 'Further reading' at the back of this book. The chapter concludes by looking at the possibility of conflict between duties to the employer and professional duties.

RELATIONSHIP BETWEEN EMPLOYEE AND EMPLOYER

At the heart of the relationship of employee and employer is a contract of employment. There is a legal right for all employees to receive written particulars of this contract and to be notified of any changes. In the past most NHS employees had been subject to the terms and conditions negotiated through the Whitley Council machinery for NHS staff. Little opportunity was available for local bargaining. Since the establishment of NHS trusts after the NHS and Community Care Act 1990, local bargaining has been encouraged, so there is likely to be competition between trusts for health professionals. The full implications of this change are yet to be appreciated and felt. The basic principles of contract law apply to the contract of employment.

Formation

A contract of employment does not come into being until there has been an offer by one side which has been accepted by the other. The acceptance can be subject to a condition precedent; for example the contract may not come into existence until a condition is met, that is, it might be subject to satisfactory references or medical examination. Alternatively it may commence but be subject to a condition subsequent, that is, the employee may commence work but if checks with the police prove that the person is unsuitable, then the contract will come to an end (see below).

Terms of the contract

These may arise from:

- express terms agreed between the parties;
- local terms and conditions already agreed with health professionals in similar posts, which the new employee is asked to accept;
- national terms and conditions which are still current;

- statutory rights (listed below) which are laid down by Act of Parliament or Regulations which the employer must accept as part of the terms and conditions of the contract of employment; or
- implied terms: these are terms which the law sees as part of the contract of employment, even though they are not agreed explicitly between the parties.; they include the duty of the employee to act with reasonable care and skill and to obey the reasonable instructions of the employer; and the duty of the employer to take reasonable care of the health and safety of the employee by employing competent staff, using a safe system of work, and by ensuring safe premises, plant, and equipment.

Statutory rights are:

- written statement of particulars;
- itemized statement of pay;
- maternity benefits and rights relating to pregnancy;
- payment and limitations on deductions;
- time off work to take part in trade union activities (unpaid); if a trade union official, to undertake trade union duties and training (paid); to search for work in a redundancy situation (pay for at least 2 days); to work as member of a local authority, statutory tribunal, or health authority, as a Justice of the Peace, or as a school governor (unpaid);
- holidays (Bank Holidays);
- patents;
- guarantee payments;
- unemployment benefit;
- redundancy; and
- medical suspension payment.

Performance of the contract

Each party has a duty to fulfil the terms of the contract binding upon it. For one party to threaten strike action is a threat to be in breach of contract. Even a threat to work to rule has been held to be a threat to breach a contract, on the basis that the employee is not intending to cooperate with the employer.

Breach of contract

If the employee is in breach of contract, the remedy of the employer is to use the disciplinary machinery. Thus an oral warning may be given, or a first written warning, or a final warning. In cases of serious or gross misconduct there could be immediate dismissal if all the facts are known, or a suspension of the employee until an investigation has been carried out.

If the employer is in breach of contract, the employee could choose whether to treat the contract as continuing and bargain for compensation, or to regard the contract as at an end by reason of the employer's conduct. The latter is known as a constructive dismissal. The employee who has the requisite length of continuous service would be able to apply to the industrial tribunal claiming remedies for unfair dismissal. If the employee alleges that he or she has been injured as a result of the employer's failure to fulfil their duties in relation to the health and safety of the employee he or she could claim compensation for the harm; he or she could also claim that he or she has been constructively dismissed by the failure of the employer to fulfil its fundamental duty of care, which is an implied term in the contract of employment, in relation to safeguarding his or her health and safety.

Termination of the contract

BREACH OF CONTRACT

As has been seen, either party is entitled to see the contract as at an end as a result of the breach of contract by the other.

PERFORMANCE OF A FIXED-TERM CONTRACT

If the contract is for a fixed term then the passage of that term will end the contract. The failure to renew a fixed term contract is defined as a dismissal in employment legislation. The parties can, however, agree to waive the right of the employee to apply to an industrial tribunal for unfair dismissal because the employer has failed to renew a fixed-term contract.

NOTICE TO TERMINATE THE CONTRACT

Either side may give notice to terminate the contract. The period of notice can be agreed between the parties, can be the statutory terms set down in the employment protection legislation, or can be what would be considered to be reasonable at common law.

FRUSTRATION

Certain events which were not considered by the parties at the time the contract was agreed may result in the contract ending by operation of law: being sent to prison, blindness, and being prohibited from law from driving a car may all frustrate the contract. It thus ends without notice being given by either party.

EMPLOYMENT WITH CHILDREN

The employer has a duty of care to child patients to ensure that only persons suitable for work with children are appointed. The employment of unsuitable persons who cause harm to the child patients could result in the employer being held directly liable to the parents for the harm which has resulted from their negligence. Thus the criminal activities of Beverly Allitt in causing the deaths and harm to children in a paediatric unit have shown the importance of screening for personality disorders. In addition, the possibility that potential applicants have criminal convictions must be checked.

Beverly Allitt

At Grantham and Kesteven General Hospital between February and April 1991 Beverly Allitt, an enrolled nurse, caused the deaths of four children and caused harm to nine others. The Regional Health Authority set up its own inquiry into the situation and an independent inquiry chaired by Sir Cecil Clothier was appointed by the Secretary of State.[1] The latter reported in 1994 and a summary of its main recommendations is shown below. The recommendations relate to the recruitment and selection of staff, the role of the occupational health department and the procedures to be taken when the unexpected death of a child or untoward event takes place. The Health and Safety implications are considered in Chapter 16.

The Clothier inquiry recommended that:

- for all those seeking entry to the nursing profession, in addition to routine references, the most recent employer or place of study should be asked to provide at least a record of time taken off on grounds of sickness;
- in every case coroners should send copies of postmortem reports to any consultant who has been involved in the patient's care before death, regardless of whether they were demanded under rule 57 of the coroner's rules 1984;
- the provision of paediatric pathology services should be reviewed to ensure that such services are engaged in every case in which the death of a child is unexpected or clinically unaccountable, whether the postmortem examination is ordered by a coroner or in routine hospital practice;
- no candidate for nursing in whom there is evidence of a major personality disorder should be employed in the profession;
- nurses should undergo formal health screening when they obtain their first posts after qualifying;

- the possibility should be reviewed of making available to Occupational Health departments any records of absence through sickness from any institution which an applicant for a nursing post has attended or been employed by;
- procedures for management referrals to Occupational Health should make clear the criteria which should trigger such referrals;
- further consideration should be given to using in practice the criteria for detecting the presence of a personality disorder and monitoring for it (i.e. the suggestion of the Chairman of the Association of NHS Occupational Physicians);
- consideration should be given to how GPs might, with the candidate's consent, be asked to certify that there is nothing in the medical history of a candidate for employment in the NHS which would make them unsuitable for their chosen occupation;
- the Department of Health should take steps to ensure that its guide 'Welfare of Children and Young People in Hospital' is more closely observed;
- in the event of failure of an alarm on monitoring equipment, an untoward incident report should be completed and the equipment serviced before it is used again; and
- reports of serious untoward incidents to district and regional health authorities should be made in writing and through a single channel which is known to all involved.

Disclosure of criminal convictions of potential staff

The need to protect children from staff and others caring for them was highlighted in 1984 with the conviction of Colin Evans for the murder of Marie Payne. This led to a Home Office chaired review on the disclosure of criminal convictions of those with access to children. As a consequence of the recommendations in the review, the Government set up arrangements for checks to be made with local police forces in many circumstances before staff or volunteers are taken on to work with children. The circular published emphasizes that the new procedure for checking is not a substitute for normal employment procedure, including the seeking and taking up of references and any requirement that applicants should declare all convictions.

A check with the police is only to be made once the preferred candidate has been selected. 'Such checks must not form part of any interview short listing procedure.'

The 1988 guidance[2] on police checks covers:

- persons on whom checks should be made;
- when checks should be requested;
- information given in response to a checking request determining the relevance of convictions;
- how checks are to be requested;
- police reporting of convictions;
- police indemnity; and
- action to be taken now.

The guidance included the specimen of a form to be used for a police check.

Subsequent guidance[3] was issued which updated the advice issued in 1988. The purpose of the revision is:

- to change the access procedures to reflect the post-reform NHS organization;
- to change the role of the nominated officer;
- to change the description of persons on whom checks may be made and the definition of what constitutes substantial access to children;
- to highlight the importance of verifying the identity of prospective employees;
- to describe the police check and timescale for the police reply;
- to provide a suggested statement of policy about relevant offences;

- to replace the specimen form to be used for requesting a check;
- to revise the form of indemnity; and
- to cover information about citizens from other countries.

DISCIPLINARY PROCEDURES

An employee who is guilty of misconduct or incompetence could face disciplinary proceedings brought by the employer. This is so whether or not all the elements of negligence for the basis of a claim for compensation are satisfied. Thus it may be that a health professional has given the wrong medication to a child. Fortunately, however, the child does not suffer harm. In such a case neither the child nor the parents would succeed in an action for negligence because harm has not been established. However, the health professional is guilty of misconduct and could be disciplined.

PROFESSIONAL REGISTRATION AND ACCOUNTABILITY (SEE ALSO CHAPTER 4)

Most health professionals have registered status under such registration bodies as the General Medical Council (doctors), the UKCC for Nursing, Midwifery and Health Visiting, and the Council for Professions Supplementary to Medicine (chiropodists, occupational therapists, physiotherapists, pharmacists, orthoptists, medical scientific laboratory officers, and dieticians). Two new professions have recently been given registered status: osteopathy (1993) and chiropractic (1994). Other groups such as psychologists and speech therapists do not have registered status. They set their own standards and professional disciplinary machinery outside the framework of the Council for the Professions Supplementary to Medicine.

The Government is at present undertaking a review of the legislation which led to the establishment of the Council for the Professions Supplementary to Medicine.

Each profession has its own code of professional conduct. If a member fails to comply with this code, professional conduct proceedings may lead to the removal of this professional either from the register, if their profession has registration status, or from the list of recognized practising professionals.

The UKCC for Nursing, Midwifery and Health Visiting, perhaps by reason of the number of its registered practitioners, has by far the most frequent number of professional conduct hearings. Its jurisdiction is wider than that of the civil courts; misconduct by a practitioner (i.e. conduct unworthy of a nurse, midwife or health visitor) may include aspects of conduct which would not found an action for compensation. Thus the failure of a nurse practitioner to wear the appropriate clothing, and failure to follow the correct procedures may lead to professional conduct proceedings, but they would not necessarily lead to a claim for civil compensation. They may lead to disciplinary proceedings by the employer; however, inconsistent decisions may result from the employer's disciplinary hearings than from the professional conduct proceedings.

Thus, following an untoward incident, for example a practitioner administers the wrong dose of a drug, the employer might issue a final written warning, but the practitioner might retain his or her post, whereas the Professional Conduct Committee might remove the practitioner from the register in which case, of course, the practitioner would automatically forfeit his or her registered post. Reference should be made to the works in the 'Further reading' for the constitution of the professional conduct committee and the way in which it operates.

The disciplinary procedures of the employment and the professional conduct proceedings of a registered health care professional or those operated by the nonregistered health care professionals (see Chapter 4) parallel the work of the civil and criminal law in making the practitioner accountable for his or her professional practice (see Chapters 13 and 16).

CONFLICT BETWEEN EMPLOYERS AND PROFESSIONAL DUTIES

In recent years there has been growing concern at the possibility that the instructions given by employers might clash with professional duties owed to the patient. As we have seen, every employee must obey the reasonable instructions of the employer, but what if the employer expects the health professional to work with inadequate resources or in circumstances which endanger the safety of the patient? Most health professionals have to abide by a code of professional conduct which requires them to take steps to ensure the safety of the patient and report to an appropriate person any potential hazards. Some trusts have included as part of the contract of employment that they have with their professional employees the requirement that these employees follow the appropriate code of professional conduct. If this is included, there should not be a conflict between the instructions of the employer and the professional standards the employee is expected to follow. The UKCC has recently recommended clauses to be included in NHS agreements to maintain high standards of professional practice.[4]

A child health professional might find that as an advocate of the patient, he or she is required to raise matters of concern with management about resources. This process has been called 'whistle-blowing'. Staff who raise such issues are entitled to be protected from any victimization, and employers are required by the Department of Health to establish an internal procedure whereby concerns can be made known to management without the employee suffering any detriment. Many clauses in the code of professional conduct of the nurse require the nurse to raise with an appropriate person concerns over the health and safety of patients and colleagues. (Clauses 8, 11, 12, and 13 all require the practitioner to report any concerns on health and safety matters to an appropriate person.) Failure to do so could result in the registered practitioner facing proceedings for professional misconduct. Reference should be made to Chapter 6 and the laws relating to confidentiality, as this is an area which has caused concern in relation to whistle-blowing. Some trusts have required employees to agree to confidentiality clauses, whereby they cannot make known concern to outside agencies. These have been called 'gagging clauses'. Staff who have raised issues relating to patient care with outside organizations have then been held to be in breach of the duty of confidentiality owed to the employer. It is essential that the procedure for raising concerns with internal management is followed to protect the safety of patients and staff and at the same time that of the member of staff who brings the concerns to the attention of senior management.

If the employer includes obedience to the code of professional conduct in the contract of employment, there should be a harmony between the duties expected of the health professional by the Registration bodies, the employment duties required under the contract of employment, and the duties required under the common law for the duty of care in the law of negligence. For example, for the registered nurse practitioner Clause 2 of the code of professional conduct illustrates the standard of care: 'ensure that no action or omission on your part, or within your sphere of responsibility, is detrimental to the interests, condition or safety of patients and clients.'

REFERENCES

1 The Allitt Inquiry: *Independent inquiry chaired by Sir Cecil Clothier into the Beverly Allitt events.* London: HMSO; 1994.

2 HC(88)9; HN(FP)(88)3; HOC 8/88; WHC(88)10

3 WHC(94)61

4 UKCC Registrar: *Council Proposed Standards for Incorporation of Contracts for Hospital and Community Health Care Services [Letter 27/95].* London: UKCC; 1995.

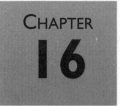

Health and safety

The purpose of this chapter is not to look at the laws relating to health and safety in general, but rather to consider the specific aspects of health and safety in relation to the child. The reader is referred to general works on health and safety for the main principles.[1] This chapter will look at:

- the liability of the occupier in relation to the care of children, as visitors or trespassers;
- the duty under the Health and Safety at Work Act 1974 and subsequent regulations to undertake a risk assessment and regulations relating to manual handling;
- duty of the employer to safeguard the health and safety of the employee as an implied duty under the contract of employment;
- the regulations relating to the control of substances hazardous to health;
- protection of children from dangerous staff, bogus professionals, and kidnapping;
- Munchausen by proxy;
- control of the child; and
- records.

INTRODUCTION

Statutory laws on health and safety include laws enforceable through both the criminal and the civil courts. Thus the Occupiers Liability Act 1957 creates a duty on the occupier which is enforceable through the civil courts in the same way as the duty of care which exists in the common law as part of the law of negligence (see Chapter 13). In contrast, the Health and Safety at Work Act 1974 and the subsequent regulations are enforceable in the criminal courts, usually by the Health and Safety Inspectorate. The health professional should also be mindful of their professional codes of conduct, many of the clauses of which relate to the duty of the professional to look out for the health and safety of their clients and colleagues. Failure to observe these codes could result in professional conduct proceedings which ultimately could, in extremely serious situations, lead to the health professional being removed from the register.

OCCUPIERS LIABILITY ACTS 1957 AND 1984

These Acts are enforceable in the civil courts if harm has occurred to a visitor (1957 Act) or trespasser (1984 Act).

Occupiers Liability Act 1957

This Act places a duty of care upon the occupier (of whom there may be several) to take care of their visitors.

OCCUPIER

The occupier would be the person in control of the premises. This would normally be the NHS trust for hospital property and the ward sister would be acting as the agent of the occupier for the safety of her ward. There can, however, be several occupiers. For example if painters, employed by independent contractors, come onto the premises, they may also be in occupation of the premises and could be responsible for harm which occurs as a result of their lack of care.

VISITOR

A visitor is a person on the premises with the express or implied consent of the occupier. In the context of hospitals the term would therefore include patients, staff, visitors, tradesmen, and anyone else with a bona fide reason to be there and who is not excluded by the occupier (see below).

THE NATURE OF THE DUTY OWED

The duty is set out in section 2(2) of the Act: 'The common duty of care is a duty to take such care as in all the circumstances of the case is reasonable to see that the visitor will be safe for the purposes which he is invited or permitted by the occupier to be there.'

Section 2(3) clarifies the duty further for specific circumstances: 'The circumstances relevant for the present purpose include the degree of care, or want of care, which would ordinarily be looked for in such a visitor, so that (for example) in proper cases:

a an occupier must be prepared for children to be less careful than adults; and

b an occupier may expect that a person, in the exercise of his calling, will appreciate and guard against any special risks ordinarily incident to it, so far as the occupier leaves him free to do so.'

When children come onto hospital premises, there is therefore a clear duty to take into account that they cannot be expected to exercise the same care for themselves as an adult. The staff must take into account their lack of foresight, the fact that they may be impetuous, may not be able to read warning notices, and, even if they can, may not take any notice of them. Consider the following case.

MARTIN V MIDDLESBROUGH CORPORATION[2]

A schoolgirl slipped and was injured by broken glass. The injury occurred in a school playground and the broken glass was probably part of a milk bottle. The defendants, the local education authority, were liable because, in the court's opinion, there should have been better arrangements for disposing of the empty bottles. The standard of care required of the defendants, who owed the common duty of care under the Occupiers Liability Act 1957, was stated to be that of 'a prudent parent in relation to his own children'.

The same principle would apply to the safety of the child on hospital premises. Thus, if there were extremely hot pipes and radiators on the ward, special precautions would have to be taken to protect children. It is necessary to undertake a risk assessment of the safety of the premises, the equipment, and the systems of work, from the perspective of the child patient (see below for risk assessment). Particular difficulties can arise if, as a result of a shortage of beds, a child has to be accommodated on an adult ward. If the child is able to move around the ward, special care must be taken.

Difficulties can also arise if parents are present on the ward with their child. They can be expected to act reasonably in protecting their child from dangers which are obvious to an adult. There may, however, be a dispute as to who at any given time was responsible for the child. The establishment of a system whereby the parent has a duty to notify the ward staff if they are leaving the child unattended is essential and would probably be seen as part of the occupier's duty of care.

A study has been undertaken by the Child Accident Prevention Trust[3] into accidents to children in hospital wards. It collected standardized information about accidents on children's wards from a range of paediatric units in order to identify major factors associated with accidents, to propose measures to reduce the frequency and severity of accidents, and to identify areas, if any, which require more detailed study. Such a study would then be undertaken. In their analysis of the accidents, they most frequently occurred between 0800 and 1159 hours. Thirty-five individual locations were identified; the main ward was the site most frequently involved, and falling the most frequent type of accident in that location (41.7% of all accidents were caused by a fall). Most frequently it was the head that was injured. The Trust concluded that many accidents in this study could have been prevented. The recommendations of the Child Accident Prevention Trust and the Royal College of Nursing on accidents to children in hospitals are listed below.

- Correct equipment should be used in every case and makeshift arrangements should not be permitted.
- Both staff and parents should be made aware of the equipment that is in use and the correct method of installing it.
- There should be proper facilities for the storage of equipment and toys, and these should be used when items are not needed.
- Beds should be replaced with the High-Lo type, and these should be kept in the low position unless the high position is actually required.
- One member of the ward team should be made responsible for safety.
- All nursing staff should review information about safety and accident prevention received during the basic training as part of their induction to the ward.
- Other staff (e.g. medical staff, health care assistants, clerical staff) should receive basic safety training as part of their induction to the ward.

The principle is that all reasonable care must be taken, and below are suggestions by the Child Accident Prevention Trust for making the ward a safe environment for children.

- Can you see clearly? Are trolleys or furniture blocking your view of the playroom and the ward?
- Are all the windows closed?
- Are electrical outlets covered?
- Are flexes from fans, televisions, telephones and so on out of reach?
- *Are toys stored away properly?*
- Have toys been checked so that broken toys are thrown away?
- Are doors to kitchens, cleaners' rooms, and disposal rooms shut?
- Are all drugs, disinfectants, and cleaning fluids stored away?
- Are all sharp items out of reach?
- Is the temperature of the unit between 21 and 24°C?
- Are cots well away from radiators?
- Are the sides up on empty cots?
- *Are all cot sides up?*

EXCLUSION OF THE VISITOR

It was noted above that the definition of visitor included a person present with the express or implied consent of the occupier. Occupiers can control whom they wish to be on the premises. They can also lay down the conditions for the continued presence of the visitor. Thus it is lawful for the hospital managers to state that no patient or visitor can bring onto the premises certain specified substances such as alcohol or drugs. Should the visitor refuse to observe such requirements, then he or she becomes a trespasser and can be asked to leave. If he or she refuses, the occupier can use reasonable force to evict him or her.

This may be important in the care of children in certain circumstances; for example, when:

- there is a dispute between parents on the hospital premises and the ward manager considers that they should leave the ward;
- an adolescent brings alcohol onto the ward against the express views of the ward manager; or
- aggressive and boisterous friends accompany an adolescent into a hospital.

In such cases, the visitors of the patient can be asked to leave. If it is the patient who is causing difficulties, the patient could be asked to leave, but here it would be a question of balancing the risks of harm to the patient against the dangers of their continued presence on the ward, taking into account other ways of controlling the situation.

Occupiers Liability Act 1984

The 1957 Act does not cover the situation relating to trespassers. Until the 1984 Act was passed the law relating to the nature of the duty owed to a trespasser was according to the common law (i.e. the decisions of judges).

Whether a duty is owed by the occupier to trespassers, in relation to risks on the premises, depends upon the following factors listed in section 1(3) of the Act. These are:

- if the occupier is aware of the danger or has reasonable grounds to believe that it exists;
- if the occupier knows or has reasonable grounds to believe that the other is in the vicinity of the danger concerned or that he may come into the vicinity of the danger (in either case, whether the other has lawful authority for being in that vicinity or not); and
- the risk is one against which, in all the circumstances of the case, he may reasonably be expected to offer the other some protection.

In applying these factors to decide if a duty is owed to a trespasser, it would be rare for a duty to be owed to an adult. There is, however, more likely to be a duty owed to a child trespasser. Thus, for example on hospital premises, if a child is expressly told that he or she cannot go through a particular door or into another section of the hospital and he or she disobeys those instructions, he or she becomes a trespasser for the purposes of the Occupiers Liability Acts. It is likely that a duty would then arise under the 1984 Act.

THE NATURE OF THE DUTY OWED TO TRESPASSERS

The 1984 Act defines a duty of care owed to a trespasser in section 1(4), as: 'The duty is to take such care as is reasonable in all the circumstances of the case to see that he does not suffer injury on the premises by reason of the danger concerned.'

The duty can be discharged by giving warnings, but in the case of children, this may have limited effect, depending upon the age of the child.

The following is an example of a situation in which the 1984 Act would be relevant.

TRESPASSING CHILD

A 5-year-old child with a chronic illness, who required frequent hospital admissions for intravenous therapy, was allowed to wander around the ward. Unnoticed, he went into the treatment room which he knew was out of bounds and drank some of the disinfectant which was in a cupboard. It would probably be held that the occupier owed a duty under the Act – the occupier was aware of the dangers in the treatment room, knew of the possibility of children entering it, and should have taken care to offer protection to the child. In such circumstances, in view of the age of the child, there would also be a duty of care under the laws of negligence to the child in respect of supervision by staff of his activities while on the ward.

HEALTH AND SAFETY AT WORK ACT 1974 AND THE REGULATIONS

The Health and Safety at Work Act 1974 is enforced through the criminal courts by the Health and Safety Inspectorate who have the power to prosecute for offences under the Act and the Regulations, and who have also powers of inspection and can issue enforcement or prohibition notices. Since the abolition of the Crown's immunity (by the National Health Service Amendment Act 1986) in relation to the health and safety laws, prosecutions and notices can be brought against the health authorities. Trusts do not enjoy any immunity from health and safety legislation.

Thus in a recent case, it was reported that Frenchay Healthcare NHS Trust was fined £15 000 by Bristol Magistrates over the death of an 81-year-old patient who fell from his bed onto a hot radiator pipe.[4]

The basic duty on the employer under the Health and Safety at Work Act 1974 is set out in section 2(1) below.

- It shall be the duty of every employer to ensure, so far as is reasonably practicable, the health, safety and welfare at work of all his employees.

Section 2(2) of the 1974 Act gives examples of the various duties which must be carried out but these do not detract from the width and comprehensiveness of the general duty.

Section 7 of the Act also places a specific responsibility upon the employee in the form of a statutory duty upon the employee:

- to take reasonable care for the health and safety of him or herself and of others who may be affected by his or her acts or omissions at work;
- as regards any duty imposed on his or her employer or any other person, to cooperate with him so far as is reasonable to enable that duty to be performed or complied with.

It is also a criminal offence for any person to interfere with health and safety measures according to section 8 of the Health and Safety at Work Act 1984. 'No person shall intentionally or recklessly interfere with or misuse anything provided in the interest of health, safety or welfare in pursuance of any relevant statutory provisions.'

The duties under the Health and Safety at Work Act are also owed to nonemployees, such as the general public or, in the context of health care, patients and their visitors.

Section 3(1) states: 'It shall be the duty of every employer to conduct his undertaking in such a way as to ensure, so far as is reasonably practicable, that a person not in his employment who may be affected thereby are not thereby exposed to risks to their health and safety.' A similar duty is placed upon self-employed people.

The effect of this wide duty to the public as well as the duty of care owed at common law to individual persons (see Chapter 13) is that the health authority or hospital trust must take major action to prevent harm to visitors or patients or employees, even if this may mean closing a unit. Such a decision would be preceded by a risk assessment in which the dangers of remaining open would have to be balanced against the loss of the facility if the unit was to close. Thus in one of the largest Scottish teaching hospitals, Ninewells Hospital in Dundee, the special care baby unit was closed to admissions on Monday 27 February 1995 after an outbreak of bacterial infection in which one baby died and three became ill. At the time the decision was made to close it, the unit was treating 13 premature and sick babies. The baby who died was suffering from a lung infection caused by Klebsiella. The hospital stated that, 'Medical and nursing staff have worked very hard and taken extraordinary precautions to limit the infection.' The other babies on the unit were put into quarantine and were screened. An outside consultant was to be appointed to undertake a further review and to make recommendations.[5]

HEALTH AND SAFETY REGULATIONS 1992

New regulations came into force on 1 January 1993 as a result of European Directives and are listed below.

- Management of Health and Safety at Work Regulations 1992
- Provision and Use of Work Equipment Regulations 1992
- Manual Handling Operations Regulations 1992
- Workplace (Health, Safety and Welfare Regulations) 1992
- Personal Protective Equipment at Work Regulations 1992
- Health and Safety (Display Screen Equipment) Regulations 1992

The effect of these regulations is to identify clearly the responsibilities placed upon employer and employee in the work context. The duties owed and the measures that must be taken to reduce the risk of harm protect not only employees but also the general public. Thus Regulation 3(1) of the Management of Health and Safety at Work Regulations 1992 requires: 'Every employer to make a suitable and sufficient assessment of (a) the risks to the health and safety of his employee to which they are exposed whilst they are at work; and (b) the risks to the health and safety of persons not in his employment arising out of or in connection with the conduct by him of his undertaking, for the purpose of identifying the measures he needs to take to comply with the requirements and prohibitions imposed upon him by or under the relevant statutory provisions.'

This risk assessment is at the heart of the provision of a safe place for the care of sick children and all staff must cooperate in its implementation.

The duty also applies to independent health professionals such as independent midwives and physiotherapists. Regulation 3 paragraph (2) requires every self-employed person to make a suitable and sufficient assessment of (a) the risks to their own health and safety to which they are exposed while they are at work; and (b) the risks to the health and safety of persons not in their employment arising out of or in connection with the conduct by them of their undertaking, for the purposes of identifying the measures they need to take to comply with the requirements and prohibitions imposed upon them by or under the relevant statutory provisions.

Duty to review the assessment

There is a duty under regulation 3(3) to review the assessment when there is reason to suspect that it is no longer valid or there has been significant change in the matters to which it relates.

If more than five people are employed, there must be a record of the findings of the assessment and any group of employees identified as being especially at risk.

Thus the regulations will apply to GP practices in which more than five people are employed.

Manual handling

It might be thought that those who work with children would be unlikely to have concerns with manual handling, yet those who work with the physically handicapped child can be at great risk from back injuries. So, too, can those who work with younger children or even babies, as even if the weight which they have to carry or move is not great, they may find that because of fixed cot sides, or other equipment which does not take into account the necessary bending of staff, damage to staff can occur. They should therefore be aware of the manual handling regulations and ensure that they are implemented both in the care of children in institutions and in the community.

THE MANUAL HANDLING REGULATIONS

The Manual Handling Regulations came into force on 1 January 1993. Guidance is provided in the form of a code of practice by the Health and Safety Executive and, in addition, a working group set up by the Health and Safety Commission has produced a booklet on guidance on manual handling of loads in the health services.[6] This document is described as 'an authoritative document which will be used by health and safety inspectors in describing reliable and fully acceptable methods of achieving health and safety in the workplace'. Part of this health services specific guidance material relates to staff working in the community.

Content of the regulations
The duty under the regulations can be summed up as follows.

- If reasonably possible, avoid the hazardous manual handling.
- Make a suitable and sufficient assessment of any hazardous manual handling which cannot be avoided.
- Reduce the risk of injury from this handling so far as is reasonably practicable.
- Review the assessment.

For full details of the Regulations and the guidance issued by the Health and Safety Commission reference must be made to their publications.

The Regulations, like the Health and Safety Act 1974, are enforceable through the criminal courts in a prosecution initiated by the Health and Safety Inspectorate. Their powers to inspect, and issue enforcement and prohibition orders, are important in preventing harm arising.

CIVIL CLAIMS FOR BACK INJURIES

If injuries have occurred and compensation is required, the person harmed or their representative would bring a civil action alleging negligence by the defendant or the defendant's employees. There has recently been an increase in litigation claims for back injuries to health employees. Sizeable awards have been made where it has been established that the employer was in breach of the duty of care owed to the employee and as a result harm has been caused to the employee (see below and also Chapter 13). Breach of the regulations can also give rise to claims for compensation in the civil courts.

DUTY OF THE EMPLOYER AS AN IMPLIED TERM OF THE CONTRACT OF EMPLOYMENT

It was noted in Chapter 15 that some of the terms in the contract of employment are implied by the law. These include the obligation of the employer to safeguard the health and safety of the employee by employing competent staff, setting up a safe system of work and maintaining safe premises, equipment, and plant. The employee must obey the reasonable instructions of the employer and take reasonable care in carrying out the work. Thus, as has been seen in the discussion on manual handling above, the employee may have a claim for breach of contract by the employer if his or her back has been injured as a result of failures on the employer's part in not providing the appropriate training or equipment.

CONTROL OF SUBSTANCES HAZARDOUS TO HEALTH

Although all health workers have responsibilities under the Regulations concerning the control of substances hazardous to health, those professionals caring for the child have specific risks to bear in mind in carrying out the assessments required by law.

The five stages set out in the guide issued by the Health and Safety Executive are shown below.[7]

- Gather information about the substances, the work and the working practices.
- Evaluate the risks to health.
- Decide what needs to be done.

- Record the assessment.
- Review the assessment.

There must be clarity over who has the responsibility of carrying out the assessment, but the guidance emphasizes the importance of involving all employees in the assessment.

All potentially hazardous substances must be identified: these will include domestic materials, such as bleach, toilet cleaner, window cleaner, and polishes; and office materials, such as correction fluids and the medicinal products in the treatment room.

An assessment has to be made for each substance as to whether it could be inhaled, swallowed, absorbed or introduced through the skin, or injected into the body (such as needles).

The effects of each route of entry or contact and the potential harm must then be identified, as must the persons who could be exposed and how.

Once this assessment is complete, decisions must be made on the measures necessary to comply with the regulations and who should undertake the different tasks. In certain cases, health surveillance is required if there is a reasonable likelihood that the disease or ill effect associated with exposure could occur in the workplace concerned. Thus the administration of cytotoxic drugs should be accompanied by strict procedures for protecting staff from exposure and monitoring staff regularly. Similarly, staff who care for HIV positive children or those with AIDS should be given the opportunity to be checked for infections.

Mangers should ensure that the employees are given information, instruction, and training. If parents are involved in the use of hazardous substances in caring for their child, they too should be given all the necessary information.

Records should show the results of assessment, the action that has been taken and by whom, and that the situation is being regularly monitored and reviewed.

PROTECTION OF CHILDREN FROM DANGEROUS STAFF, BOGUS PROFESSIONALS AND KIDNAPPING

Allitt situation

In 1993 and 1994 all paediatric units were put on the alert after the crimes of Beverly Allitt, the kidnapping of Abbie Humphries, and several cases of bogus professionals attempting to treat or remove patients. Although in one sense their actions give rise to different issues, in each one the role of the management and that of each individual health professional caring for the child should be considered. The legal implications of the Beverly Allitt case are discussed further in Chapter 15 in relation to the contract of employment. In the context of this chapter, health professionals should note that even though they are unlikely to encounter an Allitt situation, they must still be aware of the possibility that a member of staff could be responsible for harming patients.

Such incidents could occur in a midwifery unit, nursery or special care baby unit or any unit, of a hospital or community. The Clothier inquiry, which was set up to investigate the deaths and injuries caused by Beverly Allitt, admitted that, even if all the recommendations were to be implemented, 'no measures can afford complete protection against a determined miscreant. The main lesson from our Inquiry and our principal recommendation is that the Grantham disaster should serve to heighten awareness in all those caring for children of the possibility of malevolent intervention as a cause of unexplained clinical events.'

What is clear is the need for far greater management control over staff, their sickness records and information concerning their present physical and mental health.

Staff too should be encouraged, as a result of the recent freedom of speech circulars, to raise their concerns with management without the fear of reprisals or victimization. High standards of care should be identified and linked with an unwillingness to accept changes in the child's condition as an inevitable consequence of being ill. Complacency is the biggest danger.

Security against intruders and bogus professionals

In 1990 a woman posing as a health visitor snatched a 1-day-old baby from St Thomas' Hospital, London (the Griffiths case). In Nottingham in 1994,[8] Abbie Humphries, a 4-hour-old baby in a maternity ward, was handed to a person pretending to be a nurse and claiming that she wished to take the baby for a hearing test. It was several weeks before she was arrested. The incident led to a review of security measures in special care baby units, maternity units, and hospitals generally.

In another incident in 1994,[9] it was reported that a failed medical student had been convicted of masquerading as a trainee doctor on a hospital ward for 3 weeks, during which time he carried out physical examinations upon patients, took patients' histories and performed blood pressure tests. He was eventually discovered when a nurse became suspicious when he tried to prescribe two antibiotics for a patient on a diabetic ward.

Such incidents are now foreseeable. The obligation upon hospital managers is to ensure that all reasonable measures are undertaken to prevent bogus staff or intruders kidnapping or harming patients. What would be considered to be reasonable?

Some trusts are now exploring the possibility of introducing new measures. These are:

- electronic tags on young babies and children;
- identity cards for staff;
- electronic identity tags for staff;
- locks on all main entrances; and
- security guards on all entrances.

The costs of these measures are considerable. However, the decision on the reasonableness of what could have been done will take into account the cost of the precautions which could have been taken against the value of such measures in preventing the risk of harm. If a trust were to be sued after the abduction of a child or baby, in its defence it would have to establish what measures it took to prevent that occurrence and show the reasonableness of what it did against the unreasonableness of measures that the plaintiff might allege should have been taken to prevent the abduction. The records of the assessment undertaken and the resulting action that has been taken are important in establishing the trust's defence. The trust is not liable for the actions of intruders, kidnappers, and other criminals. It is, however, liable if it failed to take reasonable measures to protect patients from the reasonably foreseeable harm which such persons can cause.

All staff have a major role to play in being alert to possible dangers and ensuring the highest standards of practice. They also need to explain to parents and relatives the reasons for some restrictions imposed to improve security.

MUNCHAUSEN BY PROXY

Munchausen by proxy, whereby an adult deliberately creates symptoms to gain medical attention for him- or herself and his or her child, is now recognized as a possible cause for the child being admitted to hospital. The syndrome was first described by Professor Roy Meadow in 1977 at St James Hospital, Leeds and the term 'Meadow's syndrome' is now used by some paediatricians to describe the condition.

Child professionals therefore need to be alert to the possibility that a parent or other adult is causing harm to the child. However, the suspicion that such a situation exists can give rise to considerable ethical and legal issues, as listed below.

- What if there is only a suspicion and no evidence yet present to justify reasonable belief?
- How can evidence be obtained?
- What action can be taken to prevent the parent caring for and therefore harming the child?

(Reference should be made to Chapter 9.)

Concern has recently arisen as a result of the use of videos in hospitals to film parents with their children. Terry Thomas[10] considers the ethical issues in using covert video surveillance to film parents who are suspected of injuring their children. He described how these cameras can provide evidence of parents deliberately injuring the child, for example by suffocation or by administering poisonous substances. Volunteer nurses with special training continuously watch the screens and keep written records of what they see. They initiate prompt intervention if a child looks likely to suffer from harm. The paediatric team at North Staffordshire Hospital, Stoke-on-Trent, has produced a protocol on how covert video surveillance might best be implemented.[11] Terry Thomas points out that there is nothing illegal about covert video surveillance, and video-cassettes of captured incidents have been used successfully in court as prosecution evidence; he cites an example in 1991 when a jury at Croydon Crown Court took 5 hours to reach a majority verdict on a 19-year-old Bristol woman who has been charged with cruelty to a child.[12] No case has yet been taken to the European Court of Human Rights on the grounds that covert video surveillance violates article 8 of the European Convention on Human Rights, which states that everyone has the right to respect for their private and family life.

In discussing the ethical issues, Terry Thomas suggests that the secrecy surrounding covert video surveillance is contrary to the spirit of the Access to Health Records Act (see Chapter 8) and the Patient's charter. He questions whether this evidence is necessary to protect the child, especially if there is already evidence of child abuse. Liberty (formerly the National Council for Civil Liberties) has called for statutory regulation on covert video surveillance. Terry Thomas concludes that: 'At best covert video surveillance is a valid technique for helping to protect children. At worst, it is an unnecessary invasion of privacy using a new piece of technology – the video camera – that has simply gone in search of a 'problem' to solve.'

In his discussion of the ethical issues raised by the use of covert video surveillance in the investigation of suspected child abuse and Munchausen by proxy syndrome, Donald Evans[13] concludes that there is an undeniable element of research involved in the procedure and that the welfare of all those subjected to surveillance would be best protected by the submission of the protocol to an independent committee for ethical assessment (see page 177).

CONTROL OF THE CHILD

Child professionals sometimes have difficulty in controlling children on the wards and protecting their health and safety. The very physically ill may of course be confined to bed, but other children who are encouraged to be ambulant may provide staff with behavioural and management problems. This can become particularly distressing in psychiatric units or units for the care of those with learning disabilities. It may also present a problem in the care of those children with a chronic condition, who require regular admissions for treatment in hospital. The difficulties in maintaining discipline which some schools experience can thus also be a problem for paediatric units. This is compounded by the greater dangers which can exist for a child in a hospital context. The health professional cannot necessarily rely upon the parents to control their child, as they may not be present with the child the whole time and even if they were, they may not be in control.

Corporal punishment

If the health professional is acting in place of the parent (in locus parenti), he or she has, in theory, the right to discipline the child with corporal punishment. In a recent case a registered child minder was refused registration under the Children Act 1989 on the grounds that she would not undertake not to smack a minded child; she was therefore automatically considered to be not fit to look after children under the age of 8 years. Her position was that she wished to reserve for herself an ability to smack gently if appropriate and only if the parent wished it. She appealed to the Magistrates Court against this refusal to register her, and won. The local authority appealed to the Family Division and lost. The Family Division held that there was nothing in the Children Act 1989, nor, the guidance and regulations, that required a local authority to take an inflexible policy on the issue of corporal punishment. If they adopted that policy, a person could appeal against a refusal of registration and the Magistrates could then consider all the evidence. The Family Division held there were no grounds for changing the decision of the Magistrates.[14]

In spite of this theoretical power, the use of corporal punishment should be avoided. The professional could face a civil action for trespass or a criminal action for assault or grievous bodily harm. Dismissal after disciplinary proceedings may also occur. In the *Sunday Times*, 20 November 1994, it was reported that a nurse employed by Salford Health Authority who had been dismissed after she smacked a troublesome child failed in her application for unfair dismissal. She had worked at the Royal Manchester Children's Hospital for over 20 years.

It might, however, in certain extreme situations, be necessary to prevent the child from carrying out a particular activity by using physical measures, such as restraining the child from hitting another or entering the treatment room. In such cases the force used should be consistent with the circumstances and reasonable to effect the purpose. Any excess force could be deemed an assault.

A UN committee has attacked the UK for defending the right of parents to smack their offspring and accused the Government of failing to improve children's health, education, and living standards.[15] The report by the UN Committee on the Rights of the Child recommended that physical punishment of children in families and in public schools should be prohibited in law. It stated that physical punishment was banned by an international convention signed by the UK. (The report's recommendations are not binding and there is no international body to ensure that governments comply.) The association known as EPOCH – End Physical Punishment of Children – has consistently fought to end smacking within the home and institutions and has produced a pamphlet 'The No Smacking Guide to Good Behaviour' designed to assist parents avoid smacking. This may be of value to health professionals caring for children. Reference ought also to be made to the report of the Gulbenkian Commision on Children and Violence,[16] chaired by Sir William Utting, which condemned smacking of children by parents, advocating positive discipline in place of counter-productive punishments. The practical support it recommends to assist parents in controlling the child would also be of great value to health professionals working with children.

In some very serious situations it may be necessary to ask the parents to take the child home; however, this would have to be balanced against the risks involved in discontinuing care. It may be relevant in the care of the older child, who can be reasoned with and told the terms on which he or she can receive treatment. Sometimes, especially in units for medium- or long-term treatment, staff may require additional training for caring for children with behavioural problems. If management seems unsympathetic to such needs, evidence should be collated of the specific difficulties and dangers which arise. If possible, multidisciplinary action should be taken to identify the specific problems and discuss how they can be resolved. It may be, for example, that a specific person or professional is able to establish a good rapport with the child and thus assist in controlling the situation. The powers which exist in relation to children with a mental disorder are discussed in Chapter 21.

RECORDS

Under the Health and Safety legislation certain accidents and incidents must by law be reported directly to the Health and Safety Executive and be recorded. These include fatal accidents, major injury accidents, and reportable lost time accidents. The latter category includes accidents which are reportable because of the type of injury and those which are reportable because of the cause of the accident.

The health professional should, however, ensure that even if the accident is not reportable by law, a record is kept of the occurrence and action taken to prevent a reccurrence. Reference should be made to the publication of the UKCC on standards for records and record keeping. Should litigation or any other court procedure arise, the clarity and comprehensiveness of the records will be a vital element in establishing the causes of the harm and the actions that were taken. Records are not, of course, proof of the truth of what is stated within them, but the person who wrote them would be questioned on the weight which can be attached to them by the court for accuracy and relevance. Reference should be made to the advice of the UKCC of Nursing, Health Visiting and Midwifery on records and record keeping.[17] The essential elements set out in paragraph 13 are of value to all health professionals. The Audit Commission[18] has recently published a study of medical records. Even though it relates to hospital records, its conclusions and recommendations are relevant to the community. It supports the extension of the patient-held records schemes, including some of the new initiatives such as smart cards, but it points out that many of the basic improvements contained in the report need to be in place before radical solutions are contemplated (see Chapter 8).

CONCLUSION

The health and safety of patients and staff is of prime concern to any health organization. Duties in relation to health and safety are included in a variety of statutes and the common law; some are enforced through the criminal courts, others enable claims for compensation to take place in the civil courts. In addition, all employees have responsibilities in their contract of employment for health and safety and all registered practitioners will also owe duties set by their registration bodies through Codes of Professional Conduct which relate to health and safety (see Chapter 15).

REFERENCES

1 Salvage J, Rogers R: *Health and Safety and the Nurse.* London: Heinemann; 1988. [See also: Salvage J: *Nurses at Risk: Guide to Health and Safety at Work.* London: Heinemann; 1988. Dimond BC: *The Legal Aspects of Midwifery.* Hale: Cheshire: Books for Midwives Press; 1994: pp173–189. Dimond BC: *The Legal Aspects of Nursing, edn 2.* Hemel Hempstead: Prentice Hall; 1995: pp182–202.]
2 (1965) 63 LGR 385.
3 Child Accident Prevention Trust and Royal College of Nursing: *Accidents to Children on Hospital Wards.* London: Child Accident Prevention Trust; 1992.
4 *Times* 7 March 1995.
5 *Times* 1 March 1995.
6 Health and Safety Commission: *Guidance on Manual Handling of loads in the Health Services.* London: HMSO; 1992.
7 Health and Safety Executive: *A Step-By-Step Guide to COSHH Assessment.* London: HMSO; 1993.
8 *Times* 2 July 1994.
9 *Times* 6 May 1994.
10 Thomas T: Under surveillance. *Health Serv J* 1995, 104:24–25.
11 Staffordshire Area Child Protection Committee: *Guidelines for the multi-agency management of patients suspected or at risk of suffering from life-threatening abuse resulting in cyanotic-apnoeic episodes.* Staffordshire Hospital Trust, Staffordshire Social Services and Staffordshire Police; 1994.
12 Hospital filmed mother trying to stop baby breathing. *Independent* 30 October 1991.
13 Evans D: The investigation of life-threatening child abuse and Munchausen syndrome by proxy. *J Med Ethics* 1995, 21: 9–13.
14 London Borough of Sutton *v* Davis [1994] 1 FLR 737

15 Barnwell R: News report. *Times* 28 January 1995.

16 Utting W: *Report of the Gulbenkian Commission on Childhood Violence.* London: Calouste Gulbenkian Foundation: 1995.

17 UKCC: *Standards for records and record keeping.* London: UKCC; 1993.

18 Audit Commission: *Setting the records straight: a study of hospital medical records.* London: HMSO; 1995.

Legal issues relating to substance abuse

Health professionals who care for the adolescent child are increasingly likely to encounter children who have problems with drink, solvent abuse, drugs, or a combination of these. They have to answer such questions as those listed below.

- Can I exclude a child from the hospital?
- Can I prevent visitors coming in with some or all of the following: drink, drugs, solvents?
- What are my powers for searching a patient or visitor?
- If I discover drink or drugs can I remove them from the patient or visitor without their consent?
- What are the laws relating to those who are recognized as being addicted to drugs?

Information is available from the Department of Health[1] who can, on request, provide the addresses and telephone numbers of local contact points. This chapter looks at the laws in this area and seeks to answer the above questions.

DRINK

Under the age of 5 years a child can only be given alcohol in an emergency or as part of medical treatment (Children and Young Persons Act 1933 section 5; Criminal Justice Act 1967 section 92(1) Schedule 3, Part 1). At other ages, the provisions listed below apply.

- Above 5 years of age a child can drink alcohol in private.
- At 14 years of age a child can go into a public house, but not to drink or buy alcohol (Licensing Act 1964 section 168(8)).
- At 16 years of age a child can go into a public house and drink beer, port, cider or sherry with a meal in a part of the establishment that has been set aside as a dining area or restaurant and is not a bar. He or she cannot, however, buy these products (Licensing Act 1964 section 169(4)).
- At 18 years of age a person can buy and drink alcohol in a public house or licensed premises.

Drink on hospital premises and the powers of the occupier

Hospitals can create their own rules within the general laws of the country on alcohol consumption and visitors bringing in alcohol. The normal rule would be that it is forbidden for visitors or patients to bring alcoholic drinks into hospital without obtaining the express permission of the ward staff. These rules can be enforced through the power of the occupier of any premises to lay down conditions for the entry of a person onto those premises and for their remaining on them. This is further discussed in Chapter 16 on the Health and Safety laws and in the first part of that chapter on the Occupier's Liability Acts 1957 and 1984. If visitors were to ignore these conditions then the visitors could be asked to leave, taking with them, the forbidden substances. If they refuse to go, they can be evicted with reasonable force as they have become trespassers.

If it is the patient who has brought alcohol onto the premises, he or she may be too ill to be asked to leave. However, it should be possible to remove the forbidden goods, as a condition of the patient remaining. This issue can arise in the care of the adolescent who suffers from a chronic illness such as cystic fibrosis. Their condition may require frequent inpatient admissions, yet they still want to live in the style and custom of their contemporaries. It is essential that there are clear rules laid down by the hospital or ward management in relation to their care while in hospital and that the patients understand the conditions of their stay. Ultimately, if the patient does not accept the conditions, he or she could be asked to leave. Health professionals should be aware that drinking among young children is causing 10 times more damage than drugs, but its dangers are being ignored. The Royal College of Physicians and British Paediatric Association have made 35 recommendations for tackling the issue.[2]

DRUGS[3]

Misuse of Drugs Act 1971

The Misuse of Drugs Act and subsequent legislation makes provision for the classification of controlled drugs and their possession, supply, and manufacture. The Act makes it a criminal offence to manufacture, supply, and possess controlled drugs contrary to the regulations. Controlled drugs are divided into three categories. Class A includes, among others, cocaine, diamorphine, morphine, opium, pethidine, and class B substances when prepared for injection. Class B includes, among others, oral amphetamines, barbiturates, cannabis, and codeine. Class C includes, among others, most benzodiazepines, and meprobamate.

The Misuse of Drugs Regulations 1985 divides controlled drugs into five schedules, listed below, each specifying the requirements governing activities such as import, export, production, supply, possession, prescribing, and record keeping.

- Schedule 1 – cannabis, lysergic acid, et cetera. Possession and supply are prohibited except in accordance with Home Office authority.
- Schedule 2 – diamorphine, morphine, pethidine, etc. Regulations control prescriptions, safe custody, and keeping of registers.
- Schedule 3 – barbiturates. Supply is subject, apart from phenobarbitone, to special prescription requirements.
- Schedule 4 – benzodiazepines, et cetera. These are subject to minimum control. They are not subject to safe custody and the controlled drug prescription requirements do not apply.
- Schedule 5 – drugs containing only minute strengths of controlled drugs. These are exempt from virtually all controlled drug requirements other than the retention of invoices for 2 years. Thus this category is sometimes known as 'CD Inv'.

Any patient or visitor bringing a controlled drug into the hospital without authority can be asked to leave the premises and the police could be summoned for assistance. If a patient is believed to be carrying drugs, he or she could be asked to agree to a search and, if he or she refuses, could be asked to leave the premises. If he or she is very seriously ill and in need of treatment, the forfeiture of any drugs could still be made a condition of staying on the premises.

What is the situation regarding the destruction of drugs which the patient has brought in with him? Illicitly obtained drugs may be handed over to the hospital or community staff. The Misuse of Drugs Act 1971 states that in certain circumstances, the person who receives them will not him- or herself be committing an offence.[4] These circumstances are that:

- they knew or suspected the substance to be a controlled drug;
- they took possession for the purpose of (a) preventing another person from committing an offence, or continuing to commit an offence in connection with that drug, or (b) delivering it into the custody of a person lawfully entitled to take custody of it;
- as soon as possible after taking possession they took all steps reasonably open to them either to destroy the drug or deliver it into the custody of a person lawfully entitled to take custody.

In a hospital the pharmacist would obviously be asked to take responsibility for any confiscated controlled drugs.

Drug addicts

What is the situation in relation to drug addicts? The Regulations state that a person is to be regarded as an addict 'if, and only if, he has as a result of repeated administration become so dependent on a drug that he has an overpowering desire for the administration of it to be continued' [Misuse of Drugs (Notification of and Supply to Addicts) Regulations 1973.]

The doctor must notify the Home Office Chief Medical Officer of the particulars of persons addicted to specific drugs (including cocaine, diamorphine, methadone, and opium) within 7 days of their considering, or having reasonable grounds to believe, that there may be an addiction. These particulars must include:

- name, address, sex, date of birth;
- NHS number;
- date of attendance; and
- name of drugs concerned.

If, therefore, a health professional suspects that one of his or her clients is addicted, he or she should ensure that a medical practitioner is informed and the requisite details are sent to the Home Office. Excluded from these provisions is any person receiving continued administration for treating organic disease or injury. Once a notification has been made, a further report is required at 12-month intervals.

SUPPLY TO ADDICTS

Only a doctor holding a licence from the Home Office is able to supply, prescribe or administer diamorphine, cocaine, or dipipanone to addicts. Any doctor can supply controlled drugs to addicts if the purpose is the treatment of organic disease or injury.

Two NHS prescription forms are provided for doctors to use when prescribing for addicts. The forms enable addicts to receive supplies of drugs on a daily basis. Form FP10(HP)Ad is issued by health authorities to doctors in hospital drug addiction clinics. Form FP10(MDA) is issued by the FHSA to any GP on request under NHS(GMS)Regulations 1992 SI 1992 No. 635. The form may be used for the instalment prescribing of any Schedule 2 controlled drug being used in the treatment of addiction in the patient. The prescription must state the amount per instalment and the interval between instalments. The Regulations restrict the supply to a maximum of 14 days per form.

Do nonillicit drugs have to be destroyed? Can drugs brought in by one patient be reused for another? The Code of Ethics of the Royal Pharmaceutical Society of Great Britain states that 'under no circumstances must medication brought in by patients be considered for re-use by anyone else'. If medicines are returned to the pharmacy from the wards, the pharmacist must examine them and assess their suitability for being returned to stock. This would take into account the necessary storage conditions, the condition of the pack, and the date. Sometimes it may be appropriate for the patient to take these drugs home with him or her. This must be subject to veto by the pharmacist.

The World Health Organization and the International Council of Nurses 1991 set out the components of the nurses' role in dealing with substance abuse (provider of care, counsellor or therapist, educator or resource, advocate, promoter of health),[5] and these are discussed by Anthony Sheehan.[6] He points out that nurses have a multitude of complex roles, and represent one of the best placed professional groups to assist in managing this problem. Such a variety of roles can, however, lead to legal conflicts in relation to respecting the rights of the child and the disclosure of confidential information to others in the best interests of the child.

ADDICTION IN MOTHERS AND YOUNG BABIES

At present there are no laws in this country which enable action to be taken against a pregnant woman to prevent the fetus being harmed by any drugs or other substances taken by her. Nor can the fetus be made a ward of court before it is born.

In Re F[7] the mother was aged 36 years and had suffered from severe mental disturbance since 1977. Throughout 1982 she had led a nomadic existence, wandering around Europe. She had returned in 1983 and had been settled in a flat in south London. Her only means of support was supplementary benefit. The local authority was concerned about the baby expected towards the end of January. Early in January the mother disappeared. The local authority instituted wardship proceedings. The Court of Appeal were of the opinion that they did not have the power to institute wardship proceedings for a fetus. They pointed to the difficulties of enforcing such an order against the expectant mother.

Once the baby is born, however, the local authority can seek an order taking the child into care and can use the prebirth conduct of the mother to justify the need for the child to be removed from the addicted mother.[8]

SOLVENT ABUSE

Health professionals need to know the signs of possible solvent abuse by their patients and ensure that appropriate action is taken. There is evidence from the deaths from solvent misuse, that solvent sniffing is increasing and the Department of Health advice to parents[9] estimates that in the average home there are over 30 sniffable products, including lighter fuel, aerosol sprays, correcting fluids, dry-cleaning fluids, and petrol. The Intoxicating Substances Supply Act 1985 makes it an offence to supply to a young person under the age of 18 years a substance which the supplier knows, or has reason to believe, will be used to achieve intoxication.

Health professionals should ensure that they have the relevant training to identify children at risk and that there are policies in place for taking appropriate action.

REFERENCES

1 Further information is available from: Information Officer, Department of Health, Skipton House, 80 London Road, Elephant and Castle, London SE1 6LW.

2 Royal College of Physicians and British Paediatric Association: *Alcohol and the Young*. London: Royal College of Physicians; 1995.

3 Merrills J, Fisher J: *Pharmacy Law and Practice*. Oxford: Blackwell Scientific Ltd; 1995. [See also Appelbe SE, Wingfield J: *Pharmacy Law and Ethics*. London: Pharmaceutical Press; 1993.]

4 Merrills J, Fisher J: *Pharmacy Law and Practice*. Oxford: Blackwell Scientific Ltd; 1995: p143.

5 World Health Organization and the International Council of Nurses: *Nurses responding to Substance Misuse*. Geneva: WHO/ICN; 1991.

6 Sheehan A: Nurses' role in relation to substance misuse. *Br J Nurs* 1992, 1:167.

7 In Re F (in utero) 1988 2 All ER 193.

8 In Re D (a minor) v Berkshire County Council and others 1987 1 All ER 20

9 Department of Health: *Solvents: a Parent's Guide. The Signs. The Dangers. What to Do*. London: HMSO; 1994 [See also Department of Health: *Drug and Solvent Misuse: a Basic Briefing*. HMSO; 1993.]

CHAPTER

18

Child health care and complementary medicines

'Complementary' is defined as: completing: together making up a whole... of medical treatment, therapies, etc...' (*complementum* from *com-* intensive and *-plere* to fill).[1] Complementary medicine is thus seen to work in parallel with orthodox medicine. The BCMA states that therapy groups which it represents advise and encourage patients to see their doctor whenever appropriate. Complementary therapy, however, cannot be seen as outside the NHS, and it is open to any GP to arrange for a complementary therapist to offer NHS treatment within his or her practice. This also applies to fundholding practices which can purchase complementary therapies for their patients.[2]

In 1991 the Consumers Association reported that one in four of their readers visited an alternative or complementary therapist, double the number found in a survey in 1986.[3] The increasing use of complementary medicines in health care has been facilitated by the internal market and the fact that GP fundholders are able to purchase services for their patients from outside the NHS and therefore take advantage of the use of complementary or alternative therapy. This chapter looks at:

- the place of such therapies in child care;
- the consent of the child;
- the standard of care which should be provided; and
- the implications to health professionals of the use of complementary therapies.

WITHIN THE NHS

In 1993 the National Association of Health Authorities and Trusts[4] published the report of a survey undertaken on the use of complementary therapies within the NHS. The survey of district health authorities, FHSAs, and GP fundholders of their attitudes towards the availability of complementary therapies in the NHS was supplemented by a questionnaire to the Royal Colleges, medical organizations, patient representative organizations, and complementary therapy bodies on their view of the role of complementary therapies within the NHS.

Over 50% of respondent district health authorities, FHSAs and GP fundholders considered that some complementary therapies should be available on the NHS. Those who did not were influenced by:

- lack of proven effectiveness;
- lack of proven cost effectiveness;
- resource constraints and priorities;

- fears about uncontrolled demands on NHS resources; and
- lack of demand from the public or from GPs.

Acupuncture received the greatest support from those responding, almost 100% of FHSAs considering that it should be available on the NHS; osteopathy was the next most popular; then homoeopathy, chiropractic and aromatherapy had support from less than 25%; reflexology had less than 5%.

Figures on availability within the NHS showed that 15% of the FHSAs had approved a policy on complementary therapies and 44 of the FHSAs (55 had been approached) had given approval to health promotion clinics which wholly or partly used complementary therapies. Acupuncture was the most common therapy to have been given approval and was mainly used in smoking cessation and pain relief clinics. In the main, district health authorities were funding complementary therapies on an individual basis as extracontractual referrals. Forty-three per cent of district health authorities had contracts for complementary therapies with either NHS providers or providers in the private sector. Some authorities refused to fund extracontractual referrals for complementary therapies whereas others would only fund them if the conventional therapies had failed to produce satisfactory results. The survey of GP fundholders showed that complementary therapies could be used for: chronic back pain, osteoarthritis, rheumatoid arthritis, hay fever, anxiety, insomnia, obesity, smoking, peptic ulcer, and mature onset diabetes.

The report concludes that well over £1 million was spent on complementary therapies in 1992. In general, funding complementary therapies is not given a high priority. There is a lack of agreement about the effectiveness of individual therapies compounded by a general lack of information about therapies, appropriate training and qualifications, cost-effectiveness, and current regulations on commissioning such therapies. The report recommends the following action.

- Research into the effectiveness of complementary therapies
- Evaluation of complementary therapy services currently available within the NHS
- Research into the cost–benefit of complementary therapies
- Development of standards for training and qualification
- Wide dissemination of guidelines, research findings, and general information

The National Association of Health Authorities and Trusts report fails to look at the extent to which children are receiving complementary therapies for their care whether inside or outside the NHS. However, it is apparent that if there is a growing use of complementary therapies by adults, they are likely to make use of such treatments for their children, especially in such chronic conditions as asthma and skin allergies, and other conditions which are not easily cured by conventional medicine. The treatment of children with nonconventional medicine raises several legal issues.

CONSENT OF THE CHILD

Exactly the same principles for consent would apply as in the case of conventional medicine, which are discussed in Chapter 6. The child, if Gillick-competent, could give consent in his or her own right. For the 16- or 17-year-old child the Family Law Reform Act 1969 would apply.

CONSENT OF THE PARENT

The parent could also give consent on behalf of the child. However, the parent can only give consent if the treatment is in the best interests of the child. This can cause some difficulties in relation to complementary and alternative therapies. In conventional medicine the courts have applied the standard of the reasonable professional, known as the Bolam test,[5] that is, the test as to whether there has been negligence or not is the standard of the ordinary skilled person exercising and professing to have that special skill (see Chapter 13).

STANDARD OF CARE IN COMPLEMENTARY MEDICINE

How would standards in complementary medicine be defined to establish whether parents had acted in the best interests of the child?

Experts from the field

Therapists with membership of the British Complementary Medicine Association would have known standards on which their senior members could give evidence. Codes of practice and protocols have been developed by the schools that offer training in complementary medicine therapies. Respected members of the therapy in dispute would be called upon to give evidence as to what standard could have been expected of the reasonable therapist. If, for example, parents decided that conventional therapy was not working on the asthmatic condition of their son and took him off the drugs prescribed within the NHS and consulted a homoeopathic specialist, how could it be determined whether they were acting in the best interests of the child or were at risk of harming the child?

If the child's asthma deteriorated, there could either be:

- an action by the parent on the grounds that the homoeopathist was in breach of his or her duty of care to the child and caused harm to him or her; or
- an action by the local authority to ensure that the child obtained what was deemed to be the correct treatment.

The parents would have to show that no reasonable homoeopathist would have acted in the way in which this one did. They would also have to show that it was the actions of the complementary therapist which caused the harm to the child; this might be difficult given that the child is already suffering from a serious condition.

In contrast, expert witnesses for the homoeopathist would give evidence that the defendant acted in accordance with the practice of any reasonable practitioner exercising and professing to have those special skills. In the final analysis the judge would determine whether the defendant failed to comply with the expected standard.

In relation to the possible action against the parents, it is possible that if they discontinued conventional treatment against all reasonable advice, and thereby caused harm to the child, they could face prosecution. A case is discussed in Chapter 6 (page 62) in which parents who discontinued insulin treatment for their diabetic daughter in favour of their own preferred treatment were convicted of causing her death.[6]

THE CHILD HEALTH PROFESSIONAL AND COMPLEMENTARY MEDICINE

The child health professional can be involved in two ways.

First, he or she may be caring for a child whose parents wish (or for a child who wishes) for treatment to be with complementary therapies. This means that the health professional must ensure that he or she knows sufficient about the therapy in question to understand the impact that it may have on any conventional treatment and vice versa.

Second, the health professionals may be trained in a specific complementary therapy and wish to give the benefits of this to the patient. In this situation they must ensure that they have the consent of their employer to work within their own field of complementary therapy as part of their usual work as a conventional medicine practitioner. For example, a paediatric nurse might decide to follow up an interest in acupuncture. The nurse should not, however, practise this within his or her job unless the employer's consent has been obtained. Failure to obtain this consent could mean that the nurse was considered to be acting outside the course of employment should harm occur to the patient, and the nurse could then be held personally liable. In contrast, if the nurse were acting with the employer's specific permission or knowledge, the employer would probably be regarded as vicariously liable for any harm that the nurse had caused (see Chapter 13 on negligence for discussion on vicarious liability).

It is also essential that the health professional should obtain the consent of the parent or child, or both, if he or she is proposing to practise his or her complementary medicine skills in parallel with his or her orthodox practice. Obtaining consent also includes giving full information about the suggested treatment and advising of the risks of any possible harm.

CONCLUSION

There seems little doubt that the interest in and the practise of complementary medicine will continue to grow. Health professionals caring for children might find that they come under pressure from parents wishing alternative therapies to be tried out if orthodox medicine appears to have failed. The health professional should ensure that he or she obtains all appropriate advice on any contraindications between conventional medicine and alternative medicine within the same patient and advises the child and parent accordingly. At the same time, many health professionals in the NHS may wish to develop skills in alternative therapies and give their patients the benefit of these. Employers should draw up procedures to protect both the patient and the health professional in relation to the use of complementary therapies.

REFERENCES

1 British Complementary Medicine Association: *Pamphlet*. London: BCMA; 1994.
2 Department of Health: *Press release*. London: HMSO; 3 December 1991.
3 Quoted in Cameron-Blackie G: *Complementary Therapies in the NHS*. Birmingham: National Association of Health Authorities and Trusts; 1993.
4 Cameron-Blackie G: *Complementary Therapies in the NHS*. Birmingham: National Association of Health Authorities and Trusts; 1993.
5 Bolam *v* Friern HMC 1957 2 All ER 118.
6 *Times* News Report 6 November 1993. [See also, *Times* editorial: A right to life: parents cannot condemn their children to die. 8 November 1993.]

Teaching and research

Research is becoming a significant area in the work of the health professional. Pressure is increasing to ensure that practice in every field of professional work is research based, and that, as part of their post-registration continuing education, health professionals are taking part in research. Several of the ethical cases described in the book by Jim Richardson raise issues relating to research and teaching, and these will be discussed in the context of the relevant law.

This chapter examines the legal rights of the child in the context of student carers, and research projects involving their care.

TEACHING

In the case of a reluctant subject, Sonia, a 14-year-old, is being treated for a complicated congenital cardiac defect. She is being treated in a new paediatric cardiac unit in a university hospital. Her consultant visits her on one occasion with six medical students. He wishes the students to examine her and listen to her heart sounds and she refuses. The grandmother, who accompanied her, puts considerable pressure upon her, but Sonia is adamant. At one stage the consultant says: 'Everyone who comes as a patient to a university hospital must accept that part of their care will involve the instruction of student doctors and nurses.' Is this the law?

The answer is that it may be, but it depends upon the circumstances. A patient is a visitor in a hospital and the occupier can state the terms on which the patient is treated. The patient is entitled to receive the standard of the reasonable practitioner according to the Bolam test (see Chapter 13, page 117). Rarely, however, is it promised that treatment is to be provided by a specific individual. If students, in what ever profession, are being trained, it is essential that they have the appropriate supervision and only tasks within their competence are delegated to them. A patient would probably not have the right to insist upon being treated by qualified staff only.

However, there is a difference between being treated by students under supervision and being used as an object for student teaching. Certainly, it is accepted by the Department of Health that a patient in a teaching hospital can refuse to be examined by medical students and most teaching hospitals in their patient information leaflets would make it clear to patients that although they hope that patients will cooperate with the teaching of students, they will not be obliged to take part. In addition, in the situation described in the case study, six students all wished to hear the girl's heart. Her right to privacy was forgotten and there was little concern for her dignity. Neither of these values are at present legally enforceable but it is hoped that most professionals would accept the need to recognize both. A compromise could have been reached whereby the patient agreed to allow one student to hear her heart.

It must be emphasized that if the patient is given treatment by a student who is not yet qualified, the patient is entitled to receive the standard of care of a competent qualified practitioner.[1]

HEALTH CARE RESEARCH

The Department of Health, the British Paediatric Association, and the Royal College of Nursing have issued advice on research on children.

Department of Health advice[2] in its guidance on the establishment of local research ethics committees emphasizes that research proposals should only involve children if it is absolutely essential to do so and the information required cannot be obtained using adult subjects. It is in harmony with the advice of the British Paediatric Association[3]

Royal College of Nursing[4]
This guidance sets out the ethical principles that underpin research and these are listed below.

- Doing good to people (beneficence)
- Doing no harm to people (nonmaleficence)
- Trust (principle of fidelity)
- Justice (principle of being fair)
- Respecting people as autonomous persons
- Veracity (truth telling)
- Confidentiality

The Royal College of Nursing provides practical advice to nurses undertaking research, nurses in positions of authority in which research is to be carried out, and nurses practising in settings in which research is being undertaken.

In relation to children the guidelines suggest that the assent of children over 7 years of age should usually be sought directly. It is submitted, however, that more important than stating a specific age is the determination of the competence of the child as the discussion below will illustrate.

INSTITUTE OF MEDICAL ETHICS

In 1986, a working group set up by the Institute of Medical Ethics to look at medical research with children published its results.

Its recommendations are summarized below.[5]

- No research should be carried out on children unless there is a clear need and no other route to the relevant knowledge available.
- The Helsinki standards should prevail.
- Consent must be given and can be withdrawn at any time.
- Parents should be seen as the trustees of the interests of their children.
- All proposals should be submitted to a local research ethics committee.
- No financial inducements should be offered.

THE BASIC PRINCIPLES ON CONSENT

Children aged 16 and 17 years
The Family Law Reform Act 1969 gives the 16 or 17-year-old the right to give consent to medical and dental treatment. The word 'treatment' includes anaesthetic and diagnostic procedures. It does not give explicitly a statutory right for the minor aged 16 or 17 years to consent to participation in research. However, on the basis of the House of Lords decision in the Gillick case[6] and in keeping with the philosophy underlining the Children Act 1989 of maximum participation of children in decisions if they have the intelligence and maturity to make a valid decision, a researcher would probably be able to undertake research on the basis of the consent

of a minor aged 16 or 17 years if the latter had the maturity and understanding to make a competent decision.

Section 8(3) of the Family Law Reform Act 1969 enables any other consent to treatment, which would have been valid before the passing of the Act, to continue to be relied upon. Thus the parent's consent to treatment for a 16- or 17-year-old would be valid. However, as the Act is restricted to treatment, this provision cannot be relied upon in relation to nontherapeutic research on a 16- or 17-year-old. Unless the 16- or 17-year-old is able to give consent on his or her own behalf to participation in such research, the research should not involve that person. In the case of therapeutic research, if the 16- or 17-year-old is unable to give consent or refuses to do so, but the parents are prepared to do so, it is a question of the benefits to be derived from the treatment and whether the refusal of the minor should be overridden. It would seem necessary for the court to become involved as happened in the case of Re W (see Chapter 6).

The child aged under 16 years

The Medical Research Council issued guidance[7] on the ethical conduct of research on children in 1991. It suggested the following safeguards.

* Children should only take part in research if the relevant knowledge could not be obtained from adults.
* All projects must be approved by the appropriate local research ethics committee. (This is discussed below.)[8]
* Children should either have given consent or consent should have been given on their behalf by a parent or guardian.

Therapeutic research can be carried out only if in the parents' opinion the benefits likely to accrue to the child outweigh the possible risks of harm, and participation is therefore in the child's best interests. Nontherapeutic research should only be carried out if there is negligible risk to the child and it is therefore not against his or her interests. When a child has sufficient understanding to consent, his or her consent should be sought. It would still be advisable to seek parental consent as well.

The Department of Health in its guidelines for local research ethics committees (see below) gives similar advice to that of the Medical Research Council shown above.

Since the Gillick case, more weight has been given to the ability of the under 16-year-old to give a valid consent. This has been reinforced by the Children Act 1989 which gives to the child who is of sufficient understanding to make an informed decision the right to refuse to submit to a medical or psychiatric examination or other assessment (section 43(8) and section 44(7)) and to treatment (Schedule 3, paragraph 4(4a) and 5 (5a)).

THE ROLE OF THE LOCAL RESEARCH ETHICS COMMITTEES

The Department of Health has requested each health authority to ensure that a local research ethics committee is set up to examine research proposals.[9]

Any NHS body asked to agree a research proposal falling within its sphere of responsibility should ensure that it has been submitted to the appropriate local research ethics committee for research ethics approval.

The role of the local research ethics committee is defined as being 'to consider the ethics of proposed research projects which will involve human subjects' and to advise the NHS body concerned. It is the NHS body which has the responsibility of deciding whether the project should go ahead, taking into account the ethical advice of the local research ethics committee. The latter are not 'in any sense management arms of the District Health Authority'. The local research ethics committee is comprised of multidisciplinary members including lay persons.

The guidelines require the local research ethics committee to be consulted for any proposal which involves:

- NHS patients, including those private sector patients treated under contract;
- fetal material and in-vitro fertilization involving NHS patients;
- the recently dead in NHS premises;
- access to the records of past or present NHS patients; or
- the use of, or potential access to, NHS premises or facilities.

The local research ethics committee MUST be consulted but the NHS body must also give permission before the project can proceed. The local research ethics committee can also advise other non-NHS bodies such as private sector companies, the Medical Research Council, and universities.

The research guidelines for local research ethics committees recommend that research proposals should only involve children if it is absolutely essential to do so and the information required cannot be obtained using adult subjects. Different principles apply according to the age and mental capacity of the child. They state that local research ethics committees should note that those acting for the child can only legally give their consent provided that the intervention is for the benefit of the child. If those acting for the child are responsible for allowing the child to be subjected to any risk (other than one so insignificant as to be negligible) which is not for the benefit of that child, it could be said that they were acting illegally.

NONTHERAPEUTIC RESEARCH

If the child has the mental competence to understand the risks and purpose of the research, then it is possible that he or she could give a valid consent to participation in it. If the risks are significant, it is unwise to rely upon the child's consent. Nor, however, in such circumstances could there be justification in the parents giving consent to submit the child to the possible risk of harm. A parent can only give consent to what is in the child's best interests; can it ever be said that nontherapeutic research, which will have no direct or indirect benefit to the child but carries a risk, could be in the child's best interests? The alternative argument is that the child might benefit from an altruistic act. This might be so, but it would be preferable for the child to consent in his or her own right, rather than for the parents to do so on his or her behalf. The local research ethics committee guidelines state that those acting for the child can legally only give their consent provided that the intervention is for the benefit of the child. 'If they are responsible for allowing the child to be subjected to any risk (other than one so insignificant as to be negligible) which is not for the benefit of that child, it could be said they were acting illegally.' They also state that: 'It should be noted that the giving of consent by a parent or guardian cannot overrule the refusal of consent by a child who is competent to make that decision.' This was written before the decision in Re W (a minor) in which the refusal of a 16-year-old suffering from anorexia nervosa to have treatment was overruled by the court. However, if the minor's refusal to give consent to participation in a research project is overruled, it would have to be shown that the therapeutic benefits of the research justified the intervention in the minor's best interests.

MENTALLY DISORDERED MINORS

Exactly the same rules would apply for the protection of these patients as apply in the case of minors under 16 years of age. If there is the possibility that they have the capacity to give consent to participation in research, then their consent could be given. It is unlikely, however, if the parents could give consent on their behalf unless there were clear therapeutic benefits to the person from the research.

The proposals of the Law Commission on decision-making on behalf of mentally incapacitated adults, if implemented, should ensure that such persons are protected against research which is not in their best interests.[10]

Case study on research

A case study in Jim Richardson's book discusses the situation of an 11-year-old boy named Albert who suffered from a rare metabolic disorder. His father heard of some research in France into the disease, which offered prospects of improvement in Albert's condition. However, after an initial stay in France, Albert decided that he did not wish to take part in the research. What are the legal implications?

First, research should not be performed upon children unless there is no risk or a minimal risk of harm and there is a benefit to the child. This means that the research should have some therapeutic value for the child. In Albert's case it appears that there is benefit to him from the research but the potential risks are not clearly spelt out.

Second, the parent could give a valid consent, in the circumstances set out in paragraph 1 and, if the child is Gillick-competent, the child's consent should also be obtained.

Third, if a Gillick-competent child refuses to take part in the research, it should probably not go ahead unless there is overwhelming therapeutic benefit to the child and the parent gives consent. It is not clear whether Albert at the age of 11 years is Gillick-competent. If he is and it can be established that the research is not significantly in his best interests, he should be allowed to refuse.

Fourth, all research projects should be placed before a local research ethics committee and its consent should be obtained. Its consent does not, however, remove the need to obtain the consent of the parent or child, or both.

INFORMATION TO SUBJECT

It is essential that before the researcher obtains consent for the research from the parent or child, full information on the risks and benefits should be given. There are considerable advantages if this is in writing. Many concerns arise from the work of the research, and many have legal implications. These are considered in a book, *Nursing and Research*, in the chapter titled 'Legal Aspects of Research'.

The researcher should also be aware of potential litigation arising from research. At present the law of negligence requires the person harmed to prove that the harm has been caused by fault on the part of the defendant or his or her employees. The Pearson report recommended that compensation should be paid without proof of fault to those volunteering to take part in research; however, this recommendation has not yet been implemented. If drugs trials are involved, pharmaceutical companies offer compensation on the basis of strict liability.

CONFIDENTIALITY

The principles of maintaining confidentiality, which are discussed in Chapter 7, also apply to the information obtained from research. Information that identifies the subjects of the research should only be disclosed with the consent of the person concerned. The exceptions discussed in Chapter 7 would, however, apply.

GENERAL ROLE OF THE HEALTH PROFESSIONAL IN RELATION TO RESEARCH ON CHILDREN

The health professional should see him- or herself as the protector of the child if research is being planned. He or she may be involved in a variety of ways, from simply caring for the child who is the subject of the research to being actively involved as a researcher. Whatever the degree of involvement, the health professional should ensure that the research has been discussed by the local research ethics committee and that there is clear consent by the parent or child, or both, and that they have been given suitable and sufficient information about the project.

If the health professional is the researcher as well as the carer of the child, he or she should be aware of the dangers of permitting pressures from wanting a successful research outcome to take precedence over the interests of the child, and the importance of ensuring that at any time the child must be allowed to withdraw from the research. All health professionals should ensure that their practise is research-based. The Department of Health announced[11] the establishment of a new National Centre for Evidence-Based Child Health in the Department of Paediatric Epidemiology at the Institute of Child Health, Great Ormond Street Children's Hospital. It will be a resource in the field of education and research, enabling health professionals to make use of the best and most up-to-date evidence in their clinical decisions. Other centres are to follow.

REFERENCES

1 Nettleship v Weston 1971 3 All ER 581. [A passenger is entitled to expect the standard of care of the reasonable motorist even when the driver is only a learner.]
2 Department of Health: *HSG(91)5. NHS Management Executive Local Research Ethics Committees – Health Service Guidelines.* London: HMSO; 1991.
3 British Paediatric Association: *Ethics Advisory Committee, August 1992. Guidelines for the Ethical Conduct of Medical Research Involving Children.* London: British Paediatric Association; 1992.
4 Royal College of Nursing: *Ethics related to Research in Nursing.* London: Scutari Press; 1993.
5 Gillick v West Norfolk and Wisbech AHA and the DHSS 1985 3 All ER 402.
6 Nicholson R (ed): *Medical Research – Ethics, Law and Practice.* Oxford: OUP; 1986.
7 *Bulletin of Medical Ethics,* 76 March 1992.
8 Dimond B: The legal aspects of research. In de Raeve L: *Nursing and Research.* London: Bailliere Tindall; 1996 [in press].
9 HSG(91)5 Chapter 4 pages 16
10 Law Commission: *Report No. 231 – Mental Incapacity.* London: HMSO; 1995.
11 Department of Health: *Press release.* London: HMSO; November 1995.

PART 4

SPECIAL SITUATIONS

This final part looks at some special situations relating to the health care of the child. The first chapter considers specific issues that arise from the care of the child at home. The next looks at the situation in which a child suffers from a mental disorder and needs to be accommodated outside the home. The care of the terminally ill child is then considered along with the law relating to letting die and consent to treatment in those circumstances. The legal issues of health promotion, including screening and vaccinations, follow, and the final chapter looks at the law relating to sexual activity and reproduction.

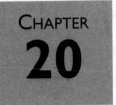

Child care in the community

INTRODUCTION

It is a fundamental principle of all the recommendations in the charters and guidance material made in relation to the care of the child in hospital (see reports referred to in Chapter 1) that the child should be admitted only when absolutely essential and that the stay should be as short as is possible in the light of his or her clinical needs. If possible the child should be cared for on a day or outpatient basis, or in the community.

THE DEFINITION OF COMMUNITY CARE

Community care covers a wide diversity of conditions and needs. It can refer to the care of the chronically sick and disabled who do not need hospital care but require nursing to assist them to maintain a reasonable quality of life. It can also cover those acutely ill persons who may need hospitalization occasionally but can be cared for at home if the high technology equipment, facilities, and the necessary support staffing can be made available in the community. Thus the term 'hospital at home' is now a familiar one. The legal implications of both these forms of community support are important though different.

The term 'community care' was first given a definition by statute law in the NHS and Community Care Act 1990 section 46(3). The definition is confined to the provision of certain statutory services by local authorities and health authorities in relation to the provision of accommodation for those aged over 18 years, services for the elderly, mentally ill, and mothers and children, and specifically excludes the provision of services under Sections 1 and 2 of the Chronically Sick and Disabled Persons Act 1970 and related legislation.

When the term 'community care' is used in this book it is used to cover all the care provided to the child with his or her family, including the community health services.

NHS SERVICES

The NHS and Community Care Act 1990, as well as setting the framework for the internal market of the NHS with purchasers and providers and NHS trusts and GP fundholders, also introduced new measures for the assessment of needs for community care and the composition of community care plans by local authorities in conjunction with health authorities and voluntary and private sector organizations.

Guidance has recently been prepared by the Department of Health on child health in the community.[1] It recommends that purchasers should take account of the provisions of the UN Convention on the Rights of the Child in considering the principles upon which they might base their contracts for child health services. Some of the areas this guidance covers are:

- the role of child health services;
- organization of child health services;
- contracting for a combined child health service;
- information needs of a child health service;
- preschool child health services and immunization;
- health services for school-aged children (including medical and oral health);
- adolescent health;
- health visiting;
- delivery of secondary care outside the hospital;
- services for children with life-threatening diseases;
- child and adolescent mental health;
- contribution of community child health services to public health;
- assessment of health-related needs in children;
- children in need;
- children with special educational needs;
- therapy services;
- child protection; and
- services in support of local authority functions.

The guidance to purchasers of community child health services from the Department of Health aims to improve the quality and efficiency of services through 'better coordination, adoption of good practice, better targeted support, and more effective collaboration'.

If a patient is being discharged from hospital, the latter is responsible for ensuring that the appropriate assessment for continuing or community care is carried out on a multidisciplinary basis. The district nurse who is due to become the key worker of the patient should attend and play a major role in the assessment.

Confusion has arisen over the boundaries between the responsibilities of the local Social Services authorities and health authorities and when there is a duty to provide continuing NHS care. Recent Government guidance[2] has laid down the criteria to be followed and requires health authorities to develop local policies and eligibility criteria that set out clealy the basis upon which decisions about need for NHS-funded care will be made in individual cases. The health authorities will also identify the range, type, location, and level of services that will be arranged and funded by the NHS to meet continuing health care needs in their area. Using this guidance the Government expects local agreement between health authorities, GP fundholders, and local authorities to be reached over the implementation of its giudelines.

THE HOSPITAL AT HOME

The District Nursing Association has published the result of a conference in Peterborough[3] which looked at the hospital at home services from the perspective of both the user and the provider. The user, a sufferer from Guillain–Barré syndrome, emphasized the following advantages of hospital at home: early discharge from hospital; one to one care; level of care appropriate to his changing needs; flexibility; regular exercise; continuity; keeping the family together; regaining independence. His conclusions were: 'Hospital at home enabled me to leave hospital several months early and I am certain in my own mind that this led to a faster rate of recovery than would otherwise have been the case. It reunited the family at a critical point in our children's development. However, the fundamental virtue of hospital at home is, in my opinion, that the care it provides is tailored to the needs of the patient.'

Exactly the same advantages could be spelt out in the case of the child. The needs of siblings of the sick child might be overlooked when the sick child is admitted to hospital and it is easier (though maybe not easy) to balance the conflicting pressures and demands of all children when the sick child is being cared for at home.

The district nurse recognized the benefits from the patient's perspective and also considered that the nurse obtained greater job satisfaction, as in addition to 'hands-on care' the nurse had an assessing and planning function and managerial role to play. She considered that resources were used to the full. The district nurse was seen as the key worker cooperating closely with other community professionals as necessary: the physiotherapist, the occupational therapist, and GP. She was contacted after the GP had accepted medical responsibility for admitting the patient to hospital at home and she then arranged a case conference with the medical ward sister, the hospital at home/hospital liaison sister, the district nursing sister, the hospital occupational therapist, community and hospital physiotherapists, and the patient's service manager. After this case conference, she saw the patient in hospital and, after an initial assessment, a preliminary plan of care was formulated with a timetable prepared for the first week at home.

Other districts might have a system in which the GP does not agree to take responsibility for the patient until after the patient has been assessed by the multidisciplinary team which will be involved in his or her care.

The GP and the nurse manager also spelt out the benefits of the hospital at home from their perspectives. The GP pointed to the benefits as being: increased patient satisfaction, increased job satisfaction for the GP who is able to remain caring for the patient and use his professional skills (he cited: setting up drips, passing nasogastric or gastrostomy tubes for feeding, care of tracheostomies, and pleural aspiration), improved relationships with hospitals, and advantages for the GP fundholder. He recognized the following possible disadvantages: possible increase in workload, inappropriate selection of patient, and possible lack of consultant support but these should be avoidable. He considered that hospital at home could be used to prevent admissions to hospital and to facilitate early discharge from hospital.

The nurse manager stated that at present the following conditions were required before hospital at home could be implemented for any patient.

- The patient is admitted to or remains in hospital.
- The consultant agrees with discharge.
- The GP accepts medical responsibility.
- The district nurse accepts nursing responsibility.
- The patient and carer wish it to happen.

Other benefits not identified by the publication include reduced risk of hospital-acquired infections and retaining social security benefits which are reduced by hospital stay.

PAEDIATRIC DAY SURGERY

Paediatric day surgery, like adult day surgery, has increased over the past years. In 1988 it was estimated that 50% of general surgical operations on children were performed as day cases.[4] Elizabeth Norris[5] examines the demands which this can make on both the physical and psychological resources of parents, and emphasizes that the nurse must see the parents as integral members of the care team. 'Parents should be encouraged to care for their child in the postoperative period thus giving them the confidence to deal with their child after discharge.' The Organization Caring for Children in the Health Service has drawn up 12 quality standards associated with day surgery.[6] These were designed on the basis of a review of the literature on day surgery and also on the results of a survey of Royal Colleges, professional and voluntary organizations, individual consumers, health authorities, and experts.

Reference should also be made to the charter drawn up by the National Association for the Welfare of Children in Hospital 1985.[7,8]

LIABILITY

GP and practice staff

The GP is not an employee but an independent contractor who has a contract for services with, at present, the FHSA; however, from 1 April 1996 it will be with the Health Authority in the District. He or she employs practice staff for whose negligence he or she is vicariously liable. If he or she is a fundholder he or she may also purchase services from the NHS trust and other bodies, including secondary (i.e. hospital) care and community care. He or she would not be vicariously liable for the negligence of those professionals who supply the services that he or she has purchased.

Nurse prescribing

The Scope of Professional Practice (see Chapter 4) has enabled the development of nursing practice to take place beyond the traditional boundaries, and prescribing by nurses in the community is now being tested out in eight pilot areas as a result of changes in the legislation enabling appropriately trained community nurses and health visitors to prescribe.[9] Practice nurses who are qualified as community nurses or health visitors will be able to prescribe after training, once the scheme is extended to the whole country. The list of drugs from which the nurse can prescribe is printed with the British National Formulary (BNF).

Practice Nurse and scope of professional practice

The GP would be vicariously liable for any harm caused by a nurse of the practice who goes beyond his or her field of professional competence. The GP may also be personally liable if he or she has delegated tasks to the nurse inappropriately.

The decision of a GP to send the practice nurse to see a baby whose parents were concerned about her feeding and vomiting was challenged by the parents. The baby was 6 weeks premature with feeding problems and had stayed on in hospital in 1979 for 2 weeks after the mother had been discharged. The baby and mother were seen by another doctor in the practice on 27 July 1980 and a note was made about the baby's problems of feeding and vomiting. The mother telephoned for the doctor on 3 August 1980 because there had been no improvement in the baby's condition. The doctor sent the practice nurse who diagnosed a nose infection and sniffles and recommended the administration of boiling water. It was later found that the baby was suffering from septicaemia from the delay in admitting her to hospital. The mother claimed that the doctor should have visited, not the practice nurse.[10]

The claim failed. The court held that the doctor should be judged by the standard of the ordinary reasonably competent general practitioner (i.e. the Bolam test), and on the basis of this test, there was no substance in the criticism of the doctor failing to attend himself and instead sending the practice nurse.

Clearly every situation must be decided on its own merits and there should be protocols in each practice covering visits by practice nurses.

Legal liability of other professionals and parents

The possibility of the parents (and the child) coping at home with conditions which in the past would have required hospital admission raises issues over the legal liability of professional or parent if things go wrong.[11] One example of the treatments now frequently administered at home rather than in hospital is the administration of intravenous antibiotics to children with cystic fibrosis. Susan Gill[12] identifies advantages to the child in receiving care at home, and the role of the nurse in exercising her professional judgment and responsibility in the decision relating to home treatment, and supporting the family in the home. She quotes several different home care schemes in which there are different programmes for achieving the common goal of teaching the parents to be competent and safe in carrying out a procedure. The selection of the families is crucial to the success of home care and, in an article on intravenous therapy at home in cystic fibrosis, Ellis sets out criteria for choosing suitable families.[13]

What could go wrong and what possible disputes could arise? The following is suggested.

- The child suffers an adverse reaction and the parents do not know how, or fail, to take appropriate action.
- The vein tissues, and does permanent damage to the child.
- An infection develops in the cannula site as a result of bad control of infection practice.
- The cannula comes out and the parent tries to replace it and causes harm to the child.
- The wrong dose of drug is given.
- The drugs are given in the wrong order.
- Air is introduced into the vein.

It is of crucial importance that instruction and training given by the hospital staff to the parents cover all such possibilities. Clearly the more that is given in writing the more difficult it would be for the parents to challenge the hospital over its failure to cover certain topics. It is essential that the parents should receive such instruction before the child initially leaves hospital. The health professionals should be confident that the parents or the child, or both, are capable of managing the delegated tasks.

EXCLUSION OF LIABILITY

Would the fact that the parents had signed a form which declared that they had been appropriately instructed be an adequate defence for the hospital to rely upon if harm were to occur? The answer is probably no, unless everything reasonable had been covered by the instructor. If the instructor had been negligent in what was covered (e.g. in leaving out vital information or in giving wrong information) the form would not protect the professional (or employer) from liability in negligence. This is because the Unfair Contract Terms Act 1977 prevents persons excluding themselves from liability for their negligence if personal injury or death were to occur (see Chapter 13).

What support should be provided to the parent? What right of action would the parents have if, once they had returned home with the child, they were not visited by any health professional, whether GP, health visitor, district nurse, or community paediatric nurse?

In some cases such a visit may not be necessary. Provided that the parents have had sufficient instruction and support, and provided that they know how to seek help, and from whom, in the event of difficulties occurring, it may not be necessary to provide any regular professional visits to the home. If the recommendations of the specialist advisory report on cystic fibrosis are implemented and each child is in contact with a specialist regional service, it should be possible for clear protocols to be developed to prevent many of the foreseeable risks.

HOME SUPPORT

It is not possible to cover all the many clinical conditions that may be cared for at home which can have legal implications for professionals and parents. Three treatments will be discussed.

- Self-administration of medicine
- Enteral nutrition
- Enuresis management

Self-administration of medicines

Children who have the capacity are encouraged to administer their own medications, even preparations requiring intravenous administration. Self-administration can take place on hospital wards and in the community, but the topic is considered in this chapter for convenience.

An article by Beverley Hancock[14] that recommends the benefits of self-administration of medicines and sets out the procedures to be followed is predominantly concerned with the benefits to the elderly patient, but all that she states could apply to the Gillick-competent child who, with supervision, is able to understand the need for treatment. A study by Elizabeth Robinson[15] on parents' attitudes to self-medication by their asthmatic children who were in primary schools revealed that the parents' anxiety concerning the taking of medication at school is greater than the child's, and many of them were not prepared to relinquish control. It was when the school was most proactive in implementing a health-promoting policy, that the parents accepted a greater degree of self-management by the child in school than in the home. Not surprisingly, too, the parents' attitudes varied considerably with the level of communication between parents and their child's teacher and head teacher. Clear recommendations arose from the study for teacher training, support groups being formed for parents, more information being provided, and the recording of medication at school.

In a case study of a young man who had failed to take his insulin, Marilyn Gallichan[16] describes the myths that the young man believed about the effects of diabetes, and how these undermined his compliance with the treatment regime. She shows that by developing a therapeutic relationship with him it was possible to develop his understanding of the disease and therefore to enhance his future prospects. In that case the young man was aged 20 years but had suffered from diabetes since he was 11 years old. Exactly the same principles should underlie the care of the younger child.

Enteral nutrition

Just as the discharge of patients still on intravenous antibiotic administration is not uncommon, so patients with enteral nutrition may also be cared for in the community. The development of home enteral nutrition (HEN) is discussed by Helen Arrowsmith.[17] She analyses the benefits and criteria by which which patients are deemed suitable for HEN, and the preparation that must be made before the patient is discharged. Crucial in the preparation is the training procedure and programme, and the parts played by the dietitian, the ward nurse and the nutrition nurse specialist. Although the paper is not directly concerned with the enteral feeding of children, similar criteria would have to be applied as were used in the determination of intravenous treatment at home in cystic fibrosis (see above). A discharge procedure lists the stages which should be followed to ensure the safety of the patient.

Management of enuresis in children

A study to review the enuresis service provided by the Community Unit of Oxfordshire Health Authority[18] showed that more staffing was necessary; many staff had gained their knowledge by experience and from books and had not had formal training. The sweeping statement that 'we need more training, more equipment and more expertise' seems to sum up the majority of comments. Respondents repeatedly stressed the need for a clinic, with trained staff, and pointed out the cost implications of the present system. Recommendations include the need for guidelines on minimum standards for treating nocturnal enuresis and regular audits.

CONCLUSION

The number of sick children being cared for at home is likely to continue increasing. Health professionals must appreciate the pressures and demands that this can make upon the family and ensure that excellent communications are established and that the family has the maximum support and instruction for all the activities that will be undertaken at home instead of in hospital. Protocols for home care for an ever-increasing variety of treatments and serious and chronic conditions need to be developed in association with parents, children, and other authorities such as education and social services. GPs and the primary health care team should be part of the group devising the protocols. Records should be kept of the information and care that is given. These will be essential in the event of litigation. The guidance issued by the Department of Health (see beginning of this chapter) should be followed.

REFERENCES

1 Department of Health: *Child health in the Community: A Guide to Good Practice.* London: HMSO; 1995. [Consultation draft March 1995.]

2 Department of Health: *HSG (95)8; LAC (95) 5 NHS Responsibilities for meeting continuing health care needs.* London: HMSO; 1995.

3 MacKenzie A (Ed): *Hospital at Home.* Edinburgh: District Nursing Association; 1991.

4 Campbell IR, Scaife JM Johnstone JMS: *Psychological Effects of Day-Case Surgery Compared with Inpatient Surgery.* 1988.

5 Norris E: Care of the paediatric day-surgery patient. *Br J Nurs* 1992, 1:547–551.

6 Thornes R: *Just for the Day: Caring for Children in the Health Services.* London: National Association for Children in Hospitals (NAWCH); 1991.

7 NAWCH: London; 1985.

8 Thornes R: *Just for the Day: Caring for Children in the Health Services.* London: National Association for Children in Hospitals (NAWCH); 1991.

9 Dimond BC: *The Legal Aspects of Nurse Prescribing.* [Special supplement to *Primary Health Care.* Merck Dermatology and Royal College of Nursing; January 1995.]

10 Stockdale *v* Nicholls [1993] 4 Med LR 191.

11 Dimond B: Parental Acts and Omissions. *Paediatr Nurs* 1990, 2:23–24.

12 Gill S: Home administration of intravenous antibiotics to children with cystic fibrosis. *Br J Nurs* 1993, 2:767–770.

13 Ellis JM: Let the parents give the care: IV therapy at home in cystic fibrosis. *Professional Nurse* 1989, 4:589–592.

14 Hancock B: Self-administration of medicines. *Br J Nurs* 1994, 3:996–999.

15 Robinson E: Parents' attitudes to self-medication by their asthmatic children. *Br J Nurs* 1994, 3:651–656.

16 Gallichen M: Educating a young man to comply with his insulin treatment. *Br J Nurs* 1994, 3:1017–1021.

17 Arrowsmith HL: Discharging patients receiving enteral nutrition. *Br J Nurs* 1994, 3:551–557.

18 Paterson H: Management of enuresis in children. *Br J Nurs* 1993, 2:418–424.

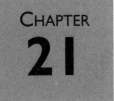

The mentally disordered child

Recent research suggests that record numbers of children under the age of 10 years are being treated in hospital for mental illness caused by family breakups, poor parenting, and increased pressures at school. Figures from the Department of Health show an increase of 50% in the children aged under 10 years admitted to a mental hospital over the past 3 years. More than 1000 are now being treated for psychosis. A similar picture exists for those between the ages of 10 and 14 years.[1] The Samaritans have reported that the increase of mental illness is mirrored by rising suicide rates among people aged 15–24 years.[2] Clearly health professionals must be alert to the possibilities of a child suffering from mental illness, including those children who are referred to them for physical causes.

There are many ways for a child identified as suffering from a mental disorder of arranging care. Only rarely will compulsory powers to transfer the patient to secure accommodation be necessary to ensure that the child receives the necessary treatment. Secure accommodation can be provided under the Mental Health Act 1983 or the Children Act 1989. This chapter covers both Acts and explains the differences between the use of the different kinds of legislation. Inevitably, only a summary can be given here of the main laws relating to the care of the mentally disordered child and the reader requiring further information is referred to the works cited in the Further Reading; In particular, the guide provided by the Children's Legal Centre.[3] Reference should also be made to the Guide provided by the Action for sick children for purchasers and providers of mental health care for children and young people.[4] The Department of Health has recently issued a consultation document[5] on guidance on child health in the community and this includes a section on child and adolescent mental health. It estimates that between 10 and 20% of children will at some time have a mental health problem which will require help.

The routes into receiving inpatient psychiatric care include:

* detention under the Mental Health Act 1983;
* admission to psychiatric hospital as an informal patient with the consent of the parent (not necessarily with the consent of the child); and
* admission under the powers given by the Children Act 1989.

Each will be considered in turn but it must be remembered that admission to a unit would usually be regarded as the last line of action and every endeavour would be made for the child to obtain any necessary treatment in his or her own home.

MENTAL HEALTH ACT 1983 AND THE PERSON AGED UNDER 16 YEARS

The philosophy of the Mental Health Act 1983 is that admission to a psychiatric hospital should be avoided if there is alternative treatment and care available outside, and compulsory admission should not be used if the patient will agree to be admitted as an informal patient or if alternative services outside the hospital are obtainable.

The Act draws a dividing line between patients who are aged under 16 and those aged 16 years and over in certain respects, as shown below.

- A person aged 16 years and over who is capable of expressing his or her views can make arrangements for informal admission (section 131(2)). This means that like any other adult entering a general hospital or psychiatric unit on a voluntary basis he or she can agree to treatment and discharge himself or herself even if contrary to medical or nursing advice.
- If a person aged under 16 years is compulsorily admitted to hospital under the Mental Health Act 1983, the managers must refer that patient to the Mental Health Review Tribunal every year if the patient has not had a hearing on the basis of their own application or that of the nearest relative. This contrasts with the situation of the person aged 16 years and over who must be referred to the Mental Health Review Tribunal by the managers after the first 6 months and then at least every 3 years if there has not been a hearing (section 68(2)).
- A child aged under 16 years cannot be placed under guardianship (section 7(1)).
- If a child is in the care of the local authority, the nearest relative for the purpose of the Mental Health Act is the local authority, unless the child is married (section 27).

DETENTION UNDER THE MENTAL HEALTH ACT 1983

What are the features of the Mental Health Act which should be borne in mind if detention under the Mental Health Act is being contemplated by the professionals as opposed to the use of the Children Act 1989? Reference should be made to the Act itself,[6] the code of practice issued by the Department of Health,[7] and other works to be found in Further Reading.

First, a person must be suffering from mental disorder, as defined in the Act, to be compulsorily detained. The definition is contained in section 1.

Second, compulsory detention must be on the basis of the medical recommendations of two doctors. At least one of these must be a doctor who has had special training in psychiatry (known as a section 12 doctor); at least one of the doctors should have had prior acquaintance with the patient. The section for admission for assessment enables the patient to be detained for up to 28 days (section 2); the admission for treatment enables the patient to be detained initially for up to 6 months. In an emergency, if it is not possible to obtain the recommendations of two doctors, an admission can be made under section 4 on the same grounds as section 2 but on the basis of only one medical recommendation. It may not be possible to obtain a section 12 doctor or one who knows the patient. The emergency admission can last up to 72 hours and it is to enable an application based on the recommendations of two doctors to be made. Section 3, admission for treatment, cannot be used if the nearest relative objects to an application being made. Under section 2 the nearest relative should be consulted over the admission but cannot prevent the compulsory admission.

Third, under section 3, admission for treatment, the two doctors must agree upon and specify at least one form of mental disorder. If the specified form of mental disorder is psychopathic disorder or mental impairment, they must declare that they are satisfied that treatment in hospital is likely to alleviate or prevent a deterioration of the patient's condition. This has become known as the 'treatability condition'.

Fourth, the nearest relative has considerable powers under the Mental Health Act 1983 and is very specifically defined with a clear hierarchy. In the case of a child, the nearest relative would be the father or mother, whichever is the elder. If the child is married, the spouse would be the nearest relative. The rights and powers of the nearest relative are:

- to make application for admission of the patient: under section 2 for assessment, or section 3 for treatment, or section 4 for emergency admission for assessment;

- to make application for the patient to be placed under guardianship section 7;
- to be consulted by the approved social worker and to object to an application by an approved social worker for admission for treatment or for a guardianship order;
- to be notified of application for admission for assessment and in an emergency sections 2 and 4; and
- to discharge the patient from compulsory admission under section 2 or 3 but give 72 hours notice to the managers of such an intention. During this time the responsible medical officer can examine the patient and give to the managers a report certifying that the patient, if discharged, would be likely to act in a manner dangerous to other persons or to him- or herself. The effect of this report is to bar the discharge of the patient. The barring of discharge automatically gives to the nearest relative the right to apply to a Mental Health Review Tribunal for the discharge of the patient to be considered if the patient is admitted for treatment (section 3).

Appeals against detention

There are several ways in which the patient can appeal against his or her detention.

- The patient and nearest relative can apply to the Mental Health Review Tribunal at specified intervals against the compulsory admission.
- The patient can also apply to the hospital managers who have the power to discharge the patient under section 23. This power can only be exercised by at least three of the nonexecutive directors or co-opted members of the trust Board. Executive members of the trust Board do not have this power and, unlike the other statutory duties of the managers under the Act, the power to discharge cannot be delegated to officers to act in their place.
- The responsible medical officer can at any time discharge the patient from his section by notifying the managers of that decision.

The fact that the patient is no longer under a section does not necessarily mean he or she is discharged from the hospital. He or she can remain as an informal patient.

Managers' duties and powers

The Act places many duties upon the managers, and these are:

- to accept a patient and record admission using Form 14 (regulation 4(3));
- to give information to detained patients (section 132);
- to give information to the nearest relative unless the patient requests otherwise (section 132(4));
- to give information to the nearest relative of the discharge of the patient unless the patient requests otherwise (section 133(1));
- to inform the nearest relative of the continued detention of the patient once a report from the responsible medical officer has been received (section 25(2));
- to discharge the patient if appropriate (section 23(2)(b));
- to refer the patient to a Mental Health Review Tribunal (section 68(1)(2));
- to transfer a patient (section 19(3), section 19(1A), regulation 7(2), and regulation 7(3));
- to scrutinize and oversee the documentation and consider whether to give their consent to rectification; and
- to oversee generally the care and treatment of the detained patient.

In addition, the managers have overall responsibility for the care of all patients and therefore would also be responsible for the care of the informal patient; this includes the duty to ensure that a complaints procedure is in place; the managers would form part of the appeal mechanism.

As explained earlier under Appeals against detention, the only duty that cannot be delegated is the decision whether to discharge the patient from the section.

Mental Health Act Commission

In 1983 a body was established to act as a watchdog over the care of the detained patient. This is the Mental Health Act Commission which is composed of about 90 different professionals and lay members who visit the detained patients and investigate their complaints if the patients are not satisfied at the response to their complaints obtained from the management. In addition commission members can investigate any complaint about the exercise of powers and duties under the Act. The Secretary of State has the power to extend their jurisdiction to cover the informal patient; but at present there is little likelihood, given the situation of public expenditure, that this would be done. The Mental Health Act Commission should therefore visit children who are detained under the Act and this should provide an additional form of protection for the child.

Patients' rights

Every detained patient has the right to be informed of the provision under which he or she is detained, the provisions relating to appeals against detention, and the role of the Mental Health Act Commission and other provisions of the 1983 Act. The duty is placed upon the managers to provide this information; they must ensure that information is given both by word of mouth and also in writing. They also have a duty to notify the nearest relative of the same information, but the patient has the right to request that the information is not given to the nearest relative. The managers have to take such steps as are practical to ensure that the patient understands. The fact that the patient is a child must be taken into account to achieve understanding, as must any handicap such as deafness or blindness.

Treatment provisions

A patient who is detained under the Act may in certain circumstances be given treatment without his or her consent. This also applies to detained children who are under 16 years of age. The provisions are set out below.

For the purpose of Part IV of the Act treatment for mental disorder is divided into the following categories.

- Urgent treatment, which may include all those given below (section 62 applies)
- Surgical treatment involving the destruction of brain tissue, surgical implantation of hormones for the purpose of reducing male sex drive, and other treatments which may be prescribed by the Secretary of State (section 57 covers these)
- Electroconvulsive therapy (section 58 applies)
- Medication given for the first 3 months after the patient is detained (section 63 applies)
- Medication given after the first 3 months of medication being administered (section 58 applies)
- All other treatments (section 63 applies)

In summary, the opinion of a second doctor appointed by the Mental Health Act Commission is required if the detained patient is unable to give a valid consent or refuses to give consent for treatment by drugs after the first 3 months of drugs being given, or for electroconvulsive therapy. In the case of a detained child who is incapable of giving consent, there is no provision for the parents to give consent on behalf of the child. If the child is an informal patient, the parents can give consent to treatment.

The provisions of Part IV of the Act do not apply to the patient who is detained under a section which only lasts up to 72 hours.

Medication can be given compulsorily for up to 3 months under the direction of the responsible medical officer. After that time, if the patient is incapable or refuses to give consent, treatment can only be given with the agreement of a second opinion appointed doctor (SOAD). The latter is appointed by the Mental Health Act Commission and is independent of the patient's doctor. The SOAD must consult the patient's nurse and another professional who is neither nurse nor doctor but who is concerned with the treatment of the patient, and can decide what treatment can be given without the consent of the patient. If a child is detained under the Act and comes under the provisions dealing with compulsory treatment, the parent would not be able to give consent on the child's behalf and if consent is necessary, and the child is unable to consent in his or her own name, a SOAD would have to be called.

Documentation

The statutory requirements on the documentation must be stringently complied with. Section 15 of the Act enables the managers to give consent to rectification of certain errors, such as failure to delete appropriately or failure to complete with the full name, within 14 days of the receipt of the documents. Errors, however, such as a failure to keep to the time limits set in the Act, failure to sign the form, and failure of the doctors to agree to one specific form of mental disorder (whether or not they mention another) cannot be rectified even within the 14 days and such errors would invalidate the application and admission. Most managers have established scrutiny systems for both the administrative and medical aspects of the documentation.

Leave of absence

Section 17 enables the responsible medical officer to grant leave to a detained patient. There is no requirement that this should be in writing though the code of practice recommends that it should be. Leave can thus be given as part of a treatment plan leading to eventual discharge from the section and ultimately discharge from hospital. There is no requirement as to where the patient would stay; such decisions are entirely in the hands of the responsible medical officer. He or she may, for example, decide that the patient should remain in some form of custodial care, though possibly of less secure conditions than the patient is usually kept in, or decide that the patient could have overnight leave to stay with their family. At present the time limit for which section 17 leave can be given is 6 months. The Mental Health (Patients in the Community) Act 1995, among other provisions, extends the time for which Section 17 leave is available to up to 1 year, from 1 April 1996.

Aftercare

If a child has been detained under section 3, there is a statutory duty placed upon the health authority and the local Social Services authority under section 117 of the Act to make plans and provision for aftercare in association with any voluntary organizations. This statutory duty is enforceable at the request of the patient (see the case of R v Ealing District Health Authority ex parte Fox[8]). This duty is in addition to those duties set out under the NHS and Community Care Act 1990 which requires an assessment to be made for community care provision. The statutory duty under section 117 continues until both authorities are satisfied that the patient is no longer in need of those services.

Conclusion

It can therefore be seen that placing the child who is mentally disordered under the Mental Health Act 1983 gives to the child certain protection which he or she would not have were he or she to be admitted as an informal patient. However, there are some weaknesses and limitations which will now be analysed.

LIMITATIONS OF THE MENTAL HEALTH ACT IN RELATION TO THE COMPULSORY ADMISSION OF A CHILD

The Mental Health Act 1983 only applies to and protects inpatients (with the exception of section 117, see above, and guardianship, which is not available to a child under 16 years). It has little application to care in the community and only comes into effect with the compulsory admission of a patient into hospital. Only section 17, which enables the patient to be given leave of absence, applies to the patient in the community. The courts have, however, stated that this section cannot be used to bring the patient back into hospital if they are refusing to take their medication, nor can compulsory admission be used if there is no evidence that the patient needs to be detained in hospital.[9] The weaknesses in the Act have led to Government action to introduce new legislation. The Mental Health (Patients in the Community) Act 1995 introduces a new power of supervised aftercare which will enable certain patients to be placed under this order and to be subject to certain conditions. The Act also amends section 17 by enabling leave of absence to be given for 12 months and section 18 by enabling the recall of a patient who has absconded up to 6 months after the absconsion.

Although treatment is regulated under Part 4 of the Act as far as consent to treatment is concerned, there is no statutory regulation for the use of seclusion. The code of practice issued by the Department of Health, which does not have legal force but guides practice, sets out suggestions for the use, monitoring, and review of seclusion. However, failure to follow these guidelines would not necessarily amount to illegal action, and research on the use of seclusion would suggest that more needs to be done to control it. It may, for example, be used on informal patients.

The fact that the code of practice is advisory and not mandatory diminishes its value for the protection of patients. Although the best managements may ensure that it is being observed, few sanctions are available against those who ignore its good advice.

Stigma

It has to be accepted that admission into a mental hospital still carries a lifetime stigma and compulsory admission even more so. This fact must be borne in mind by those who may see advantages in the mentally disordered child being admitted under the Mental Health Act 1983. Once the patient has ceased to be detained, those limitations on his or her civil rights, such as voting, will end, but the stigma will not necessarily do so. The existence of a stigma was commented upon in the case of Re W[10] in which Lord Donaldson said: 'The provisions of the Mental Health Acts were not considered in any detail in the course of the argument. Suffice it to say that in some circumstances they authorise treatment despite the objections of the patient, whether minor or adult. Probably they would have had no application to J (the child in this case), but even where they are applicable it may be in the long term interests of the minor that if the same treatment can be secured upon some other basis, this shall be done. Although mental illness should not be regarded as any different from physical illness, it is not always so viewed by the uninformed and the fact that in later life it might become known that a minor had been treated under the Acts might redound to his or her disadvantage.'

No Rehabilitation Act

Unlike the offender who can rely upon the Rehabilitation of Offenders Act for offences to be wiped away after a specified period (except in relation to a large number of exempt employments), there is no such rehabilitation period for those who have been identified as suffering from a mental disorder, whatever their current condition and prognosis. Nor is there any statutory protection against discrimination as exists for sex and race. The difficulties of being rehabilitated and avoiding the stigma are likely to be increased by the exceptional circumstances of the murders committed by Beverly Allitt.[11] The recommendations of the

Clothier Committee[12] may increase the problems for those who have suffered in the past from mental disorder and not just those who suffer from personality disorders.

ADMISSION TO PSYCHIATRIC HOSPITAL AS AN INFORMAL PATIENT

What, however, of the possibility of informal admission for the child?

The child aged 16 years and over

We have seen above that a child aged 16 years and over who is capable of expressing his or her own wishes can be admitted as an informal patient to a psychiatric hospital (section 131(2)). This applies even though there are persons with parental responsibility for him or her. Although section 131 specifically refers to the possibility of informal admission for treatment, the right of informal admission covers all reasons, including assessment as opposed to treatment (see Kirklees case discussed below).

If the child aged 16 years and over refuses to consent to admission as an informal patient – could he or she be admitted against his or her will but still remain outside the Mental Health Act 1983? The answer is yes and this is the situation which occurred in the case of Re W.[13] This is discussed in detail in Chapter 6. As can be seen, in that case the court held that the refusal of a minor aged 16 or 17 years could be overridden in certain circumstances.

In that case the minor aged 16 years who needed life-saving treatment for anorexia was compelled against her will to accept treatment in a special clinic. The court emphasized that the refusal by the minor was an important consideration in making clinical judgements and for parents and the court in deciding whether themselves to give consent. Its importance increased with the age and maturity of the minor. It was therefore held that the court in the exercise of its inherent jurisdiction to protect minors, had power to override the refusal of the girl to consent to particular treatment for her condition of anorexia nervosa. The local authority and the aunt who shared responsibility with it were therefore authorized to move her to a particular medical unit against her wishes and to give consent to the proposed treatment.

The child aged under 16 years

What about a child who is under the age of 16 years; can the parent give a valid consent for the admission of the child, contrary to the wishes of the child, without the child being admitted under the Mental Health Act 1983?

This was answered in the affirmative in a recent case. The facts in this case were as follows.[14]

A child, aged 12 years, was taken into care by the local authority on 2 November 1989 and placed in an assessment centre. Her behaviour was violent and disrupting to the extent of breaking windows, deliberately cutting herself with glass, and threatening to throw herself out of the window. Her behaviour became so self-destructive that eventually, on 17 November 1989, she was admitted by the local authority to hospital for an assessment to be made of her needs. In the event, she absconded from the hospital on 4 December 1989 and was ultimately returned to the centre. She applied for judicial review of the council's decision to place her in hospital, a declaration that the decision was ultra vires and unlawful, and damages for unlawful imprisonment, on the ground that, as there had not been a compulsory admission under Part III of the Mental Health Act 1983 and she was not a person needing treatment for mental disorder within the provisions of section 131(1) of the Act, there was no power under the Act and no residual power of common law to arrange for her voluntary admission. The judge dismissed the application and the child appealed to the Court of Appeal which upheld the judge's findings on the following grounds.

There was nothing at common law to inhibit or restrict the admission of a voluntary patient to hospital for assessment. There had never been any doubt that an adult patient might lawfully be admitted for assessment provided that he or she consented, and that in such a situation, the hospital would have a complete answer to a claim for damages for false imprisonment. As the voluntary admission of a patient for assessment was lawful at common law, it could not become unlawful by virtue of section 131, notwithstanding the fact that the Mental Health Act 1983 made no provision for voluntary admissions for the purpose of assessment. The position was no different for a minor as the local authority, having decided that the child was not competent in the terms set out in the Gillick case[15] to accept or reject treatment, was competent to assent on her behalf under the powers contained in section 10 of the Child Care Act 1980.

The decision of the Court of Appeal is clearly correct. Just as a parent could agree to the admission of a child for an appendectomy, so the parent can agree to admission for psychiatric care. However, in practice there are strong reasons why admission under the Mental Health Act 1983 may be preferable in spite of the limitations and weaknesses spelt out above, as it does provide a considerable armoury of protection for the patient, such as the second opinion appointed doctor, the appeals to managers, and Mental Health Review Tribunals, and so on, which are discussed above. It could also cause difficulties for staff if some of their child patients were protected by the Mental Health Act 1983 and treatment could therefore only be given against their will in certain defined circumstances, whereas other children who were in hospital with the consent of the parents could be given treatment against their will on the basis of parental consent.

CHILDREN ACT 1989

The basic principles of the Act in relation to the responsibilities of the parents and the rights of the child are set out in Chapters 1, 2, 3, and 9.

The Act attempts to create a partnership between parents, children, and the local authority. If a child is suffering from a mental disorder, initial efforts will be made to ensure that appropriate care and treatment can be provided without the use of any powers of compulsion. The local authority has a duty under the 1989 Act to take reasonable steps designed to avoid the need for children within their area to be placed in secure accommodation. Schedule 2 paragraph 7 is shown below.

Every local authority shall take reasonable steps designed:

- to reduce the need to bring:
  a   proceedings for care or supervision orders with respect to children within their area;
  b   criminal proceedings against such children;
  c   any family or other proceedings with respect to such children which might lead to them being placed in the authority's care; or
  d   proceedings under the inherent jurisdiction of the High Court with respect to children
- to encourage children within their area not to commit criminal offences; and
- to avoid the need for children within their area to be placed in secure accommodation.

In some extreme circumstances, however, it may be necessary to restrict the liberty of a child. The liberty of children can only be restricted in accordance with the provisions set out in section 25 of the Children Act 1989, the Children (Secure Accommodation) Regulations 1991, and the Children (Secure Accommodation) No. 2 Regulations 1991.[16] Reference should be made to the guide by Wyld and Carlton 'Family Emergency Procedures'.[17]

Section 25(1), the use of accommodation for restricting liberty, is set out below.

- Subject to the following provisions of this section, a child who is being looked after by a local authority may not be placed, and, if placed, may not be kept, in accommodation provided for the purposes of restricting liberty ('secure accommodation') unless it appears:

a that (i) he has a history of absconding and is likely to abscond from any other description of accommodation; and (ii) if he absconds, he is likely to suffer significant harm; or

b that if he is kept in any other description of accommodation he is likely to injure himself or other persons.

The Secretary of State is given power to specify the maximum period that a child may be kept in secure accommodation without the authority of the court; 72 hours has been specified.

Section 25 applies to accommodation provided by an NHS hospital, private hospital, and by local education authorities. It does not apply to persons detained under the Mental Health Act 1983; however, it would apply to children admitted to mental hospital who are not detained under the Mental Health Act 1983.

Application to the court

A local authority, health authority, or person running the residential care home, nursing home or mental nursing home that wishes to keep the child in secure accommodation for longer than 72 hours must apply to the court.

The court must satisfy itself that those making the application have shown that the statutory criteria in section 25(1) or, in the case of children charged or convicted of specified offences, Regulation 6 have been met and must have regard to the principles of section 1 of the Act (set out in Chapter 1 of this book). The court must also be satisfied that making an order is better than making no order at all. The court must also appoint a guardian *ad litem* for the child unless it is satisfied that it is not necessary to do so in the interests of the child.

The court must specify the maximum period that the child may be kept in secure accommodation. For nonremand cases, the maximum periods a court may authorize a child to be kept in secure accommodation for are: 3 months, on first application to the court (Regulation 12); 6 months, for any further application to the court to continue to keep that child in secure accommodation (Regulation 13).

Medical or psychiatric examination or assessment

The Children Act 1989 enables a child to refuse to submit to a medical or psychiatric examination or assessment in certain circumstances. Under section 43 (emergency protection order), section 44 (child assessment order), and section 38(6) (interim care or supervision order) the court can make a direction for examination or assessment, but the child who is of sufficient understanding to make an informed decision can refuse to submit to examination or assessment. However, it is possible for the High Court in the exercise of its inherent jurisdiction to override the child's refusal to consent under section 38(6).

SOUTH GLAMORGAN COUNTY COUNCIL V W AND B[18]

The facts of this case are given in full to illustrate the complexity of the situation that can arise when a child is manifesting severe behavioural problems. In this case, after the divorce, custody of all three children was granted to the father, with reasonable access to the mother, who did not see the youngest child, a girl now aged 16 years and the subject of these proceedings, on any regular basis until recently. The eldest boy had psychiatric problems and lived as a recluse in the family home. The younger boy refused to attend school or to leave his bedroom for a long period, but was at this point assisted by the local authority to lead an independent life. Since her admission to secondary school, the youngest child had begun to show signs of disturbances. Her attendances at different schools being sporadic, she was referred to an adolescent unit, where she was assessed by a consultant child-and-adolescent psychiatrist and educational psychologist as having an average intelligence quotient. After several admissions to the adolescent unit, she was discharged into the care of her father and her aunt, who agreed that she should attend school regularly and be supported by the social services department. On her refusal to attend school, she was made the subject of several interim care orders which were eventually opposed by the family. Proposals to rehabilitate the girl finally changed to long-term foster care. The girl was assessed by yet another consultant child-and-adolescent psychiatrist, who found no trace of any psychiatric abnormality or of a psychotic or personality disturbance, which had occurred in her family. The guardian *ad litem* appointed for the girl recommended a care order in favour of the local authority, but providing for her to attend school from her father's house. After further failures to attend school she was placed under the local authority's supervision for 18 months and returned home. She continued to miss school, confining herself to her room, becoming demanding, domineering, and obsessive. She then effectively barricaded herself in her room refusing entry to certain persons and becoming verbally abusive. She was seen by another child psychiatrist who recommended her removal to the adolescent unit in her own best interests. A later attempt to persuade her to open the door by a social worker and psychiatrist failed. An application for an emergency protection order was refused by the magistrates. She was seen by another psychiatrist, who could not persuade her to leave her room. Eventually the local authority commenced care proceedings with the reappointment of a guardian *ad litem,* who reported that the child was beyond the control of the father. The judge made an interim care order with directions under section 38(6) of the Children Act 1989 for the child to receive a psychiatric examination and assessment and, if necessary, to be treated at an adolescent unit and to remain there during the assessment. She did not consent to go to the unit, so leave was granted to the local authority under section 100(3) to bring proceedings to invoke the exercise of the inherent jurisdiction, on the grounds that the child was likely to suffer significant harm if that action was not taken. The girl did not consent, despite pleadings and encouragement for over 2 hours by social workers and the guardian. The local authority now applied for various orders under the inherent jurisdiction, essentially asking for judicial consent to the proposed treatment and assessment and leave for the girl to be removed from her home for that purpose. The child was represented by her guardian *ad litem.* The mother supported the guardian, but the father opposed the application. The medical evidence pointed to immediate, urgent, and vigorous assessment and therapy. The judge found that the child was of sufficient understanding to make an informed decision about medical examination or psychiatric examination or other assessment.

The following was held.

- There was inherent power under the parens patriae jurisdiction to override the refusal of a minor, whether over the age of 16 years or under that age, to submit to assessment and medical examination and treatment if it was in her best interests, and notwithstanding that she was of sufficient understanding to make an informed decision about medical examination or psychiatric examination or other assessment.
- In an appropriate case, in which other remedies within the Children Act 1989 had been exhausted and found not to bring about the desired result, there was jurisdiction to resort to other remedies, and the particular remedy at present was that of providing authority for doctors to treat the child and authority, if it was needed, for the local authority to take all necessary steps to bring the child to the doctors so that she could be assessed and treated properly.
- On the basis of the facts, the child must be admitted to the adolescent unit in her own interest without any further delay. Leave would be granted to the local authority to take the necessary steps for the child to be assessed and treated.

The case illustrates the extent of attempts by the local authority to avoid the necessity for removing the child compulsorily. It can also be noted that there was no use of the powers under the Mental Health Act 1983. The essential requirement before there can be admission under the Act is that mental disorder should be present and the early psychiatric examinations suggested that there was no evidence of psychiatric disorder.

For a full consideration of the powers open to the local authority, reference should also be made to Chapter 3 in which other powers under the Children Act are discussed.

LINK BETWEEN THE MENTAL HEALTH ACT 1983 AND THE CHILDREN ACT 1989

Notification

Section 85(1) of the Children Act states that if a child is provided with accommodation by any health authority or local education authority for a consecutive period of at least 3 months; or with the intention, on the part of that authority, of accommodating him or her for that period, the accommodating authority shall notify the responsible authority.

The authority must also be notified when the accommodation ends.

DUTY OF LOCAL AUTHORITY AFTER NOTIFICATION
When the local authority has been notified, it must, under section 85(4):

- take such steps as are reasonably practicable to enable them to determine whether the child's welfare is adequately safeguarded and promoted while he or she is being accommodated there, and also consider the extent to which (if at all) it should exercise any of its functions under the Act.

If the child is admitted to accommodation in a residential care home or mental nursing home, under section 86 there is a similar duty on the accommodating authority to notify the local authority as there is under section 85. The local authority has powers of entry and it is an offence to obstruct it.

Under Section 116 of the Mental Health Act 1983, if a child who is in the care of the local authority by virtue of a care order under the Children Act 1989, is admitted to a hospital or nursing home in England or Wales (whether for treatment for mental disorder or for any other reason), the authority shall arrange for visits to be made to him or her on behalf of the authority, and shall take such other steps in relation to the patient while in the hospital or nursing home as would be expected to be taken by his or her parents.

Application to the Family Proceedings Court

Under section 25 of the Children Act and its regulations, there must be an application to the Family Proceedings Court within 2 hours of a child being placed in accommodation if liberty is to be restricted beyond that time (see above for section 25). This duty does not, however, apply if the child is detained under the Mental Health Act 1983.

If the child is a ward of court, the permission of the High Court is necessary to restrict the liberty of the child.

AFTERCARE

Both health authorities and local authorities have duties under the NHS legislation to provide care for the patient after discharge. A child who suffers from mental disorder would come under the provisions of the Chronic Sick and Disabled Persons Act 1970. This requires a local authority social services department to meet the needs of such a person by providing services to him or her. The services identified in section 2 include the provision of practical assistance for that person in the home (see Chapter 5).

CONCLUSION

It must not be assumed that this chapter is laying down any rules as to which is the most appropriate path to be taken in the care of the child suffering from mental disorder: that must remain a professional decision based upon the detailed circumstances of the child's situation and diagnosis. The aim has simply been to show the various routes that can be taken in law to detain compulsorily a child for assessment and treatment of a mental disorder. All have their strengths and weaknesses and it is essential that those professionals caring for the child are acquainted with the legal provisions and differences.

At present it would appear that the route of the child's care and treatment depends not upon the intrinsic differences between the different kinds of legislation but upon the nature of the professionals who are brought in to assist with their care. This can affect not only the diagnosis of the child's condition and the treatment and care necessary, but also, depending upon the professional's background, the route used to provide protection for the child. A review is being undertaken to consider the relationship between the Mental health Act and the Children Act for the care of the child suffering from mental disorder.

REFERENCES

1   Cohen J: Mental Illness among children jumps 50%. *Sunday Times* 19 March 1995: p7.
2   Emma Borton, reported by Cohen J: Mental Illness among children jumps 50%. *Sunday Times* 19 March 1995: p7.
3   Harbour A, Ayotte W (Eds): *Children's Legal Centre Mental Health Handbook: A Guide to the Law Affecting Children and Young People, edn 2*. London: Legal Centre; 1994.
4   Kurtz Z: *With Health in Mind: Mental Health Care for Children and Young People*. London: London Action for Sick Children and South West Thames Regional Health Authority; 1992.
5   Department of Health: *Child health in the community: a guide to good practice*. London: HMSO; 1995. [Consultation draft March 1995.]
6   Jones R: *Mental Health Act Manual., edn 4*. London: Sweet and Maxwell; 1994.
7   Department of Health: *Code of Practice of the Mental Health Act, revised edn*. London: HMSO; 1993.
8   R *v* Ealing District Health Authority ex parte Fox [1993] 3 All ER 170.
9   R *v* Hallstrom ex parte W; R.v.Gardener ex parte L [1986] 2 All ER 306.
10 Re W (a minor) (Medical Treatment) [1992] 4 All ER 627.
11 Inquiry chaired by Sir Cecil Clothier: *Report*. London: HMSO;1994.
12 These are given in Chapter 15, p153.
13 Re W (a Minor) (Medical Treatment) [1992] 4 All ER 627, [1993] 1 FLR 1.
14 R *v* Kirklees Metropolitan Borough Council ex parte C Court of Appeal [1993] 2 FLR 187.
15 Gillick *v* West Norfolk and Wisbech Area Health Authority and another [1986] AC 112, [1985] 3 All ER 402.
16 Department of Health: *The Children Act 1989 Guidance and Regulations*. London: HMSO; 1991.
17 Wyld N, Carlton N: *Family Emergency Procedures*. London: London Legal Action Group; 1993.
18 South Glamorgan County Council v W and B [1993] 1 FLR 574.

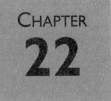
Terminal illness and death

This chapter will consider seven issues in relation to the dying child. These are:

- the extent of the duty to maintain life;
- the involvement of the courts;
- 'not for resuscitation' orders;
- the rights of the parent;
- the rights of the child;
- the care of the dying child; and
- registration of death.

INTRODUCTION

Care of the dying can be extremely stressful for staff and the care of dying children even more so. Health professionals need to know the legal framework within which they work. They need to know the extent to which the law requires them to prolong life in the terminally ill child and when the court is likely to become involved; they must be aware of the rights of the parent and, even, the rights of the child, to refuse or insist upon treatment. They also need to be aware of the standards of care that are recommended for the care of the chronically sick and dying child. Finally, they need to know the practicalities of dealing with death, such as certification, registration, and so forth, so that the parents are given accurate information and are referred to the appropriate agencies with minimum hassle. Reference should be made to the guidance issued by the Department of Health on child health in the community which includes a section on services for children with life-threatening illnesses.[1] It cites the charter published by the Association for Children with Life-Threatening or Terminal Conditions and Their Families (see below) and cites some of the examples of good practice in the care of these children including those suffering from AIDS and who are HIV positive.

THE EXTENT OF THE DUTY TO MAINTAIN LIFE

The care of neonates and children can sometimes present health care professionals with the problem of whether there is a duty in law to carry out every possible procedure known to science in order to save the life of a baby and child or whether the law enables a person to be allowed to die.

Voluntary euthanasia
Voluntary euthanasia means the killing of a person with that person's consent. This is unlawful. It could amount to murder, which is punishable on conviction by life imprisonment.

Alternatively, if the act amounts to assistance in a suicide bid, then it is illegal under section 2(1) of the Suicide Act 1961, shown below.

- A person who aids, abets, counsels, or procures the suicide of another or an attempt by another to commit suicide, shall be liable on conviction on indictment to imprisonment (up to 14 years).

Even if the parents wish a grossly handicapped baby to die, any professional who intentionally speeded up the process of death could be guilty of causing the death of the child. In the case of R v Arthur,[2] a paediatrician was prosecuted for attempting to cause the death of a grossly handicapped baby who was suffering from Down's syndrome and who had other disabilities when he prescribed dihydrocodeine and nursing care only. Dr Arthur was, however, acquitted by the jury. The judge stated that: 'There is no special law in this country that places doctors in a separate category and gives them extra protection over the rest of us... Neither in law is there any special power, facility or license to kill children who are handicapped or seriously disadvantaged in an irreversible way.'

In contrast, at the other end of life, Dr Nigel Cox[3] was convicted when he prescribed potassium chloride to a terminally ill patient, and was sentenced to a year's imprisonment which was suspended for a year. He also had to appear before disciplinary proceedings of the Regional Health Authority, his employers, and the General Medical Council.

The Select Committee of the House of Lords[4] has reported that there should be no change in the law to permit euthanasia. This is also the view put forward by the Law Commission in its recent report.[5]

Do these cases mean that it is never lawful to permit a patient to die whatever the circumstances of his or her condition? The answer is that the law does not expect constant medical intervention, whatever the prognosis, and that in certain circumstances it is legally permissible to let die. A distinction is, however, drawn between letting die and killing.

An example of the court permitting a child to be allowed to die is the case of Re C.[6] In this case a baby was born suffering from congenital hydrocephalus and had been made a ward of court for reasons unconnected with her medical condition. The local authority sought the court's determination as to the appropriate manner in which she should be treated should she contract a serious infection, or should her existing feeding regimes become unviable. A specialist paediatrician assessed C's condition as severely and irreversibly brain damaged, the prognosis of which was hopeless. He recommended that the objective of any treatment should therefore be to ease suffering rather than prolong life. Although not specifying the adoption or discontinuance of any particular procedures, he further advised consultation with C's carers as to the appropriate method of achieving that objective. The judge accepted this report and approved the recommendations as being in her best interests. He initially made a very restrictive order to treat the child to die. But these words 'to die' were changed to 'to allow her life to come to an end peacefully and with dignity.'

The official solicitor who had been appointed guardian *ad litem* of the child appealed to the Court of Appeal on the grounds that the judge had no jurisdiction and was plainly wrong in the exercise of his discretion to make an order that the hospital be at liberty to treat the minor to die. The Court of Appeal varied the judge's order and substituted the words: 'The hospital do continue to treat the minor within the parameters of the opinion expressed by [the specialist paediatrician] in his report of 13/4/1989 which report is not to be disclosed to any person other than the health authority.'

In the case of Re J,[7] in contrast with that of Re C, the baby, a ward of court, was not at the point of death. However, the prognosis was not good and although he was expected to survive a few years he was likely to be blind, deaf, unable to speak, and to have serious spastic quadriplegia. The judge made an order that he should be treated with antibiotics if he developed a chest infection but if he were to stop breathing he should not receive artificial ventilation. The official solicitor on behalf of the child appealed against the order on the grounds that unless the situation was one of terminal illness or it was certain that the child's life would be intolerable, the court was not justified in approving the withholding of life-saving treatment. The court held that the court can never sanction positive steps to terminate the life of a person. However, the court could direct that treatment without which death would ensue need not be given to prolong life, even though the person was neither on the point of death nor dying. The court had to undertake a balancing exercise in assessing the course to be adopted in the best interests of the child, looked at from his point of view and giving the fullest possible weight to his desire, if he were in a position to make a sound judgment, to survive, and taking into account the pain and suffering and quality of life which he would experience if life was prolonged and the pain and suffering involved in the proposed treatment.

Peter Ellis suggests[8] that in such dilemmas as in the case of Baby J 1990: 'the only conclusion that one can come to in a case like this is that there is no right decision... I would suggest that Daniel and his mother should be the primary decision-makers, as long as they are fully informed of all possible outcomes. After all, Mrs Stoneham is the child's mother and there can be no stronger motivation than love for making a right decision.'

Unfortunately, although this might be so in the majority of cases, it will not always been so and the courts, as is illustrated in the case of Re J 1992 (see below), have made it clear that the decision should be in the hands of the health professionals, that is, the doctors.

INVOLVEMENT OF THE COURT

When should the consent of the court be obtained to take action? There are probably many occasions in practice when a patient is allowed to die without court approval being obtained.

In the case described by Jim Richardson,[9] Sally and Joe Woods have a boy, Toby, who is born prematurely and is found to be suffering from several abnormalities, including duodenal atresia that will need surgery, and he may also have Down's syndrome. He requires transfer to a regional unit if he is to survive but there are concerns about whether he could withstand a journey of 65 miles. He survives for 8 days on a ventilator in the small hospital. On the ninth day his cardiac functioning is deteriorating and his intake of fluids intravenously is ended. A ventilator is required in the short term for a baby with a good prognosis. Can Toby be taken off his?

As Toby is dying, it could be argued that a few hours would not make any difference and such a case is unlikely to come before the courts. In practice, if the doctors, the parents, and the rest of the multidisciplinary team are agreed about the prognosis of the child and whether aggressive treatment is appropriate, there is unlikely to be a court hearing. The baby or child will be allowed to die and 'nature to take its course'.

Withholding of artificial feeding has, however, been a matter for court intervention as the Tony Bland case shows.

Tony Bland case[10]

The House of Lords had to decide if it was lawful to permit artificial feeding to be discontinued in the case of a patient in a persistent vegetative state (Airedale NHS Trust v Bland). The patient was a victim of the football stadium crush at Hillsborough and it was established that although he could breathe and digest food independently, he could not see, hear, taste, smell or communicate in any way, and it appeared that there was no hope of recovery or improvement. The House of Lords decided that it would be in the best interests of the patient to discontinue the nasal gastric feed and he was later reported as having died.

The House of Lords recommended that if any similar decisions were required to be made in the future there should be application before the courts.

A court in Bristol gave consent in a similar case a few months after the House of Lords' decision in Tony Bland's case.[11]

A practice note on withdrawal of medical treatment from a patient in a persistent vegetative state was issued by the Official Solicitor in March 1994 for such situations.[12] It is summarized below.

- The termination of artificial feeding and hydration for patients in a persistent vegetative state will in virtually all cases require the prior sanction of a High Court Judge.
- The Medical Ethics Committee of the British Medical Association issued guidelines on treatment decisions for patients in a persistent vegetative state in July 1993. Current methods of diagnosing a persistent vegetative state are not infallible and such a diagnosis should not be considered confirmed until the patient has been insentient for at least 12 months. Before then, as soon as the patient's condition has stabilized, rehabilitative measure such as coma arousal programmes should be instituted.
- Applications to court should be by originating summons issued in the Family Division of the High Court seeking a declaration in the form set out in paragraph 4 below. The application should follow that laid down for sterilization cases as set down in F v Berkshire Health Authority[13] and in the practice note of May 1993.[14]
- Sets out the wording of the originating summons.
- The case should normally be heard in chambers and the judgment given in open court.
- The applicants may be either the next of kin or the relevant health authority or NHS trust (which in any event ought to be a party). The views of the next of kin are very important and should be made known to the court in every case.
- The official solicitor should be invited to act as guardian *ad litem* of the patient.
- There should be at least two neurological reports on the patient, one of which will be commissioned by the official solicitor. Other medical evidence, such as evidence about rehabilitation or nursing care, may be necessary.
- The views of the patient may have been previously expressed, either in writing or otherwise. The High Court exercising its inherent jurisdiction may determine the effect of a purported advance directive as to future medical treatment. The patient's previously expressed views, if any, will always be a very important component in the decisions of the doctors and the court.
- Members of the official solicitor's legal staff are prepared to discuss persistent vegetative state cases before proceedings have been issued. Contact with the official solicitor may be made by telephoning 0171-911-7127 during office hours.

Court is not always the most appropriate forum for coming to decisions in cases of dying children. Legislation may follow the Law Commission's recommendations on decision-making and the mentally incapacitated adult; however, this does not apply to the minor under 16 years of age.[16] There needs to be clarification on when the court's intervention should be sought in the care of a terminally ill child.

Can the court order doctors to treat?

In a later case,[16] J was born in January 1991 and suffered an accidental fall when he was 1 month old with the result that he was profoundly handicapped both mentally and physically. He was severely microcephalic, his brain not having grown sufficiently after the injury. He also had severe cerebral palsy, cortical blindness, and severe epilepsy. He was in general fed by a nasal gastric tube. Medical opinion was unanimous that J was unlikely to develop much beyond his present functioning, that that level might deteriorate, and that his expectation of life, although uncertain, would be short. The paediatrician's report stated that given J's condition it would not be medically appropriate to intervene with intensive procedures, such as artificial ventilation, if he were to suffer a life-threatening event. The baby was in the care of foster parents with whom the local authority shared responsibility. The local authority applied to the court under section 100 of the Children Act 1989 to determine whether ventilation should be given to the child. The judge had regarded J's best interests as well as the interests of justice in preserving his life as both pointing in favour of the grant of an interim injunction requiring such treatment to take place. The mother supported the requirement that the hospital and doctors should be forced to put the baby on a life-support machine.

Lord Donaldson, Master of the Rolls, stated that he could not at present conceive of any circumstances in which to require a medical practitioner, or health authority acting by a medical practitioner, to adopt a course of treatment which, in the bona fide clinical judgment of the practitioner, was contraindicated as not being in the patient's best interests; such a requirement would be abuse of power, as directly or indirectly requiring the practitioner to act contrary to the fundamental duty owed by a doctor to his patient.

Lord Donaldson said that the order of the judge, ordering specific treatment to take place, was wholly inconsistent with the law as stated in Re J[7] and in Re R[17] and could not be justified on the basis of any known authority. It was also erroneous on two other substantial grounds: first, its lack of certainty as to what was required of the health authority, and second, its failure adequately to take account of the sad fact of life that health authorities might on occasion find that they had too few resources, either human or material, or both, to treat all the patients whom they would like to treat in the way they would like to treat them. It was their duty to make choices. The court would have no knowledge of competing claims to a health authority's resources and was in no position to express any view on their deployment

The Court of Appeal thus held that if a paediatrician caring for a severely handicapped baby considered that mechanical ventilation procedures would not be appropriate, the court would not grant an injunction requiring such treatment to take place.

The effect of the court's decision to set aside the judge's ruling was to leave the health authority and its medical staff free, subject to consent not being withdrawn, to treat J in accordance with their best clinical judgment. That did not mean that in no circumstances should J be subjected to mechanical ventilation.

The reluctance of the court to interfere with the decision-making of the doctors in the interests of the patient was seen in a recent case in very different circumstances. In the case of Re B,[18] in which the father of a 10-year-old girl suffering from leukaemia brought an action against the health authority for its refusal to fund a course of chemotherapy followed by a second bone marrow transplant operation (see Chapter 5. pages 41–42, for full discussion of the case), the Court of Appeal took the view that the court should not intervene in such a decision but that the health authority should follow medical advice as to what was in the best interests of the child.

The court has made it clear that decisions relating to the sterilization of a mentally incompetent adult[13] and the cessation of artificial feeding[10] require the involvement of the court, and it is likely that the need for reference in other cases may be made explicit.[19]

NOT FOR RESUSCITATION ORDERS

The legal aspects of such orders are considered by the author and the Royal College of Nursing has issued a paper for guidance.[20]

What is the legal significance of such orders in the care of the child?

A child aged 16 or 17 or one aged below 16 years who is considered to be Gillick-competent could legally give a clear indication that he or she did not wish to be resuscitated in certain circumstances. However, if such a decision were not in the best interests of the minor, it could be overruled by order of court, as occurred in the case of Re W[21] in which a girl aged 16 years refused to be treated for anorexia nervosa. If, however, the decision has been made by the minor and it is considered to be in his or her best interests, then it would be valid for all professional carers of that patient to accept that refusal of care and the instructions that the patient is not to be resuscitated.

If the child is incompetent and the decision has been made by the consultant in charge of the care of the patient that the patient should not be resuscitated, the legality of such a decision depends upon the prognosis of the child, and in dubious cases there are advantages in a declaration from the court being obtained.

Could parents give 'not for resuscitation' or 'do not resuscitate' instructions? It is clear that although the parents should be fully consulted in the decision-making, ultimately they do not have the right to refuse treatment if treatment would be in the child's best interests.

PARENTAL VIEWS

Health professionals also need to know what, if any, rights the parents have in such circumstances; if they wish the child to be allowed to die, would the professionals be acting illegally to go against their wishes? It is clear that in discussions about the future care of the child, the parents have an important part to play, but ultimately the decision whether a child should receive life-saving treatment cannot be theirs alone. If the parents refuse to give consent to treatment that, in the doctor's view, is in the best interests of the child, an application could be made to the court. (This is the situation in relation to refusal by Jehovah's Witnesses parents to consent to blood transfusions discussed in Chapter 6.) The same principles apply when the child is dying.

An example of a case where the courts refused to uphold the parents' wish to allow the child to die is seen in the case of Re B.[22] In Re B a child was born suffering from Down's syndrome and an intestinal blockage. She required an operation to relieve the obstruction if she was to live more than a few days. If the operation were performed, the child might die within a few months but it was probable that her life expectancy would be 20–30 years. Her parents, having decided that it would be kinder to allow her to die rather than live as a physically and mentally handicapped person, refused to consent to the operation. The local authority made the child a ward of court and, when a surgeon decided that the wishes of the parents should be respected, the hospital sought an order authorizing the operation to be performed by other named surgeons. The judge decided that the parents' wishes should be respected and refused to make the order. The local authority appealed to the Court of Appeal, which allowed the appeal. It stated the following.

- The question for the court was whether it was in the best interests of the child that she should have the operation and not whether the parents' wishes should be respected.
- As the effect of the operation might be that the child would have the normal span of life of a mongol, and as it had not been demonstrated that the life of a mongol was of such a nature that the child should be condemned to die, the court would make an order that the operation be performed.

Crucial to the decision in this case was the prognosis for the child.

A case study which raised the issues that surround conflict between the parents' views and those of professional staff is discussed by Lesley Lowes.[23] The case concerned the near drowning of a 2-year-old boy who was transferred from intensive care to an acute medical paediatric ward. He arrived in a comatose state and after 2 weeks of aggressive treatment in the intensive care unit, the parents agreed that he should be treated positively until he died. He received humidified oxygen via a tracheostomy, and was fed nasogastrically. He developed total extension which, although treated with physiotherapy and medication, made it difficult to position him comfortably. His parents became increasingly concerned that he was suffering, and after 6 weeks, they requested all treatment, including nasogastric feeding, be stopped to allow him to die.

The multidisciplinary team agreed that physiotherapy should be discontinued and any ensuing chest infection remain untreated, with a gradual increasing of analgesic, ensuring that he would not suffer and could die peacefully. It was decided to continue nasal gastric feeding. In spite of the decision in the case of Tony Bland,[24] the author states that the legal position is not clear. It is suggested, however, that in view of the decisions by the Courts in the cases outlined above, the legal principles are clear, the only point in doubt being in which cases the court would wish the issues to be brought before it.

The parents do not have the right to insist upon care or treatment that the doctors consider is not in the best interests of the child. As has been discussed above, the court would not order the doctors to carry out treatment on a child that the doctors considered not to be in the best interests of the child.

THE WISHES OF THE CHILD

Difficulties can arise over the extent to which the views of the child should be taken into account. Clearly, if the child is below the age of Gillick-competence, decisions can only be made on the basis of the prognosis, and the best interests in the light of that prognosis. The issues relating to the older Gillick-competent child are considered in Chapter 6. Problems can arise when the wishes of the Gillick-competent child in relation to his or her future differ from the views of the parent or health professional. The conflicts that can arise are considered in Chapter 6 on the law on consent. Here, however, we consider the issue relating to a child refusing treatment which is life-saving.

Three of Jim Richardson's case studies[25] deal with this in very different circumstances. One is discussed above in relation to neonatal care. In the second (Painful treatment) Shawn Brooker, a 9-year-old boy who is suffering from tuberculosis meningitis, has to have long-term treatment involving daily lumbar punctures and he shows increasing reluctance to have the treatment. There is no evidence, however, that he could be described as Gillick-competent and has taken on board the probability that death would follow. Therefore, despite his protests, health professionals have a duty to ensure that he receives the necessary treatment. If the parents support the boy's refusal, there would be justification in going to court to seek a specific order.

The third case (My CF is just too strong) Pamela is 9 years old and has reached the stage in her illness where she is refusing admission to hospital, physiotherapy, and, eventually, any form of treatment. She tells her father that she thinks she is going to die soon; that she feels her treatment is a waste of time and she has decided not to have any of it any more. From that moment on she stoutly refused to have any sort of treatment.

What is the legal position?

It may be that Pamela even at 9 years old is Gillick-competent, that is, that she has the capacity to understand all the issues. In balancing the continued discomfort and suffering to herself against the benefits of her being able to survive until new treatments, or a cure, or a heart–lung transplant can be made available, she has made the decision that she would prefer to end her life now.

Her parents and her health professionals may, however, disagree with her decision and consider that new treatments will shortly be available and that immediate treatment of her infections would lead to an improvement in her condition. In this situation compulsory admission to hospital and compulsory treatment is justified.

If the matter were to go before the courts, it is likely that they would be influenced by the medical reports on prognosis. In the case of Re W,[26] which is discussed in Chapter 6, even though there was evidence that the 16-year-old girl was Gillick-competent and even though she had the right to give consent to treatment under the Family Reform Act 1969 and even though the Children Act 1989 specifically requires the court to take into account the wishes of the child, according to their level of competence, the court ordered that the treatment for her anorexia must be given.

In the case of Re E[27] in 1993, a boy of 15 years and 9 months who was a Jehovah's Witness refused to have blood and this refusal was supported by his parents but the court held that he should be given it, in spite of the fact that he was so close to his sixteenth birthday (see Chapter 6, pages 56–58, for further discussion on this case).

In the case of Pamela, therefore, it is highly likely that if the health professionals were of the view that her prognosis was reasonable enough to give her a good quality of life for some time yet and, even if the parents supported Pamela's views, treatment could be given compulsorily, if necessary by court order. The health professionals have a duty to provide care according to the standard of the Bolam test (see Chapter 13) and would have to determine in the exact circumstances of Pamela's case where her interests lay.

The final point in the situation is Pamela dying and the parents asking whether they could give her all the morphine in the syringe and finish her suffering. The law on this is clear, as the Nigel Cox case cited above illustrates. To carry out such an action would be illegal. Morphine given in quantities to relieve pain and suffering is lawful even if there is a side effect that expectancy of life will be reduced; morphine given with the intention to end life is murder or manslaughter.

Further discussion on the ethical principles in withdrawing paediatric intensive care is considered by Karen Bracegirdle[28] who discusses cases in which aggressive treatment has been withdrawn and the importance of communication between parents, child, and professionals in ensuring that the child can have a peaceful and dignified death.

There is a danger that those writing of the situation from an ethical standpoint fail to pay sufficient attention to the legal rights of the parent and child in giving consent to aggressive treatment which may prolong life. For example, Karin Enskar,[29] in taking a case study of a 7-year-old girl suffering from leukaemia, discusses the choice that has to be made between intensification of chemotherapy treatment which might increase the survival rate but which has a higher risk of side effects against a less intensive regime. The author states that: 'the girl is only 7 years old and cannot be regarded as competent enough to decide which treatment will be the most appropriate.' She also says: 'Normally, parents have enough competence to be autonomous, but, in a very stressful situation, and especially where very specific knowledge is required they are not competent enough to decide upon their child's treatment.' Neither of these statements can be taken as the law in this country. The competence of the child will relate to the decision to be made and the maturity of the child in question, and it could be argued that the parents should be given sufficient information to ensure that they are capable of making the decision if the child lacks the competence.

CARE OF THE DYING CHILD

The Association for Children with Life-Threatening or Terminal Conditions and Their Families has been active in developing a Charter for the care of children, the ACT Charter for Children with Life-Threatening Conditions and their Families. Its clauses are set out below.

- Every child shall be treated with dignity and respect and shall be afforded privacy whatever the child's physical or intellectual ability.
- Parents shall be acknowledged as the primary carers and shall be centrally involved as partners in all care and decisions involving their child.
- Every child shall be given the opportunity to participate in decisions affecting his or her care, according to age and understanding.

- Every family shall be given the opportunity of a consultation with a paediatric specialist who has particular knowledge of the child's condition.
- Information shall be provided for the parents, and for the child and the siblings according to age and understanding. The needs of other relatives shall also be addressed.
- An honest and open approach shall be the basis of all communications which shall be sensitive and appropriate to age and understanding.
- The family home shall remain the centre of the caring whenever possible. All other care shall be provided by paediatric trained staff in a child-centred environment.
- Every child shall have access to education. Efforts shall be made to enable the child to engage in other childhood activities.
- Every family shall be entitled to a named key worker who will enable the family to build up and maintain an appropriate support system.
- Every family shall have access to flexible respite care in their own home and in a home-from-hospital setting for the whole family with appropriate paediatric nursing and medical support.
- Every family shall have access to paediatric nursing support in the home when required.
- Every family shall have access to expert, sensitive advice in procuring practical aids and financial support.
- Every family shall have access to domestic help at times of stress at home.
- Bereavement support shall be offered to the whole family and be available for as long as required.

A report was prepared by a Working Party on the Care of Dying Children and their Families by the British Paediatric Association, King Edward's Hospital Fund for London, and the National Association of Health Authorities in 1988.[30] The aim of the report is to guide health authority members, managers, and practitioners. The topics which are covered include a philosophy of care, the needs of the families, and the principles of care at all stages of the illness. It also covers the practical implementation of these principles, and considers the structure of existing services, emphasizing the need to improve communications and strengthen community care and the education and support of staff involved . The recommendations from the 'Care of dying children' report are summarized below.

- Every regional health authority and district health authority should produce and publish a strategy for the care of children with life-threatening conditions.
- The responsibility for the service should lie with one named officer and be included in that person's job description.
- The number of children falling into the three categories [progressive degenerative conditions for which there is no cure (e.g. cystic fibrosis, muscular dystrophy); serious handicaps which can be life threatening (e.g. Down's syndrome); life-threatening diseases where they may be a cure, but many children still die (e.g. leukaemia, and liver and heart disease] should be calculated in each district, including those receiving treatment at a regional centre.
- The adequacy of existing local services and methods of communication should be assessed, as a basis for further discussion.
- Checklists on the quality of service offered should be prepared, using the principles of care as a starting point.
- Ways of improving the continuity of the service between hospital and community, especially from the families' point of view, should be considered.
- Arrangements for the speedy transfer of information, skills, and expertise between the hospital and primary care teams should be agreed.
- A key-person system should be introduced, so that each family has help in locating services and building up a support structure.

- A domiciliary paediatric nursing service should be provided, to cover all children with life-threatening conditions, throughout the course of their illness and at the terminal stage if the home option is chosen. Access to respite care should be part of this service.
- A firm commitment should be made to keep abreast of the leaflets published by voluntary organizations and to use family or group support facilities.
- Money donated by the public to set up services and facilities for dying children and their families can form a valuable additional resource, but health authorities should never set up anything before completing the first, third, and fourth steps of these recommendations. Cooperation between districts should be considered.
- Examples are specified of excellent care for children with a life-threatening condition, and their practices might help to form models for the development of a domiciliary paediatric nursing service.
- Many children will continue to die in hospital. Health authorities should review their procedures and arrangements, so that parents are under less pressure to make quick decisions.
- Health authorities should arrange training sessions for hospital and community staff on the special needs of dying children and their families.
- Care of dying children and their families can be emotionally exhausting and a strong support system should be provided for the caring teams.

Since the recommendations were written in 1988, NHS trusts have been set up and many of the detailed recommendations would now be the responsibility of such trusts. It would fall, however, to the health authorities as commissioners to plan a strategy to ensure that the relevant services were purchased and standards set in the NHS agreements and to monitor the implementation of these standards by the providers.

REGISTRATION OF DEATH

The doctor who attended the patient during the last illness must certify the death and give the cause unless the circumstances are such that the death should be reported to the coroner. Such circumstances are:

- if the deceased was not attended in his last illness by a doctor;
- if the deceased was not seen by a doctor either after death or within the 14 days before death;
- if the cause of death is unknown;
- if death appears to be caused by industrial disease or poisoning;
- if death may have been unnatural or caused by violence or neglect or abortion or attended by suspicious circumstances; or
- if death has occurred during an operation or before recovery from an anaesthetic.

Usually the individual coroner will make the cause of death known to local doctors in respect of the notification of deaths occurring in hospital. Some, for example, may require reporting of all deaths occurring within 24 hours of emergency admission.[31]

The causes of death that would therefore be reportable to the coroner are:

- deaths resulting from a criminal offence, such as murder and manslaughter;
- suicide;
- road traffic accidents, industrial accidents, domestic accidents, etc;
- death in custody, prison, or police custody;
- deaths associated with medical treatment;
- sudden death;
- deaths after abortion, drug dependence, alcoholism;

- infant deaths where no midwife or doctor was present; and
- cot-deaths.

Until the coroner has formally notified the doctor of his or her decision in relation to the deceased, the body remains under the control of the coroner, that is, under his or her jurisdiction. The coroner has the right to request a postmortem and there can be no action taken over the body without his or her consent.

Can relatives view the body? The consent of the coroner must be obtained for the body to be viewed by the relatives.[32]

Postmortem

The relatives have no right to refuse an order by the coroner for a postmortem. This is so even when the religious views of the deceased would be against a postmortem.[33] On the other hand, if the doctor requests a postmortem when the body is not under the jurisdiction of the coroner, the person in charge of the body could refuse to give consent. In any event the requirements of the Human Tissue Act 1961 and the Anatomy Act 1984 must be followed.

Inquest

The coroner will decide whether or not to hold an inquest after receiving a report of a death. He or she is obliged by law to hold an inquest if there are reasons to suspect a criminal offence has caused the death, and in the cases of industrial accidents and diseases and deaths in prison or police custody. The existence of a general discretion to hold an inquest has been doubted.[34] The purpose of the inquest is to ascertain who the deceased was and how, when, and where the deceased died.[35] Possible verdicts are:

- natural causes;
- unlawful killing;
- killed lawfully;
- killed himself or herself (while the balance of his or her mind was disturbed);
- accidental death;
- misadventure;
- dependence upon a drug;
- nondependent abuse of drugs;
- industrial disease;
- neglect;
- want of attention at birth;
- attempted or self-induced abortion; and
- open verdict.

An open verdict indicates that there is insufficient evidence to determine the nature of the death, that is, 'The evidence did not further or fully disclose the means whereby the cause of death arose.' Once completed, the inquest cannot be resumed but the High Court has the power under section 13 of the Coroners Act 1988 to order another inquest to be held.[36]

The health professional and the coroner's court

The health professional might be required to give evidence at an inquest on the events which preceded death. He or she should be alert to this possibility. For example, a nurse may know that a child who has died in an apparent cot death situation suffered from certain symptoms before the death. This information from the nurse may be vital at any inquest into the death.

It is essential that the nurse obtains assistance from a senior manager on the statement which the coroner's office will require from him or her. If he or she is subsequently asked to attend the inquest, he or she should have assistance in preparation for this. One means of preparation is to attend an inquest before giving evidence so that the nurse can have an understanding of the geography of the court, the procedure which is followed, and the level of formality at a time when he or she is not personally involved. He or she should note that the coroner's court is known as an inquisitorial one. This means that, unlike the magistrates, crown, and civil courts in which an action is brought by one person or organization against another and the judge controls the proceedings of this adversarial system, the coroner determines the witnesses who will give evidence and the course of the proceedings, and will disallow any question which in his or her opinion is not relevant or otherwise not a proper one. The coroner can him- or herself examine the witnesses, often asking leading questions if information is not disputed to speed up the hearing. Hence the words 'inquisitorial' and 'inquest'.

If the death has been reported to the coroner, no certificate can be issued or registration take place until the coroner has made his or her decision. If he or she decides that a postmortem should be carried out, but no inquest is needed, he or she will issue Form B which is sent or taken to the registrar. The registrar will then issue the death certificate, and the certificate for disposal which is required by the undertaker before burial can take place. Authorization for cremation requires an additional medical certificate or the certificate issued by the coroner.

BIRTH AND THEN DEATH

If the baby is born alive and then dies, there must be a registration of both the birth and the death.

STILLBIRTH

A stillbirth is defined as: 'Where a child issues forth from its mother after the 24th week of pregnancy, and which did not at any time after being completely expelled from its mother breathe or show any signs of life' (section 41 of the 1953 Act as amended by section 1 of the Still Birth Act 1992). The stillbirth has to be registered as such and the informant has to deliver to the registrar a written certificate that the child was not born alive. This must be signed by the registered medical practitioner or the registered midwife who was in attendance at the birth or who has examined the body. The certificate must state, to the best of the knowledge and the belief of the person signing it, the cause of death and the estimated duration of the pregnancy (section 11(1)(a)). If the midwife is in sole attendance at the confinement, whether in a home or in a hospital, she must complete the certificate.

Alternatively, a declaration in the prescribed form giving the reasons for the absence of a certificate and that the child was not born alive could be made (section 11(1)(b)).

A stillbirth should be disposed of by burial in a burial ground or churchyard or by cremation at an authorized crematorium.

A health authority should not dispose of a stillbirth without the consent of the parents.

FETUS OF LESS THAN 24 WEEKS

No registration is necessary in the cases of a fetus of less than 24 weeks being delivered showing no signs of life. The fetus may be disposed of without formality in any way which does not constitute a nuisance or an affront to public decency. If the fetus shows signs of life and then dies, it would have to be treated as both a birth and a death.

Health professionals should be sensitive to the fact that parents may suffer the same feelings of bereavement whatever the period of gestation and should therefore arrange for counselling and support as they would if the baby were full term.

REFERENCES

1 Department of Health: *Child Health in the Community: A Guide to Good Practice*. London: HMSO; 1995. [Consultation draft March 1995.]
2 R *v* Arthur *Times* 6 November 1981
3 R *v* Cox [1993] 2 All ER 19
4 House of Lords: *Committee on Medical Ethics, Session 1993–4*. London: HMSO; 1994.
5 Law Commission: *Report No. 231 – Mental Incapacity*. London: HMSO; 1995.
6 Re C (a minor) [wardship; medical treatment] 1989 2 All ER 782.
7 Ellis P: A child's right to die: who should decide? *Br J Nurs* 1992, 1:406–408.
8 Richardson J, Webber I: *Ethical Issues in Child Health Care*. London: Mosby; 1995: pp27–34.
9 Airedale NHS Trust *v* Bland 1993 1 All ER 821.
10 Frenchay Healthcare NHS Trust *v* S [1994] 2 All ER 403.
11 Practice note [1994] 2 All ER 413.
12 Practice Note [1993] 3 All ER 222.
13 F *v* West Berkshire Health Authority [1989] 2 All ER 525.
14 Law Commission: *Report No. 231 – Mental Incapacity*. London: HMSO; 1995.
15 Re J (a minor) [wardship; medical treatment] [1990] 3 All ER 930.
16 Re J (a minor) [wardship; medical treatment] [1992] 4 All ER 614.
17 Re R (a minor) [wardship; medical treatment] [1991] 4 All ER 177.
18 Re B *v* Cambridge and Huntingdon Health Authority. *Times* Law Report 15 March 1995.
19 Dimond B: Not for resuscitative treatment. *Br J Nurs* 1992, 1:93–94.
20 Royal College of Nursing: *Resuscitation: Right or Wrong. Paper No. 000 163*. London: RCN.
21 Re W (a minor) [medical treatment] [1992] 4 All Er 206.
22 Re B (a minor) [wardship; medical treatment] [1981] 1 WLR 1421.
23 Lowes L: Ethical decision making: theory to practice. *Paediatr Nurs* 1993, 5:10–11.
24 Airedale NHS Trust *v* Bland House of Lords [1993] 1 All ER 821.
25 Richardson J, Webber I: *Ethical Issues in Child Health Care*. London: Mosby; 1995.
26 Re W (a minor) [medical treatment] [1992] 4 All Er 206.
27 Re E (a minor) [wardship; medical treatment] [1993] 1 FLR 386.
28 Bracegirdle KE: A time to die: withdrawal of paediatric intensive care. *Br J Nurs* 1994, 3:513–517.
29 Enskar K: Ethical aspects of judging alternative treatment of children with cancer. *Nurs Ethics* 1995, 2:51–62.
30 Thornes R: *The Care of Dying Children and Their Families*. Birmingham: Birmingham National Association of Health Authorities; 1988.
31 Knight B: *Legal Aspects of Medical Practice, edn 5*. London: Churchill Livingstone; 1992: p96.
32 Dimond BC: Death in the Accident and Emergency Department. *Accident and Emergency Nursing* 1995, 3:38–41.
33 R *v* Westminster City Coroner, ex parte Rainer (1968) 112 Solicitors Journal 883.
34 Ex Parte Thomas 1993 2 WLR 547 Court of Appeal.
35 Coroners Act 1988 section 11(5)(b).
36 Coroners Act 1988 section 13(1)(b).

CHAPTER

23

Health promotion: screening and vaccination

The legal issues to be covered in this chapter on health promotion include legal entitlement, duty to screen and to vaccinate, and issues relating to consent and confidentiality. Screening and vaccination can give rise to claims for compensation and these will be considered in relation to the laws of negligence and state compensation through the Vaccine Damage Payments Act 1979. Reference should be made to the Department of Health Guidance on Child Health in the Community[1] and the section on preschool child health services and immunization and the references cited in that document.

SCREENING

Consent
It can usually be assumed that participation in a screening programme will be in the best interests of the child and that a parent who gives consent for that participation would be acting in the child's best interests. This is not necessarily so however. At present there is no recognized cure for AIDS or for being HIV positive. The disadvantages that could result from a positive finding could have a stigmatizing effect upon the child and considerably disadvantage him or her without any corresponding benefits.

In addition, there can be false-positive and false-negative results from some screening programmes with consequent problems.

Genetic screening
Genetic screening for potential diseases and weaknesses has raised huge ethical and legal issues for insurance and employment and other areas of life, and the question must therefore be raised as to whether it is necessarily in the best interest for a parent to give consent for a minor to undergo a genetic screening test, which may create immense problems for him or her for the rest of his or her life.

The human genome project was proposed by Robert Sinsheimer in California in 1984 to identify the protein building blocks which shape human life. The aim is that by 2005 all three billion letters in the genetic code should be identified. The fact of identification of genetic predispositions raises huge ethical and legal dilemmas which are only just being confronted. One of the issues is the right of employers and insurance companies to insist on applicants being genetically screened.

The adult person could, of course, refuse the test but this may mean the loss of insurance cover or employment. Those who are genetically screened could be disadvantaged as a result of a discovery that he or she may have a potential susceptibility to a particular condition even though there is no certainty that that condition would in fact later develop. A request that a parent gives consent for a child to be screened raises similar issues in relation to the child being possibly disadvantaged.

At present there are no laws relating to screening other than the common law of trespass to the person and the law relating to consent which is discussed in Chapter 6. The Nuffield Council on Bioethics was established in 1991 to consider the ethical issues presented by advances in biomedical and biological research. Its first report on genetic screening was published in December 1993.[2] It recognized the difficulty in assessing individual health risks exposed by genetic screening; the complexity of the issues relating to confidentiality; the resource implications of any requirements introduced on ethical grounds; and the need for a broad framework to prevent potential eugenic abuse.

The main conclusions of the report on genetic screening are shown below.

- Adequately informed consent should be a requirement for all genetic screening programmes.
- Counselling should be readily available for those being genetically screened, and for those being tested on account of a family history of a genetic disorder.
- Health professionals should seek to persuade individuals, should persuasion be necessary, to allow the disclosure of relevant genetic information to other family members.
- Appropriate professional bodies should prepare guidelines to help with the difficult decisions over confidentiality and the passing on of information within the family.
- The Department of Health should consider, with health authorities and the appropriate professional bodies, effective arrangements for the preservation of confidentiality, particularly that of genetic registers, and should issue the necessary guidance.
- The Department of Employment should keep under review the potential use of genetic screening by employers.
- Genetic screening of employees for increased occupational risks ought only to be contemplated in specifically defined circumstances, such as if there is strong evidence of a clear connection between the working environment and the development of the condition for which genetic screening can be conducted.
- British insurance companies should adhere to their current policy of not requiring any genetic tests as a prerequisite of obtaining insurance.
- There should be early discussions between the Government and the British insurance industry about the future use of genetic data, and, pending the outcome, companies should accept a temporary moratorium on requiring the disclosure of genetic data.
- The need for improving public understanding of human genetics should be borne in mind in any review of the national curriculum and in the work of all public bodies concerned with the public understanding of science.
- Its recommendations of adequately informed consent, confidentiality and the central coordination and monitoring of genetic screening programmes should be essential to the safeguards on eugenic abuse.
- The Department of Health in consultation with the appropriate professional bodies should formulate detailed criteria for introducing genetic screening programmes, and establish a central coordinating body to review genetic screening programmes and monitor their implementation and outcome.

No action has yet been taken upon its proposals. It is suggested that the minor requires special protection from parents giving consent to genetic screening which is not necessarily in his or her best interests.

SITUATION

A child is diagnosed as having cystic fibrosis. He has two siblings and these are immediately tested to see whether they also have the disease. It is found that they are negative. It is known, however, that they have a one in two chance of being carriers of the disease. The children are now aged 4 and 6 years, respectively. Should the parents give consent for them to be tested for being carriers?

It is suggested that it is not in the best interests of the children at that time to be tested for being carriers and it would be advisable to wait until the child reached the age of 16 years or became Gillick-competent when he or she could give consent in his or her own right for a test. Being a carrier only becomes a significant issue when the person is contemplating sexual activity or having children.

Confidentiality

If the parent gives consent for the child to be screened, to whom can that information be made available? What duties of confidentiality apply?

In Chapter 7 the basic principles are set out and it is unlikely that different principles would apply for information obtained from screening for health status. However, any disclosure should be seen from the child's perspective and in relation to the child's interests.

The difficulties can be seen in a family in which members are at risk from Huntington's chorea. The fact that one member has been diagnosed as a sufferer might be kept confidential from others at risk and they may only discover their vulnerability when they themselves have had children who might become sufferers.

Negligence

DUTY OF THE PROFESSIONAL

Certain screening tests are now so well established and of such significance in the prevention of disease that there is a duty upon the health professional to ensure that the parent is offered the test at the appropriate time. To fail to do so could be evidence of negligence. Failure to ensure that a pregnant woman in a high risk group is offered screening could be evidence of a breach of the duty of care. Similarly, the health professional is under a duty to ensure that a child is given screening at the appropriate times during his or her childhood.

What is the legal situation if a professional fails to ensure that the child is given, for example, a test for congenital dislocation of the hip? Failure to detect the abnormality at an early stage could result in the child failing to walk by the appropriate time and being unable to balance on the affected leg. Remedying the deformity at a later stage may prove more difficult and traumatic for the child. Could the parents sue for failure to diagnose, claiming compensation for the additional harm that has resulted from the breach of the duty of care? The answer is yes, and the parents would probably have little difficulty in establishing that the appropriate duty of care owed to the child by the professionals was broken.

The child also has a course of action, as can be seen in a case[3] discussed in Chapter 13. In this case the deformity was not diagnosed until the child, born on 3 February 1959, was 3 years old. She issued a writ 28 years later and the judge held that she did not have the knowledge, actual or constructive, of her right of action until she was seen by a doctor in 1984 and her action was not therefore statute barred. The implications of this case are significant for health professionals, but it must be emphasized that each case, and whether it is statute barred, is determined on its own facts (see Chapter 13).

The right to be screened does not apply to all genetic diseases. For example, not all centres at present screen for such illnesses as cystic fibrosis and sickle-cell anaemia. Parents with a known genetic predisposition for these kinds of illness could probably obtain screening for the child under the NHS but there is no clear principle that all possible screening tests are available as of right. Failure to be offered the test does not therefore automatically give a parent or child a right of action in negligence if it is subsequently found that the child is a sufferer.

Campbell[4] gives examples of litigation which can arise from negligence in screening. Hypoglycaemia can be screened for but because of its known link with brain damage this could lead to litigation. What is noted in the records is therefore very important. Litigation could result from allegations that hypoglycaemia, hyperbilirubinaemia, and kernicterus have led to neurological damage.

Campbell also points out: 'Unfortunately screening tests are not infallible and they contain potential pitfalls for doctors and nurses.' They may be omitted for one reason or another at the routine time and then forgotten. They may be carried out under unsatisfactory conditions, performed incompetently, the results ignored, or there may be errors in the laboratory. There will also be false-positive and false-negative results that require follow-up and reappraisal. 'The relative responsibilities of doctors and nurses in carrying out these screening tests and in acting on the results require that clear and unambiguous policies are formulated in the hospital and community health services.'

He cites a case in which a Guthrie test was not performed. 'An infant was transferred to a medical centre for the treatment of transient respiratory distress a few hours after birth. He improved quickly and was returned to the small district hospital on the fifth day, still mildly jaundiced. It was assumed that the Guthrie test would be performed at the district hospital on the following day but the nurses there assumed that it would have been done at the main hospital prior to transfer. Nobody checked. The baby was seen regularly by his general practitioner who noted that the jaundice cleared after about six weeks. He measured the baby carefully and regularly but did not plot the measurements on growth centile charts and did not appreciate that although the infant's weight was increasing normally his head circumference and length were lagging behind. At the age of nine months it was obvious that the infant was severely delayed in development and when seen again by the paediatrician who had discharged him from the main hospital nine months earlier there were obvious clinical features of hypothyroidism.'

The case illustrates:

- grave failures in communication;
- the GP's false assumption that a test had been undertaken and that therefore the persistent jaundice was a result of breast-feeding; and
- the importance of using centile charts to identify early any subtle variations in growth.

Congenital dislocation of the hip
Litigation can result from the failure by doctors and nurses and health visitors to notice the signs of dislocation, even after the mother has expressed concern.

CHILD HEALTH SURVEILLANCE
The Government has recently emphasized the importance of child health surveillance by including in the contract for GPs, introduced in 1990, payments for GPs to take responsibility for preschool child health surveillance. The Department of Health in its guidance on child health in the community estimates that 70% of children are receiving child health surveillance from their GP.[5]

The following are the recognized screening procedures.[6]

- Neonatal examinations: review of family history, pregnancy, and birth; any concern expressed by the parents; full physical examination, including weight and head circumference; check for congenital dislocation of hips and testicular descent; inspect eyes, view red reflex of fundus with ophthalmoscope but do not attempt fundoscopy; if high-risk category for hearing defect, consider more specialist hearing tests; PKU and thyroid tests to be done at usual time.

- At discharge or within ten days: check hips again.
- At 6 weeks: check history and ask about parental concerns; full physical examination, including weight and head circumference; check for congenital dislocation of hips; enquire particularly about concerns regarding vision and hearing; inspect eyes; do not attempt hearing test but check again whether baby is in high-risk category for hearing loss and refer if necessary; give parents checklist of advice for detection of hearing loss.
- At 8 months (range 7–9 months): enquire about parental concerns over health and development; ask specifically about vision and hearing; check weight if parents so request or if indicated; look for evidence of congenital dislocation of hips; check for testicular descent; observe visual behaviour and look for squint; carry out distraction test of hearing.
- At 21 months (range 18–24 months): enquire about parental concerns, particularly regarding behaviour, vision, and hearing; confirm that child is walking with normal gait, is beginning to say words, and is understanding when spoken to; do not attempt formal tests of vision or hearing – arrange detained assessment if either are in doubt; remember high prevalence of iron deficiency anaemia at this age.
- At 39 months (range 36–42 months): ask about vision, squint, hearing, behaviour, and development. If any concerns, discuss with the parent whether the child is likely to have any special educational problems or needs and arrange further action as appropriate; measure height and plot on chart; check for testicular descent (if not checked on any other occasion since 8 months); if indicated, perform or arrange hearing test.
- At 5 years (school entry, range approximately 48–66 months): enquire about parental and teacher concerns; review preschool records; physical examination, including auscultation of heart if specific indication or if no record available to confirm previous medical care; measure height and plot on chart; check vision using Snellen chart; check hearing by 'sweep' test.
- School years: further visual acuity check at ages 8, 11, and 14 years; test colour vision using Ishihara plates at age 11 years; repeat height measurement if indicated.[7]

Failure of a health professional to offer and carry out these tests, in the absence of special justifying circumstances, could lead to an action for compensation if it can be shown that had the defect been detected earlier, greater harm could have been prevented.

DUTY OF PARENTS

Does it therefore follow that the parents have no option other than to agree to the screening being carried out? The answer must depend upon the nature of the test and the advantages to the child in being screened. For example, if the parents refuse the heel test (for phenylketonuria) and as a consequence the child is not placed on the correct diet, any subsequent child who is likely to be at risk and should therefore be tested could be the subject of an application to the courts. If, once the diagnosis is made, the correct diet is not provided for the child, this could justify intervention by the local authority to protect the child. On the other hand, screening for hearing or vision may not be life-saving and, unless there are clear contraindications, is unlikely to lead to immediate action being taken against the parents. Concerns by teachers or health professionals about the condition of the child might eventually lead to action being taken under the Children Act 1989.

The disadvantages to the child of certain forms of genetic screening are discussed above.

VACCINATIONS

Public Health law in this century has relied heavily upon prevention of diseases in childhood through immunization and vaccination. Ours system is, however, voluntary. No health professional has the right to give a vaccination or immunize a child without the consent of the parent or guardian. Even though national protection against these diseases relies upon achieving what is known as 'herd immunity', there are no compulsory powers to be invoked. Jim Richardson's book[8] spells out the increasing pressures on health staff to achieve high levels of immunization, including the fact that payment is not made until a specified rate of vaccination has been reached.

This raises several legal issues. These are:

- the nature of the consent that must be obtained before a vaccination can be given;
- the information that must be given;
- the consequences for health care staff if they fail to get consent or fail to give all necessary information;
- the consequences if harm follows the vaccination – to the staff and to the makers of the vaccine;
- the significance of risk in legal terms;
- the compensation available to the child if harm occurs; and
- the duties of the parents to ensure the child is vaccinated and whether they could be sued by the child if the unvaccinated child suffers from an illness which the vaccine was designed to prevent, or if the vaccinated child suffers from an illness or disability as a consequence of the vaccination.

In Jim Richardson's book,[9] the case of Emily Hodge is discussed. Emily is 3 months old and her parents have to make the decision as to whether she should be immunized. The mother was badly shaken as a result of her earlier contact with the health services and Emily's birth at 34 weeks after a course of fertility treatment. The parents seek out as much information as they can about the advantages and disadvantages of immunization and initially, after taking Emily to the clinic, leave without the immunization having been given. Many factors influenced this decision, including the fact that there appeared to be no opportunity at the clinic to discuss the issue further and also the fact that consent was not required to be given in writing.

The nature of the consent that must be obtained before a vaccination can be given

The Department of Health book on immunization[10] does not suggest that a consent form should be completed for immunization as consent can be considered to be implicitly agreed because the parent has brought the child to the clinic. This may not necessarily be true. However, if the health worker asks the mother to pull up the child's sleeve for the vaccine to be given, there can be considered to be an implied consent to it taking place. This would be sufficient to prevent an action for battery; it may not be sufficient to prevent an action for breach of the duty to inform under the law of negligence.

The information that must be given

The requirement in law is that sufficient information must be given to the person before consent is obtained as would be reasonable according to the standards of the reasonable professional (applying the Bolam test; see the case of Sidaway discussed in Chapter 6).

Clinics should ensure that either the health visitor or another health professional has already seen the parent to discuss all the pros and cons of the vaccination, or otherwise that time is given at the clinic for the information to be provided. This would include information in writing and by word of mouth. Time should also be taken to ensure that all contraindications to the vaccination being done at a specific time should be checked with the mother.

The consequences for health care staff if they fail to get consent or fail to give all necessary information

If there is failure by the clinic staff to check any contraindications against giving an immunization at that particular time, or if they fail to spell out the risks involved, their employer could be held vicariously liable should harm befall the child as a consequence of their failure. The child's representative would have to show that any reasonable professional would have asked relevant questions or obtained information which they failed to obtain and which, if it had been known would have led to a postponement of the vaccination.

The consequences if harm to the child follows the vaccination – the liability of the staff administering the vaccine and the makers of the vaccine

This is discussed below.

The significance of risk in legal terms

The significance of the risk of harm is a factor which the courts take into account in deciding whether professional staff have followed the reasonable standard of care. Thus if the specific situation of Emily showed that there were certain risks attached to her present state of health or to her earlier history this would suggest that the vaccination should not have been given then or ever; fault may be established and therefore higher payments would be available under the fault system.

However, the fact that it is known that there is a likelihood that a specific tiny number will be vaccine-damaged would not in itself justify a health professional not giving a vaccination, unless there were specific reasons why a particular child should not have it. Risks are balanced; the risks of harm as a result of the disease itself and the risks from immunization.

The compensation available to the child if harm occurs

This is explained below. Under the civil law fault system, the child can be compensated against all the losses and suffering that he or she has endured; under the Vaccine Damage Payments Act the sum currently stands at £30 000.

The duties of the parents to ensure the child is vaccinated and whether they could be sued by the child

IF THE UNVACCINATED CHILD SUFFERS FROM AN ILLNESS THAT THE VACCINE WAS DESIGNED TO PREVENT

For the child to obtain compensation if they suffer from an illness that the vaccine was designed to prevent, it would be necessary for the child to show that the parents were in breach of their duty of care to the child in failing to provide immunization, and that as a foreseeable consequence the child has suffered the harm the immunization should have protected him or her against. There are to my knowledge no decided cases upon it and it would seem that, as society permits parents to make this choice, and the vaccination is not compulsory, it would be reasonable for parents to decide against it. The question, of course, only becomes more than theoretical when the parents have the funds to pay out compensation or are insured against the possibility.

Failure to vaccinate on religious grounds

The headmaster of Ampleforth College, a Roman Catholic establishment, decided not to allow his pupils a combined measles and rubella vaccination in October 1994 on the grounds that the vaccine was derived in the 1960s from the tissue of an aborted fetus. He offered a measles-only vaccine to pupils. He accepted, however, that for parents who have daughters the combined vaccine is acceptable because of the established danger of rubella in pregnancy.[11] Parents would, of course, have the right to overrule the headmaster for their own children.

The Royal College of Nurses reminded its members that those who were Roman Catholic must still carry out the nationwide vaccination programme: 'We are telling nurses they have to give these jabs. Any nurse who refuses to do so would be guilty of professional negligence.'

Compensation for harm arising from vaccinations

There are three main sources of compensation. These are:

- the Vaccine Damage Payments Act 1979;
- the law of negligence; and
- the Consumer Protection Act 1987.

VACCINE DAMAGE PAYMENTS

The present system of compensation by means of civil action for negligence involves establishing fault, that is, a breach of the duty of care owed to the person injured. As can be seen from Chapter 13 it may be difficult to establish all the elements required in an action for negligence. After the recommendations of the Royal Commission on Civil Liability and Compensation for personal injuries,[12] the Government introduced the Vaccine Damage Payments Act 1979.

The rationale for this Act is that it is in the public interest for as many children as possible to be vaccinated against infectious diseases. However, on very rare occasions there can be side effects of a very crippling kind from vaccines. Therefore, if vaccine damage could be proved to have arisen from medical procedures recommended by the Government, those who suffered serious damage should be entitled to automatic compensation, to be made out of public funds. The sum payable was originally £10 000 but this has since been increased and now stands at £30 000.

The diseases covered by the Vaccine Damage Payments Act 1979 include diphtheria, tetanus, whooping cough, poliomyelitis, measles, rubella, tuberculosis, smallpox, and any other disease specified by the Secretary of State by statutory instrument.

Severe disability must be established and this is defined in section 1(4) of the Act as shown below.

- For the purposes of this Act, a person is severely disabled if he suffers disablement to the extent of 80% or more, assessed as for the purposes of Social Security legislation.

The Act also covers the situation in which a person is severely disabled as the result of a vaccination given to his mother before he or she was born (section 1(3)).

The conditions for obtaining payment under the Act are set out below.

- The vaccination was carried out in the UK or Isle of Man on or after 5 July 1948 or in the case of smallpox before 1 August 1971.
- With the exception of poliomyelitis and rubella, the vaccination was given while the person was under 18 years of age or during an outbreak of that disease in the UK or Isle of Man.
- That the disabled person was over the age of 2 years on the date when the claim was made or, if he or she died before that date, he or she died after 9 May 1978 and was over 2 years of age when he or she died.

Causation

It must be shown that the disablement is the result of the vaccine. If such causation is in dispute, the Act provides that 'the question whether the severe disablement results from vaccination against any of the diseases shall be determined for the purposes of the Act on the balance of probability.'

Time limits
A claim for payment must be made within 6 years beginning on the latest of the following dates:

- Date of the vaccination
- Date on which the disabled person attained the age of 2 years
- 9 May 1978

Referral to medical tribunal
The Secretary of State can refer to a tribunal:

- the question of the extent of the disablement suffered by the disabled person;
- the question whether he or she is, or, as the case may be, was immediately before his or her death disabled as a result of the vaccination to which the claim relates; and
- the question whether, if he or she is or was so disabled, the extent of his or her disability is or was such as to amount to severe disablement.

The Act also provides for the payments to, or for the benefit of, the disabled person and the holding of money by trustees where appropriate.

Anyone who makes any false claims commits an offence under the Act.

THE LAW OF NEGLIGENCE
In comparison with the statutory fixed sum for severe disablement, the awards which are payable by civil action for negligence are much larger. However, as is shown in Chapter 13, all elements necessary to establish liability must be shown or accepted by the defendant. The person seeking compensation must therefore show that:

- a duty of care was owed;
- this duty has been broken by a failure to follow the accepted standard of care; and
- as a reasonably foreseeable consequence of this breach harm has occurred.

Severe disablement does not have to be shown to recover compensation in the civil courts.

What happens if payment has already been paid out under the Vaccine Damage Payment Act 1979? Does this prevent a civil action taking place? The answer is no. Section 6(4) states that the making of a claim for, or the receipt of, a payment under the Act does not prejudice the right of any person to institute or carry on proceedings in respect of disablement suffered as a result of vaccination against any disease to which the Act applies. However, the fact that a payment has been made under the Act must be taken into account by the court in any civil proceedings in which compensation in respect of such disablement is awarded.

An example of an unsuccessful case brought under the civil law of negligence is discussed below.

Loveday v Renton (The Times, 31 March 1988 Queen's Bench Division.)
Mrs Loveday claimed damages on behalf of her daughter Susan, then aged 17 years, for permanent brain damage after a whooping cough vaccine was given in 1970 and 1971. The claim was brought against the Wellcome Foundation, who made the vaccine, and against the doctor who had administered it. The claim was dismissed because she had failed to show on a balance of probabilities that pertussis vaccine could cause permanent brain damage in young children. It thus failed on the issue of causation. The judge stated that if the case had not failed on the issue of causation: 'any plaintiff would face insuperable difficulties in establishing negligence on the part of the doctor or nurse who had administered the vaccine'.

Such a claim would have to be based on the ground that the vaccination had been given in spite of the presence of certain contraindications.

BEST V WELLCOME FOUNDATION *ET AL.*
In contrast to the Loveday case, a claim against the Wellcome Foundation succeeded in an Irish case in 1992. (Best v Wellcome Foundation, Dr O'Keefe, the Southern Health Board, the Minister for health of Ireland and the Attorney General 1994 5 Med LR page 81 and discussed in Medico Legal Journal vol 61 part 3 1993 page 178.)

The High Court had dismissed the plaintiff's claim because of the lack of proof of causation. However, the Irish Supreme Court held that the Wellcome Foundation was liable for the negligent manufacture and release of a particular batch of triple vaccine and that the brain damage was caused as a result. It referred the case back to the High Court on the amount of compensation. On 11 May 1993 the High Court approved an award of £2.75 million as compensation for the brain damage sustained in September 1969.

It remains to be seen if any further successful cases will be brought in the civil courts for vaccine damage. It must be stressed that in the Best case, there was evidence that the particular batch of vaccine was below standard and should not have been released onto the market. However, the contrast between the sums available if fault and causation can be established in the civil courts is clear. The Association of Parents of Vaccine-Damaged Children has been formed to give advice and support to parents.

It has recently been reported[13] that dozens of schoolchildren suffered fever and hallucinations after being given overdoses of diphtheria vaccine by medical officers in Wiltshire. Two hundred and fifty pupils aged between 14 and 15 years received incorrect doses of the vaccine during routine immunization programmes. Parents received a letter telling them of the error a week later. The vaccines were administered by the Bath and West Community NHS Trust, which conceded that mistakes had been made. The children should have been given booster injections of the diphtheria vaccine to protect them against a resurgence of the disease in Eastern Europe. Instead they received a stronger dose intended for babies. The chief executive of the trust reported that an inquiry had been started. No mention has been made of the possibility of compensation being claimed by the children or by the parents on their behalf, but they would have to show that the harm was caused by a breach of the duty of care.

IF THE VACCINATED CHILD SUFFERS FROM AN ILLNESS OR DISABILITY AS A CONSEQUENCE OF THE VACCINATION
It is highly unlikely that a parent could be liable to the child in this context unless there were clear reasons why the child should not have been vaccinated at that time or at all and the parent had failed to mention these to the health professionals before the vaccination was given. If the health professionals failed to ask the relevant questions they would share in the responsibility.

CONSUMER PROTECTION ACT 1987
A person who has suffered harm as a result of a defect in the vaccine might also be able to bring a claim under the Consumer Protection Act 1987. Fault need not be established, but the claimant would have to show that there was a defect in the vaccine. This might prove a stumbling block to a successful action.

REFERENCES

1 Department of Health: *Child Health in the Community: A Guide to Good Practice.* London: HMSO; 1995. [Consultation draft March 1995.]
2 Nuffield Council on Bioethics 1993
3 Colegrove *v* Smyth and others [1994] Med LR 111
4 Campbell AGM: The paediatrician and medical negligence. In *Medical Negligence.* Edited by Powers M, Harris N. London: Butterworths; 1994.

5 Department of Health: *Child Health in the Community: A Guide to Good Practice.* London: HMSO; 1995. [Consultation draft March 1995.]

6 Hall D (Ed): *Health of all Children: A Programme of Child Health Surveillance.* Oxford: Oxford Medical Publications; 1989.

7 Macfarlane A, Seft S, Cordeiro M: *Child health the screening tests.* Oxford: Oxford University Press; 1990.

8 Richardson J, Webber I: *Ethical Issues in Child Health Care.* London: Mosby; 1995.

9 Richardson J, Webber I: *Ethical Issues in Child Health Care.* London: Mosby; 1995: pp49–53.

10 Department of Health: *Immunisation against infectious disease, edn 3.* London: HMSO; 1992.

11 Duce R: *Times,* News Report 27 October 1994.

13 Darch M: *Times,* 25 March 1995.

CHAPTER 24

Reproduction and fertilization

In this chapter we shall cover the following areas of law.

- Family planning
- Pregnancy
- Termination of pregnancy
- Sterilization
- Human fertilization treatments and embryology
- Sexual abuse

FAMILY PLANNING

Consent of the 16- or 17-year-old

The young person aged 16 or 17 years can give a valid consent to family planning treatment under the Family Law Reform Act 1969 (see Chapter 6). In theory, the parent could also give a valid consent to treatment under section 8(3) of the 1969 Act but this is unlikely to arise.

Consent of those aged under 16 years

It is unlawful for a boy to have sexual intercourse with a girl under 16 years of age. Even though the age of consent to sexual intercourse is 16 years, health professionals caring for children and young persons are likely to be involved in providing advice and care for sexual activity below that age. In the Gillick case[1] the House of Lords agreed by a majority that a child under 16 years of age could in certain circumstances give a valid consent to treatment (see further discussion of this case in Chapter 6) and receive family planning advice from the doctor.

Criminal involvement of the health professional?

The House of Lords also held in the Gillick case,[1] by a majority, that a doctor who gave advice to an underage girl when he realized that she was having and would continue to have underage sexual intercourse, was not thereby committing the criminal act of causing or encouraging unlawful sexual intercourse contrary to section 28(1) of the Sexual Offences Act 1956. (Lord Brandon dissented holding that the provision of contraception to an under 16-year-old girl necessarily amounted to promoting, encouraging, or facilitating unlawful sexual intercourse, because it removed one of the major inhibitions to sex (i.e. the risk of pregnancy). He argued for the civil law and the criminal law to be consistent.)

Even the majority of the House of Lords emphasized that it was necessary for the doctor to make an evaluation of the child's maturity. Failure to do this and simply provide treatment without being satisfied that the child was competent could render the doctor liable to be prosecuted. This principle would apply to all health professionals who are involved in providing family planning advice to underage children.[2]

Duty to provide family planning services

Department of Health guidance has been issued on family planning provision which includes advice on services for young people.[3] It is made clear by the Department of Health that health authorities have a duty to make provision for family planning clinic services to supplement those services provided by the GPs and there should be no reduction of services to make financial savings.

UNDERAGE PREGNANCY

Health professionals must ensure that arrangements are made for the underage person to receive all necessary care. The fact that a girl is pregnant does not release her from the duty of attending school if she is within the age of compulsory schooling. Many authorities have set up units for pregnant girls of compulsory school age to continue to receive education (see Chapter 10).

There must be multidisciplinary involvement in the care of the pregnant schoolgirl, including social services advice and support. Postnatal family planning is also essential. The duty of the local authority to protect the child is discussed in Chapter 9.

TERMINATION OF PREGNANCY

The Abortion Act 1967 applies as amended by the Human Fertilisation and Embryology Act 1990. The conditions set down by the Act for a lawful termination are shown below.

- 1(1) – Subject to the provisions of this section, a person shall not be guilty of an offence under the law relating to abortion when a pregnancy is terminated by a registered medical practitioner, if two registered medical practitioners are of the opinion formed in good faith:
  a that the pregnancy has not exceeded its twenty-fourth week and that the continuance of the pregnancy would involve risk, greater than if the pregnancy were terminated, of injury to the physical or mental health of the pregnant woman or any existing children of her family; or
  b that the termination is necessary to prevent grave permanent injury to the physical or mental health of the pregnant woman; or
  c that the continuance of the pregnancy would involve risk to the life of the pregnant woman, greater that if the pregnancy were terminated; or
  d that there is substantial risk that if the child were born it would suffer from such physical or mental abnormalities as to be seriously handicapped.
- 1(2) – In determining whether the continuance of a pregnancy would involve such risk of injury to health as is mentioned in paragraph (a) or (b) of subsection (1) of this section, account may be taken of the pregnant woman's actual or reasonably foreseeable environment.
- 1(3) – Except as provided by subsection (4) of this section, any treatment for the termination of pregnancy must be carried out in a hospital vested in the Minister of Health or the Secretary of State under the National Health Service Acts, or in a place for the time being approved for the purposes of this section by the said Minister or the Secretary of State.
- 1(3A) – The power under subsection (3) of this section to approve a place includes power, in relation to treatment consisting primarily in the use of such medicines as may be specified in the approval and carried out in such manner as may be so specified, to approve a class of places. Termination in an emergency dispenses with the requirements of section 1, as shown below.
- 1(4) – Subsection (3) of this section, and so much of subsection (1) as relates to the opinion of two registered medical practitioners, shall not apply to the termination of a pregnancy by a registered medical practitioner in a case where he is of the opinion, formed in good faith, that the termination is immediately necessary to save the life or to prevent grave permanent injury to the physical or mental health of the pregnant woman.

Many teenage pregnancies are not diagnosed until late into the pregnancy, beyond the 24-week period set in section 1(1)(a). It is then only possible to proceed with a termination if the requirements of section 1 (1)(b),(c), or (d) are satisfied.

Who gives consent to the termination in respect of a girl under the age of 16 years? Provided that the girl has the maturity to give a valid consent, that is, she is Gillick-competent, she can give her consent to the termination. There would have to be the recommendations of two doctors on the appropriate forms.

What would be the situation should her parents refuse to agree to the termination? This occurred in the case of Re P[4] in which a girl aged 15 years who had already given birth to a boy was in the care of the local authority and became pregnant again. Her parents wished to prevent her from having a termination and refused to give consent. The girl herself wished to have an abortion and the requirements of the Abortion Act 1967 were satisfied. The judge, Mrs Justice Butler-Sloss, using the test that the welfare of the girl was the paramount consideration, decided that the termination could proceed. It should be noted that this decision was made before the House of Lords' ruling in the Gillick case that the professional could rely upon the consent of a Gillick-competent minor.

In the case of Re G-U,[5] a girl aged 16 years who was a ward of court became pregnant and the local authority arranged for her pregnancy to be terminated. The court held that this was the correct thing to do as it was clearly in the interests of the child. However, it emphasized that the consent of the court should have been obtained.

Failure to terminate

The courts have refused to recognize the right of a person to sue for wrongful life, that is, that had a pregnancy been terminated, that person would not now be alive.

In the case of McKay v Essex Area Health Authority,[6] Mrs McKay suspected that she might have contracted German measles early in her pregnancy. After blood tests she was wrongly informed that she was not infected and therefore did not have a termination. The baby was born disabled. An action for negligence was brought in the name of the child and also in the name of the mother. The Court of Appeal held that the child's action must fail as the court held that there was no action for wrongful life. The mother's claim, however, could proceed.

STERILIZATION

A distinction has to be made between a sterilization which is necessitated by the physical condition of the child, for example if the ovarian tubes are cancerous and a sterilization which is indicated by the social situation of the child, linked with mental incapacity.

Therapeutic sterilization

In the former case, if an operation is necessary on physical grounds and as a result sterilization would ensue, it can proceed on the basis that it is in the interests of the child. The consent of the court would not be necessary and the parents or the child herself, if over 16 years of age or Gillick-competent, could give consent.

Sterilization for social reasons

The House of Lords in the case of Jeanette[7] stated that the consent could be given by the local authority to the sterilization of a girl aged 17 years who was in their care. She suffered from a moderate degree of mental impairment and had the speech of a 2-year-old and the understanding of a 6-year-old. She had recently shown signs of sexual awareness but was incapable of understanding the process of sex, pregnancy, and childbirth. If she were to give birth she would require heavy sedation, would probably have to have a caesarian and would be likely to pick at her wounds. As an epileptic and a person of unpredictable moods, a daily course of contraceptive pills was considered to be impracticable. Her mental condition ruled out other methods of contraception. The local authority made the child a ward of court and asked the High Court to provide the necessary consent. A guardian *ad litem* was appointed and he opposed the giving of consent. The House of Lords held that consent should be given and that the sterilization operation should be carried out. The paramount consideration was the welfare of the child.

A different outcome occurred in the case of Re D.[8] In this case an 11-year-old girl suffered from Soto's syndrome, which is a condition likely to lead to neonatal abnormalities. Her mother feared that she would be seduced and would be unable to cope with a resulting pregnancy or to care for the baby. It was agreed with the doctors and gynaecologist that the operation to sterilize would go ahead, but an application was made by the educational psychologist to make the child a ward of court and prevent the operation proceeding. Mrs Justice Heilbron considered that the right of a woman to reproduce was a basic human right and as the girl was likely to have the mental capacity when older to appreciate the nature of the operation and give her consent, the operation should not proceed. Her options should be kept open.

It was emphasized that in future the declaration of the court should be sought before such an operation proceeded. Practice directions were issued in 1989.[9] (See pages 61–62 for further discussion of this case.)

HUMAN FERTILIZATION AND EMBRYOLOGY

It is unlikely that a health professional caring for a child will be involved in the procedures for treatment for fertilization or surrogacy in respect of the fertility of the child. However, the health professional may need to have an understanding of this legislation because the child may wish to have access to information about the parents.

If the child has been born as a result of treatment licensed under the Human Fertilisation and Embryology Act 1990, access to a limited amount of information can be obtained by the child from the Human Fertilisation and Embryology Authority. The child must be aged 18 years and over and receive counselling before the request is granted. A child who is 16 or 17 can receive information if he or she is intending to get married. The rights of access are further discussed in Chapter 8.

SEXUAL ABUSE OF THE CHILD

The duty of the health professional, the powers that are available, and practical guidance on the procedures that should be followed are discussed in Chapter 9.

CONCLUSION

Health professionals are likely to be involved in discussion of many of the above issues, especially with teenage patients. Reference should also be made to Chapter 7 on confidentiality and Chapter 6 on consent.

REFERENCES

1   Gillick *v* West Norfolk andWisbeck Area Health Authority [1985] 3 All ER 402.
2   Norrie K McK: *Family Planning Practice and the Law.* Aldershot: Dartmouth Publishing Co; 1992.
3   HC(86)1 [Services for young people]; EL(90)MB115 [Balance of provision in family planning services].
4   Re P (a minor)[1981] 80 Local Government Reports 301.

5   Re G-U [1984] FLR 811.
6   McKay *v* Essex Area Health Authority [1982] 2 All ER 771.
7   Re B (a minor) [sterilization] [1987] 2 WLR 1213.
8   Re D (a minor) 1976 1 All ER 326.
9   Official Solicitor's Practice Note, October 1989.

Glossary

actionable per se a civil court action can be brought without showing any harm has occurred.

actus reus the elements that make up a criminal offence (see **mens rea** for mental element).

a fortiori so much more; so much stronger.

civil noncriminal jurisdiction.

commissioning determining the health care needs of a population, specifying the services required to meet those needs, funding providers through a contractual relationship to provide those services, and working in cooperation with other agencies.

common law law derived from the decisions of judges determining individual cases. A hierarchy of courts and a system of precedents decides which decisions are binding on judges hearing future cases; as opposed to statutory law.

contributory negligence negligence by the plaintiff which has caused or further increased the harm that he or she has suffered.

criminal pertaining to the noncivil jurisdiction.

Gillick-competent a child who is deemed to have the maturity to make a decision in a particular set of circumstances. [From the House of Lords decision in the case brought by Mrs Gillick against the Department of Health *et al.*]

GP fundholders GPs who have been allocated a budget to purchase certain health care services from hospitals and community units on behalf of their patients.

hazard the potential to cause harm, including ill health and injury; damage to property, plant, products or the environment; production losses or increased liabilities.

hierarchy the courts in order of seniority: The House of Lords takes precedence over all others and its decisions are binding on lower courts.

limitation of time the rule relating to the time within which a legal action can be commenced, set by Act of Parliament. Action which is outside the time limits is known as 'statute barred'.

mens rea the mental element that is required before a person can be convicted of a criminal offence; for example, intension reckless as to outcome (see **actus reus**).

named nurse a specific nurse allocated to oversee the care of a specific child throughout their stay in hospital (primary nursing). It can also include allocating nurses for each shift (team nursing).

nebulizer a powerful device for administering inhaled drugs in the treatment of asthma and other conditions.

neonatal the first 28 days of life.

neonatal units units which provide intensive care and special care of newborn babies.

neonatal intensive care continuous skilled supervision of newborn babies (up to 28 days old and longer if necessary) by qualified and specially trained nursing and medical staff involving assisted ventilation. Intensive care is sometimes defined as including procedures other than assisted ventilation.

paediatric the branch of medicine dealing specifically with children.

paediatric intensive care continuous skilled supervision of babies and children over 28 days.

parens patriae the paternal jurisdiction of the court jurisdiction to act on behalf of minors as part of its inherent powers.

plaintiff the person who brings a civil action in the courts seeking compensation or other remedy.

precedent a decision of judges in an earlier decision, relevant to a case being heard by a court which must follow the ruling unless it can be distinguished.

presumption an assumption in law that a particular fact exists, for example presumption of innocence. Presumptions can be contradicted (ie rebutted) by evidence.

prima facie at first sight; it could be disproved by contradictory evidence or could be affirmed.

primary care health care and health services provided by GPs or primary health care teams working with them.

primary health care GPs, practice nurses, district nurses, team health visitors, school nurses, and other support staff who work with GPs.

purchasing the process of specifying health care services to be provided, negotiating with providers, paying providers which results from commissioning, monitoring and reviewing performance.

rebutted/rebuttable refers to a presumption which will cease to be relied upon if contrary evidence is established.

Registered General Nurse (RGN) a nurse qualified in adult general nursing whose name is on parts 1 or 12 of the UKCC Nursing, Midwifery and Health Visiting General Register of Nurses.

Registered Sick Children's Nurse (RSCN) a nurse qualified in nursing sick children whose name is on parts 8 or 15 of the UKCC General Register.

reviewing is used to describe activities involving judgments about performance, and decisions about improving performance. Reviewing is based on information from 'measuring' and 'auditing' activities.

risk the likelihood that a specified undesired event will occur because of the realization of a hazard by, or during, work activities or by the products and services created by work activities.

secondary care care provided following a referral from the primary care team, a hospital accident and emergency department or a maternity unit.

special care baby units units which provide special care for newborn babies. They must also be able to provide initial care of a baby before transfer for neonatal intensive care.

statute/statutory relates to laws which derive from Acts of Parliament or regulations (Statutory instruments) which are enacted through an approved system of delegated law making.

tertiary care care provided after a referral from a consultant paediatrician, surgeon or GP. It is essentially care that would not normally be provided at a district general hospital because of the relatively small numbers of children involved.

trespass to the person a civil action in law where an individual is touched, or threatened with touching, without his or her consent or other lawful justification.

ultra vires outside the powers held.

very low weight babies less than 1500 grams at birth.

Further reading

LAW

Bainham A, Cretney S: *Children – the Modern Law*. Bristol: Family Law; 1993.

Brazier M: *Medicine, Patients and the Law*. London: Penguin; 1992.

Carrier J, Kendall I: *Medical Negligence Complaints and Compensation*. Aldershot, England: Gower Publishing; 1990.

Harbour A, Ayotte W (Eds): *Children's Legal Centre Mental Health Handbook: A Guide to the Law Affecting Children and Young People, edn 2*. London: Legal Centre; 1994.

Campbell AGM: The Paediatrician and Medical Negligence. In *Medical Negligence*. Edited by Powers M, Harris N. London: Butterworths; 1994.

Cowley R: *Access to Medical Records and Reports*. Oxford: Association of Health Authorities and Trusts, Radcliffe Medical Press; 1994.

Department of Health: *The Children Act 1989 Guidance and Regulations*. London: HMSO; 1991.

Denyer RL: *Children and Personal Injury Litigation*. London: Butterworths; 1993.

Dimond BC: *The Legal Aspects of Midwifery*. Hale, Cheshire: Books for Midwives Press; 1994.

Dimond BC: *The Legal Aspects of Nursing, edn 2*. Hemel Hempstead: Prentice Hall; 1995.

Dimond BC, Barker F: *Mental Health Law for Nurses*. Oxford: Blackwell Scientific Publications; 1996.

Dimond BC: *Patients' Rights, Responsibilities and the Nurse*. Central Health Studies Quay Publishing; 1993.

Dingwall R, Fenn P, Quam L: *Medical Negligence: A Review and Bibliography*. Oxford: Oxford Centre for Socio-Legal Studies; 1991.

Freeman MDA: *The Rights and the Wrongs of Children*. London: Frances Pinter Publishers; 1983.

Hendrick J: *Child Care Law for Health Professionals*. Oxford: Radcliffe Medical Press; 1993.

Home Office: *Memorandum of Good Practice on Video Recorded Interviews with Child Witnesses*. London: HMSO; 1992.

Hoggett B: *Mental Health Law*. 3rd Edition. London: Sweet and Maxwell.

Jones R: *Mental Health Act Manual, edn 4*. London: Sweet and Maxwell; 1994.

Keane A: *The Modern Law of Evidence, edn 3*. London: Butterworths; 1994.

Kennedy A, Grubb B: *Law Materials*. London: Butterworths; 1994.

Lamb B, Percival R: *Paying for Disability: A Discussion Document on No Fault Liability*. London: Spastics Society; 1992.

Lewis C: *Medical Negligence: A Practical Guide*. Croydon: Tolley; 1992.

Markinsinis BS, Deakin SF: *Tort Law, edn 3*. Oxford: Clarendon Press; 1994.

Mitchells B, Prince A: *The Children Act and Medical Practice Family Law*. Bristol: Jordan and Sons; 1992.

Morgan D, Lee R: *Human Fertilisation and Embryology Act*. London: Blackstone Press Ltd; 1991.

Nicholson R: *Medical Research with Children: Ethics, Law and Practice*. Oxford: Oxford University Press; 1986.

Norrie K McK: *Family Planning Practice and the Law*. Aldershot: Dartmouth Publishing Co; 1992.

Powers M, Harris N: *Medical Negligence*. London: Butterworths; 1994.

Rae M: *Children and the Law*. London: Longmans; 1986.

Robertson S: *Disability Rights Handbook*. London: The Disability Alliance ERA; 1995.

Secretary of State for Social Services: *Report of the Inquiry into Child Abuse in Cleveland 1987*. London: HMSO; 1988

Smith JC, Hogan B: *Criminal Law, edn 7*. London: Butterworths; 1992.

Keenan D (Ed): *English Law*. London: Pitman; 1992.

Brazier M (Ed): *Street on Torts, edn 8*. London: Butterworths; 1988.

White R, Carr P, Lowe N: *A Guide to the Children Act 1989*. London: Butterworths; 1990.

Wyld N, Carlton N: *Family Emergency Procedures*. London: London Legal Action Group; 1993.

Wyld N: *Getting Help From Social Services: A Guide for Children and Young People on the Children Act*. London:Children's Legal Centre; 1991.

CHILD HEALTH

British Paediatric Association: *Report of a Working Party on Paediatric Intensive Care*. London: Critical Care Publications; 1987.

British Paediatric Association: *The Care of the Critically Ill: Report of a Working Party on Paediatric Intensive Care (November)*. London: Critical Care Publications; 1993.

Hall D (Ed): *Health of all Children: A Programme of Child Health Surveillance*. Oxford: Oxford Medical Publications.

Health Policy and Public Health Directorate The Scottish Office Home and Health Department: *At Home in Hospital*. Edinburgh: HMSO; 1993.

Jones T: *Medical Conditions in School Children – A Guide for Teachers*. London: Edward Arnold; 1988.

Macfarlane A, Seft S, Mario C: Child Health: *The Screening Tests*. Oxford: Oxford University Press; 1990.

MacKenzie A (Ed): *Hospital at Home*. Edinburgh: District Nursing Association; 1991.

MANAGEMENT OF CHILD CARE SERVICES/STANDARD SETTING

Association for Children with Life-threatening Diseases: *Charter 1993 Act*. Bristol: Institute of Child Health, Royal Hospital for Sick Children; 1993.

Action for Sick Children: *Putting Children First: Ten Targets for the 1990s*. London: Action for Sick Children; 1992.

Audit Commission: *Children First: A Study of Hospital Services*. London: HMSO; 1993.

Audit Commission: *Making Time for Patients: A Handbook for Ward Sisters*. London: HMSO; 1992.

Audit Commission: *Seen But Not Heard: Co-ordinating Child Health and Social Services for Children in Need*. London: HMSO; 1993.

Clincial Standards Advisory Group: *Cystic Fibrosis: Access to and Availability of Specialist Services*. London: HMSO; 1993.

Clinical Standards Advisory Group: *Childhood Leukaemia: Access to and Availability of Specialist Services*. London: HMSO;1993.

Department of Health: *Welfare of Children and Young People in Hospital*. London: HMSO; 1991.

Eskin Frada (Ed): *Good Practices in Child Health in Yorkshire – Occasional Papers in Public Health, No. 6*. Harrogate: Yorkshire Regional Health Authority; 1992.

Flekkoy A: *Children's Rights Thesis on the Norwegian Ombudsman for Children*. [PhD Thesis]. Gent: University of Gent; 1993. Cahier 13

Forfar JO (Ed): *Child Health in a Changing Society*. Oxford: British Paediatric Association, Oxford University Press; 1988.

Hogg C: *Setting Standards for Children Undergoing Surgery. Quality Review Series*. London: London Action for Sick Children; 1994.

National Health Service Management Executive: *Report of the Joint Working Party on Medical Services for Children*. London: NHS Management Executive and the British Medical Association; 1992.

Paediatric Intensive Care Society: *Standards for Paediatric Intensive Care*. London: Critical Care Publications; 1992.

Platt Committee (Report of): *The Welfare of Children in Hospital*. London: HMSO; 1959.

Rudd P, Nicoll A (Eds): *Manual on Infections and Immunisation of Children*. Oxford: Oxford University Press; 1991

South East Thames Regional Health Authority: *Better Care for Children: Commissioning Paediatric Services*. London: South East Thames Regional Health Authority; 1994.

South East Thames Regional Health Authority: *A Mandate for Children: A Guide to Commissioning Health Services under the Children Act 1989*. London: South East Thames Regional Health Authority; 1992.

PARENTS AND CHILDREN

Cleary J: *Caring for Children in Hospital: Parents and Nurses in Partnership*. London: Scutari Press; 1992.

Darbyshire P: *Living with a Sick Child in Hospital: The Experiences of Parents and Nurses*. London: Chapman & Hall; 1994.

Darley B, Griew A, McLoughlin K, Williams J: *How to Keep a Clinical Confidence*. London: HMSO; 1994.

Sutherland E, McCall Smith A: *Family Rights: Family Law and Medical Advance*. Edinburgh: Edinburgh University Press; 1990.

Thornes R: Just for the Day: *Caring for Children in the Health Services*. London: National Association for Children in Hospitals (NAWCH); 1991.

Thornes R: *The Care of Dying Children and Their Families*. Birmingham: Birmingham National Association of Health Authorities; 1988.

While A (Ed): *Caring for Children Towards Partnerships with Families*. London: Edward Arnold.

DRUGS

Appelbe GE, Wingfield J: *Dale and Applelbe's Pharmacy Law and Practice*. London: The Pharmaceutical Press; 1993.

Merrils J, Fisher J: (1995) *Pharmacy Law and Practice*. Oxford: Blackwell Scientific Publications; 1995.

RESEARCH

British Paediatric Association: *Ethics Advisory Committee August 1992 Guidelines for the Ethical Conduct of Medical Research Involving Children*. London: British Paediatric Association; 1992.

HEALTH AND SAFETY

Child Accident Prevention Trust and Royal College of Nursing: *Accidents to Children on Hospital Wards*. London: Child Accident Prevention Trust; 1992.

Department of Health: *Report of Chief Medical Officer's Expert Group—Sleeping Position of Infants: Cot Death*. London: HMSO; 1993.

Sibert J (Ed): *Accidents and Emergencies in Childhood*. London: Royal College of Physicians; 1992.

MENTAL HEALTH AND COMMUNITY CARE

Department of Health: *Code of Practice of the Mental Health Act, revised edn.* London: HMSO; 1993

Department of Health: *Working for Patients White Paper.* London: HMSO; 1989.

Department of Health: *The Health of the Nation White Paper.* London: HMSO; 1992.

Elfer P, Gatiss S: *Charting Child Health Services: A Survey of Community Child Health Services Provided by Health Authorities in England, Scotland and Wales*. London: National Children's Bureau; 1990.

Kurtz Z: *With Health in Mind: Mental Health Care for Children and Young People*. London: London Action for Sick Children in association with South West Thames Regional Health Authority; 1992.

GENERAL

Cameron-Blackie G: *Complementary Therapies in the NHS*. Birmingham: National Association of Health Authorities and Trusts; 1993.

Christian Aid Foundation: *Directory of Grant Making Trusts 1995*. Tonbridge: Christian Aid Foundation; 1995.

BIBLIOGRAPHIES

See series published by the National Children's Bureau, including:

Dinnage R, Gooch S: *The Child with Asthma*. Windsor: NFER-Nelson; 1986. [1].

Dinnage R: *The Child with a Chronic Medical Problem (Cardiac Disease, Diabetes and Haemophilia)*. Windsor: NFER-Nelson; 1986. [3]

Index